Urolithiasis: Therapy · Prevention

Edited by
Hans-Joachim Schneider

Contributions by

P. Alken
D. Bach
Ch. Chaussy
R. Hautmann
F. Hering
W. Lutzeyer
M. Marberger
E. Schmiedt
H.-J. Schneider
W. Stackl

Springer-Verlag
Berlin Heidelberg New York Tokyo

Handbook of Urology · Volume 17/II

Continuation of Handbuch der Urologie · Encyclopedia of Urology

With 127 Figures

ISBN-13:978-3-642-70714-8 e-ISBN-13:978-3-642-70712-4
DOI: 10.1007/978-3-642-70712-4

Library of Congress Cataloging in Publication Data. Main entry under title: Urolithiasis : therapy, prevention. (Handbook of urology ; v. 17/II) Includes bibliographies and index. 1. Calculi, Urinary—Treatment. 2. Calculi, Urinary—Surgery. I. Schneider, Hans-Joachim, 1931- . II. Alken, P. III. Series. [DNLM: 1. Urinary Calculi. WJ 39 U78 v. 17 no. 2] RC916.U77 1985 616.6'22 85-26162 ISBN-13:978-3-642-70714-8 (U.S.)

2122/3130-543210

List of Contributors

SCHNEIDER, H.-J., Professor Dr.
Ludwigsplatz 11, D-6300 Giessen

ALKEN, P., Professor Dr.
Urologische Klinik und Poliklinik, Klinikum der Johannes Gutenberg-Universität Mainz, Langenbeckstr. 1, D-6500 Mainz

BACH, D., Professor Dr.
St. Agnes-Hospital Bocholt, Barloer Weg 125, D-4290 Bocholt

CHAUSSY, CH., Professor Dr.
Urologische Klinik und Poliklinik der Universität München, Klinikum Großhadern, Marchioninistr. 15, D-8000 München

HAUTMANN, R., Professor Dr.
Ärztlicher Direktor der Urologischen Klinik, Klinikum der Universität Ulm, Prittwitzstr. 43, D-7900 Ulm

HERING, F., Priv.-Doz. Dr.
Urologische Klinik und Poliklinik, Kantonsspital Basel, Universitätskliniken, Spitalstr. 21, CH-4031 Basel

LUTZEYER, W., Professor Dr.
Vorstand der Abteilung Urologie der medizinischen Fakultät, an der Rhein.-Westf. Techn. Hochschule Aachen, Goethestraße 27–29, D-5100 Aachen

MARBERGER, M., Professor Dr.
Vorstand der Urologischen Abteilung der Krankenanstalt Rudolfstiftung, Juchgasse 25, A-1030 Wien

SCHMIEDT, E., Professor Dr.
Direktor der Urologischen Klinik und Poliklinik der Universität München, Klinikum Großhadern, Marchioninistr. 15, D-8000 München 70

STACKL, W., Dr.
Urologische Abteilung der Krankenanstalt Rudolfstiftung, Juchgasse 25, A-1030 Wien

Preface

Since the early days of medicine one concern of doctors has been the removal of kidney stones and prevention of recurrence. Owing to the hesitancy of progress in the prevention of initial stone formation and of relapse, however, removal of stones from the kidney and ureter were developed to highly refined techniques and they formerly accounted for a major proportion of the urological operations performed.

In the last few years developments in the treatment of kidney stones have taken a completely different turn. In the majority of cases suitable methods are available to bring about spontaneous passage of the stones, while in a smaller proportion drug-induced litholysis is possible. Stones that cannot be passed are now treated mainly with extracorporeal shockwave lithotripsy, percutaneous litholapaxy or ureterorenoscopy. These methods are often used in combination and complement each other. Nonetheless, despite the accumulating experience with the new methods there will still be situations in which stones cannot be removed except by open surgery. "Our skill as surgeons and the management of the brilliantly designed equipment would amount to nothing more than highly skilled mechanical work if they did not go hand in hand with enhanced insight into the cause of lithiasis and thus into ways of preventing it – or at least of preventing the relapse that is the lot of most patients. Otherwise, stone and machine would be keeping each other going, a symbiosis that would be thoroughly unsatisfactory for all concerned" (A. Sigel). Purposeful and controlled preventive measures after an initial episode can bring about a striking reduction in the high primary relapse rate, while attempts at general prophylaxis to prevent stones from forming at all unfortunately still have little success.

Heartfelt thanks are due to all the authors who have worked on this volume. Some of them are among the pioneers of this revolution in the treatment of urinary tract stones, and their chapters reflect the fact that they embody the greatest cumulated experience in these techniques to date. The first volume of this work has already been published. It deals with the morphology and composition of urinary tract concretions, including stone analysis, together with epidemiology, aetiology, pathogenesis, and diagnosis.

The object of this volume is to inform doctors of the present status of our knowledge relating to the treatment of urolithiasis and the prevention of relapse, so that all patients everywhere who have such stones can benefit from the options available.

I am grateful to my colleagues and friends for their stimulating ideas and critical comments, and to Mr. W. Bergstedt of Springer-Verlag for his support and patience in the preparation of the book.

Giessen HANS-JOACHIM SCHNEIDER

Contents

The Treatment of Ureteric Colic and Promotion of Spontaneous Passage. D. BACH. With 1 Figure

Surgical Treatment of Renal Calculi. M. MARBERGER and W. STACKL. With 16 Figures

Ischemia and Regional Hypothermia in Renal Stone Surgery. H.-J. SCHNEIDER. With 5 Figures

Treatment of Bladder Stones. R. HAUTMANN. With 9 Figures

Treatment of Urethral Stones. H.-J. SCHNEIDER.

Extracorporeal Shockwave Lithotripsy (ESWL) in the Treatment of Kidney and Ureter Stones. CH. CHAUSSY and E. SCHMIEDT. With 19 Figures

Drug Therapy of Urinary Calculi and Prevention of Recurrence

W. LUTZEYER and F. HERING

I. Introduction

The disease of urolithiasis has been well documented throughout medical history, as evidenced by the finding of a calculus in the famous El Amara mummy, dating back to 4,800 B.C.

Hippocrates (460 – 370 B.C.) exhibits an astonishing degree of professional knowledge in his descriptions of urolith case material. The Hippocratic Oath requires the removal of bladder calculi to be undertaken only by trained lithotomists. Hippocrates also gives detailed dietary and pharmacologic instructions for the prevention of stones. He was well acquainted with the effects of drinking cures and plant extracts, as well as with the lithogenic properties of certain dishes and the importance of maintaining a dilute urine.

Galen (131 – 201 A.D.) was the first physician to suspect a metabolic disorder at the root of stone disease, and he likewise makes dietary stipulations for the prevention of calculi.

It was, however, left to the radical changes in living conditions and nutrition brought about by the 20th century to elevate urolithiasis to the rank of an endemic disease. The same process also led to significant advances in drug therapy and prevention.

Operative treatment had previously been in the hands of wandering lithotomists, frequently quacks or charlatans, yet it was also undertaken by members of lithotomist families or of regular schools of lithotomy. Many of these were French, such as the Colots, Frère Jacques Beaulieu and Tolet. In Germany Heister, a pupil of Rau and of Frère Jacques, was at his zenith around 1750. In the 19th century Civiale was to open up the age of transurethral litholapaxy (1824), followed by Guyon and the Englishman Thompson (Napoleon III. 1873).

At this time attempts at drug therapy consisted simply of drinking cures, acupuncture (BUTT 1960) and paramedical manoeuvres such as exorcism or the wearing of jade amulets to prevent stone formation. Osler, himself plagued by uric acid stones, suggested as early as 1912 that the disease be treated by drinking distilled water. This approach was duly termed "a return to the Hippocratic method in the treatment of urinary calculi".

True successes were not in fact seen until the mid-20th century with the advent of improved stone analysis and of further understanding of the solubility properties of urolithogenic substances as a function of urinary pH. At the same time our knowledge of extrarenal metabolic disorders and their causal relationship to urolithiasis was expanding rapidly. HAMMARSTEIN (1929) gave an extensive description of the pathophysiology of stone disease, particularly of calcium oxalate lithiasis. He attributed the latter to magnesium deficiency and thus proposed magnesium therapy. A further milestone was the introduction by PRIEN and GERSHOFF (1974) of combination vitamin B_6 therapy, an approach which retains a certain validity even today. This movement was followed by widespread trials of drug therapy and prophylaxis, often on the basis of plant preparations or extracts.

In the years that followed, improved techniques of biochemical investigation opened up research into the pathophysiology of cystine and uric acid stone formation, and so allowed treatment to be more causally orientated. With certain reservations stones of the infective group are now open to a similar therapeutic approach.

On the other hand, the apparently multifactorial etiology of both calcium oxalate and calcium phosphate stones remains essentially obscure, and so treatment and prophylaxis of these conditions must still be symptomatic.

II. General Preventive Measures

General measures aimed at the prevention of stone disease should avoid or reduce the effect of known risk factors. The first principle of any dietary or drug treatment should be to avoid the precipitation of lithogenic salts or minerals by controlling their relative saturation in solution. The cardinal requirement is thus adequate urinary *dilution*. This can usually be achieved by adequate fluid intake, evenly distributed over day and night. Only a continuous intake, rather than acute bursts of drinking, will guarantee the required urinary specific gravity of <1015. At values in this range the precipitation of urinary salts is, as a rule, inhibited.

To this must be added an adaptation of life-style, both at work and in leisure periods. In other words, fluid losses due to perspiration, hot working conditions, sunbathing, saunas and various sporting activities all have to be made up for. Weight reduction and all forms of physical activity are also to be encouraged.

The figure usually quoted as a desirable fluid intake is certainly too low at 1.5–2 liters, if one considers the effects of physical labor, insensible loss (750 ml) and nocturnal urodilution.

Sensible physical activity is particularly important for those of sedentary occupation and who are under stress (pilots, locomotive engineers) (SCHMUCKI et al. 1979). In these patients overweight, often in combination with hyperuricemia, is of special significance, particularly in relation to protein-rich diet. The purine metabolism of such people is also worthy of attention (ZOELLNER 1960, 1972), and so it would appear the "affluent society" in general is connected with a number of risk factors. Indeed such a relationship between high GNP and an above average incidence of stone disease has already been described (ROBERTSON et al. 1978, 1979).

The waning of so-called waves of stone disease during both world wars represents a form of enforced mass experimentation on the prophylactic effects of a low protein, high water diet.

Climatic factors, such as heat or aridity of a given zone (Israel, Mediterranean, Stone Belts of the southern US) may also give rise to a higher urolithiasis rate in that region. Apart from factors such as increased exposure to ultraviolet light and chronic fluid loss, the latter with its inevitable effect on urinary concentration, there can be little doubt that increased intestinal calcium absorption due to raised 25-hydroxycholecalciferol levels plays a part (ELOMAA et al. 1981).

III. Special Preventive and Therapeutic Measures

1. Calcium Oxalate Calculi (Mono- and Dihydrates)

a) Diet and Fluid Intake: Quantity and Choice of Drinks

Two main factors still characterise the calcium oxalate calculus as the problem stone of our age: on the one hand its frequency and high rate of recurrence, and on the other the lack of much therapeutic effect from dietary or pharmacologic attack. Despite a number of promising hypotheses, the pathogenetic mechanism of intrarenal calcium oxalate stone formation remains obscure. It has to be said that, in view of the dominant role of hyperoxaluria in the pathogenesis of calcium stones (ROBERTSON et al. 1981), our therapeutic efforts in respect of this factor are neither clinically nor scientifically satisfactory.

One continues to come across recommendations for a relatively low dietary calcium or oxalate intake, but it is essential that such regimes be set out in table form, easily understood by the patient. Dietary restriction must not be allowed to leave the basal requirements unsatisfied, since deficiency will merely lead to increased parathyroid activity.

α) Calcium Requirements of Stone Sufferers

Three *protein hormones* regulate calcium metabolism within the body. They control intestinal absorption, skeletal resorption or deposition and renal excretion or tubular reabsorption of calcium. These hormones are *parathormone,* from the parathyroid glands, *calcitonin,* secreted by the parafollicular or C-cells of the thyroid, and the active metabolite of vitamin D, *1,25-dihydroxycholecalciferol* (Fig. 1).

The total calcium content of the human body is about 1.5% by weight, or about 1,100 g for a 70 kg man. Of this, 1% is in solution in the blood, whilst the other 99% is held in the skeleton, chiefly as calcium apatite crystals. There is a continuous exchange of calcium between blood and bone: approximately 15% of the free exchangeable calcium pool is replaced every day, of which 10% is

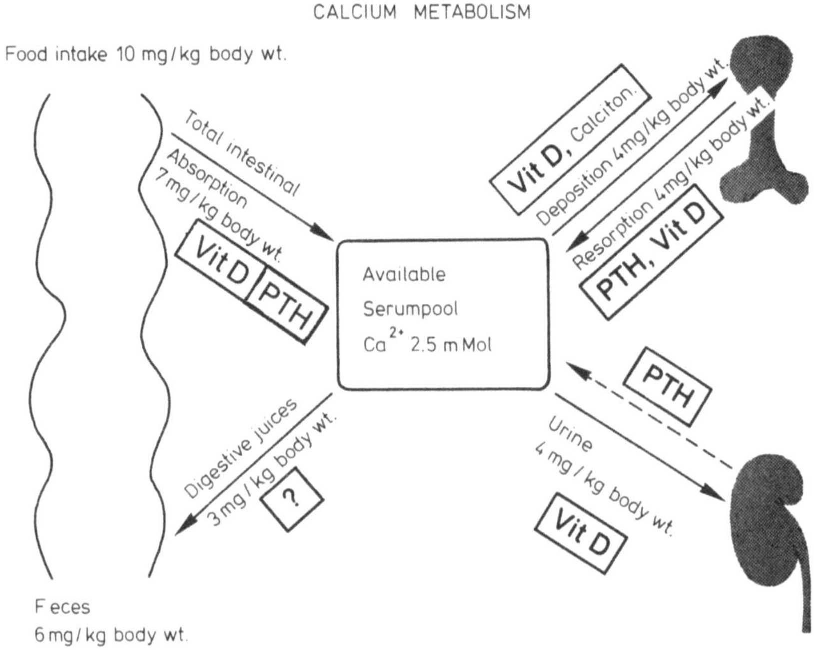

Fig. 1. Turnover and regulation of calcium in the human body

Table 1. Calcium content in the fresh of principal foodstuffs in mg/100 g

Pork	8	Butter	13
Beef	8	Rice	23
Liver	6	Spaghetti	20
Ham	9	Rye bread	43
Salami	33	Bread rolls	24
Venison	7–18	Potatoes	13
Goose	8	Milk chocolate	214
Perch	46	Cabbage	13
Herring	36	Peas	10
Cod	6	Lettuce	15
Egg yolk	140	Spinach	83
Egg white	11	Tomatoes	13
Cow's milk, 3.5% fat content	118	Dried carrots	256
Skimmed milk	123	Dried green beans	195
Condensed milk, 7.5% fat content	240	Fruit	1–3
Cream	110	Hazel nuts	225
Yoghurt	150	Almonds	252
Ice cream	135	Peanuts	67
Cheese, full fat (45% dry wt.)	830	Fruit juice	1–6
Soft cheese, demi fat (20% dry wt.)	500	White wine	10
Camembert cheese	380	Red wine	10
Cottage cheese, low fat	71	Lager beer	6

accounted for by bone turnover. Under normal conditions bone deposition and resorption are in equilibrium.

Calcium is excreted at the rate of 3% of total body content a day in the urine and 2% in the bile and pancreatic juice. The result is a daily dietary calcium requirement in the region of 10 mg/kg body weight.

These figures are necessarily approximate, since true calcium requirements will vary according to age, sex and individual factors. Calcium requirements are, for example, raised in postmenopausal osteoporosis, in osteomalacia, in pregnancy and during lactation.

In summary therefore, the calcium intake of stone patients should be matched to their 24-hour urinary calcium excretion. For women this value will be maximally 250 mg, for men nearer 300 mg.

Table 1 gives the calcium content of the principal basic foodstuffs and drinks. The highest values are found in dairy produce, so that as a rule of thumb an average sized patient with normal renal function should choose between 1 glass of milk, 1 pot of yoghurt, 1 pack of cottage cheese or a maximum of 100 g cheese daily. Fiercer restrictions or complete prohibition of dairy foods should then be unnecessary. One hazard lies in the formation of poorly soluble and poorly diffusing calcium oxalates within the gastrointestinal tract. Intestinal absorption is then grossly reduced, with 90–95% being lost unaltered in the feces as calcium oxalate salts (CASPARY 1979; HAUTMANN 1980). Only 5–10% of such oxalates get absorbed. Extreme calcium restriction results in a considerable calcium deficit and in a reduction in enteric calcium availability. Calcium is the normal biochemic partner of oxalate, and in its absence sodium or potassium complexes are formed which diffuse far more easily across the lipoprotein barrier of the intestinal mucosa. The result may be an increase in oxalate uptake of up to 40% (KLAUWERS et al. 1969; PINTO and BERNSHTAM 1978; CASPARY 1979; HAUTMANN 1980).

β) Dietary Oxalate in Stone Patients

Oxalate is the end product of endogenous metabolic pathways, is toxic in high concentration and is 90–95% excreted in the urine. Additional oxalate originating from intestinal absorption is also excreted by the kidney (ANDERSON 1967; ARCHER and DORMER 1957; COCHRAN et al. 1968; EARNEST et al. 1974; ELDER and WYNGAARDEN 1960; HODGKINSON and ZAREMBSKI 1968; HODGKINSON et al. 1973; HODGKINSON 1977; WILLIAMS and SMITH 1968; WILLIAMS et al. 1971; WILLIAMS 1976). By this means serum oxalate is kept at a low level, lying in the region of 10^{-6} to 10^{-4} mol/l, depending on the author and his chosen analytic method (HATCH et al. 1977; HODGKINSON et al. 1973). The preeminent renal pathway of oxalate elimination is glomerular filtration and a calcium concentration dependent tubular diffusion. Neither active secretion nor reabsorption have been documented (CATTEL et al. 1962; HAUTMANN and OSSWALD 1979; HODGKINSON 1977; WILLIAMS et al. 1971). Small quantities of oxalate are excreted in the digestive juices (BINDER 1974; CASPARY 1979; WILLIAMS 1976).

Table 2. Oxalate content in the fresh of principal foodstuffs in mg/100 g

Foodstuff	Oxalic acid content (mg/100 g fresh wt.)
Rhubarb	260–620
Spinach	400–800
Butter	0
Cheese	0
Eggs	0
Chocolate	60
Coffee	60–250
Tea	400–1500
Parsley	170
Apples	1.5

Table 2 shows the percentage oxalate content of basic foodstuffs and drinks. The dietary treatment of calcium oxalate lithiasis is aimed at reducing or eliminating nutritional oxalate intake. Although the poor absorption of dietary oxalate has led to doubt being expressed, such measures are nevertheless important in secondary hyperoxaluria of intestinal causation (HODGKINSON and ZAREMBSKI 1968).

Intestinal hyperoxaluria is best avoided by restricting the following: cocoa drinks, chocolate, candies, black tea (other types of tea are permitted), excessive coffee intake, spinach, rhubarb, asparagus, celery, parsley and tomatoes.

γ) Uric Acid

Patients with calcium oxalate stones who have proven hyperuricemia or hyperuricosuria should have their drug therapy complemented by a low purine diet. Offal such as liver or kidneys and excessive intake of meat or fish are to be avoided. Brassicas of any kind and alcohol in general should be reduced to a minimum.

b) Drug Therapy of Calcium Oxalate Lithiasis

α) Hypercalciuria

Definition: Hypercalciuria is excessive urinary calcium excretion, exceeding the upper limit of normal at 250 mg/24 hrs in women and 300 mg/24 hrs in men (DENT et al. 1964; HAUTMANN et al. 1978; HAYASHI et al. 1975; HERING and LUTZEYER 1979; NORDIN 1976; PAK 1973; PARFITT et al. 1964; RAPADO et al. 1976; YENDT et al. 1966). Since the values given take no account of body weight, standard computed surface, renal function or fluid intake, it is of some advantage to quote hypercalciuria in terms of the calcium-creatinine quotient.

Because the literature is devoid of data on a stone-free cohort, only limiting values can be quoted for this parameter. According to PAK (1975) the upper limit lies at 0.31 in a starved subject. The quotient is calculated from the daily calcium and creatinine excretion in g or mg, and therefore has no units.

Classification: PAK (1975) defines three types of hypercalciuria:

1. Absorptive
2. Resorptive
3. Renal

On the other hand, NORDIN (1976) recognises only two categories:

1. Absorptive
2. Resorptive

Cases of hypercalciuria that are difficult to classify, or uncertain in their etiology, are subsumed under the heading of idiopathic hypercalciuria.

(i) Absorptive Hypercalciuria

This condition is characterised by increased intestinal uptake of dietary calcium. The utilization rate of dietary calcium is higher in these patients than in a normal population. The associated pathophysiologic mechanism leads to a temporary increase in the ionised fraction of the serum calcium, resulting in suppression of parathormone secretion. The ionised calcium undergoes increased glomerular filtration, following which, and because of the reduced parathormone levels, its reabsorption in the loop of Henle and in the distal tubule is impaired. Since proximal tubular calcium reabsorption is coupled to sodium reabsorption, calcium accumulates in the loop of Henle and the distal tubule. In the latter regions, as distinct from the proximal tubule, calcium reabsorption is under parathormone control (DIRKS et al. 1976). The consequence is hypercalciuria.

Two distinct mechanisms are known to be involved in dietary calcium uptake. One is vitamin D dependent and one involves passive diffusion (ADAMS and NORMAN 1970; DE LUCA 1979; MARTIN and DE LUCA 1969; NICOLAYSON 1937; SCHACHTER and ROSEN 1959; WILKINSON 1976). Although calcium is absorbed throughout the small intestine, 90% is taken up in the duodenum and upper jejunum (HARRISON and HARRISON 1963; WILKINSON 1976). Passive diffusion is dependent on dietary calcium- and sodium concentrations (DE LUCA 1979; MARTIN and DE LUCA 1969). The term "passive" fails to take account of the fact that a carrier mechanism is needed to overcome the lipoprotein membrane of the small intestinal mucosa, and this occurs in the form of a calcium binding protein. Other authors are of the opinion that 1,25-dihydroxycholecalciferol improves the permeability of the mucosal membrane to calcium (DE LUCA 1979) (Fig. 2).

Whole body calcium depletion of whatever etiology, be it growth, pregnancy or lactation, brings in to play active transport mechanisms, even in the presence of low calcium concentrations. This mechanism presumably improves nutritional yield (DE LUCA 1979).

Active uptake of dietary calcium is under the control of 1,25-dihydroxycholecalciferol. The effect of this active form of vitamin D in turn de-

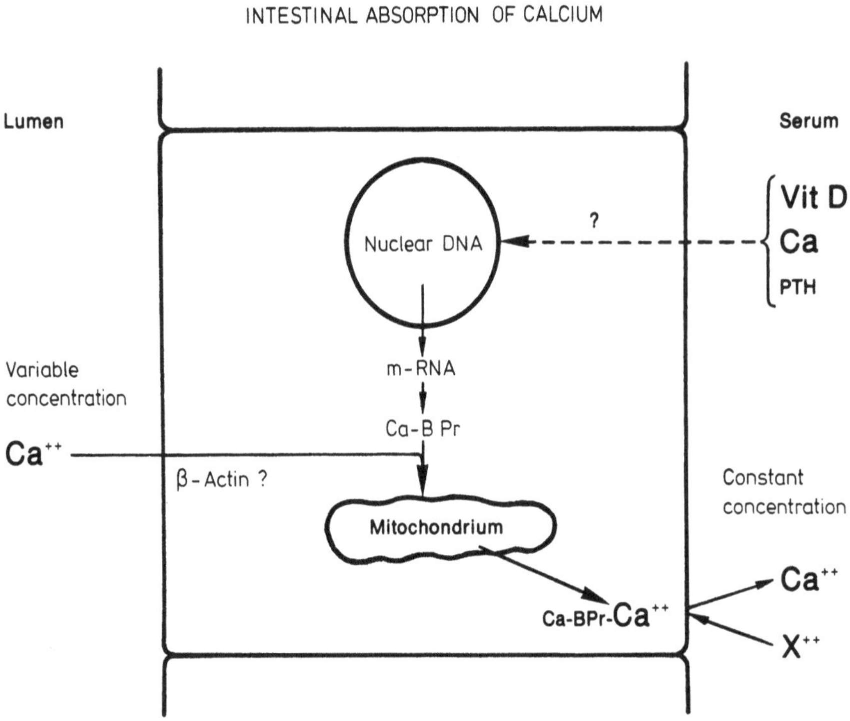

Fig. 2. The control of calcium uptake from the gut

pends on adequate serum parathormone levels (DE LUCA 1979; WILKINSON 1976).

In patients with absorptive hypercalciuria there is an increase both in uptake by diffusion and in active uptake of dietary calcium, irrespective of intestinal calcium levels or of the body's requirements. The exact mechanism of this inappropriate activity is not yet clear. 1,25-dihydroxy-cholecalciferol probably plays a key role (WILKINSON 1976). In addition to phosphate depletion, patients with absorptive hypercalciuria have been demonstrated to have increased levels of 1,25-dihydroxycholecalciferol (HAUSSLER et al. 1977). It appears fairly certain that their enterocytes exhibit an enhanced response to normal serum 1,25-dihydroxycholecalciferol levels.

(ii) Resorptive Hypercalciuria

The term resorptive hypercalciuria also refers to a state of increased daily calcium excretion. The latter is, however, independent of dietary intake (NORDIN 1976; PAK 1975; ROBERTSON 1976; YENDT and COHANNIM 1973). Hyperparathyroidism, the principal cause of resorptive hypercalciuria, also gives rise to increased intestinal calcium absorption. Central to the pathophysiology of hyperparathyroidism is a disturbance in the normal equilibrium of bone mineral deposition and resorption in favor of demineralization. Degradation of skeletal apatite gives rise to a transient hypercalcemia and hyperphosphatemia, both calcium and phosphate being eliminated via the kidneys. Raised parathormone levels (primary hyperparathyroidism), however, result in only moderate hypercalciuria, since parathormone acts on the loop of Henle and the distal convoluted tubule to promote reabsorption of calcium. This process goes hand in hand with a far more marked hyperphosphaturia.

The *classical* form of *resorptive hypercalciuria* occurs in *primary hyperparathyroidism:* In this condition relatively autonomous secretion of parathormone proceeds independently of serum calcium levels and results in osteoclastic breakdown of the skeleton. The physiologic equilibrium of deposition and resorption then ceases to pertain. Other syndromes leading to resorptive hypercalciuria include osteomalacia, osteoporosis, prolonged immobilization after injury or surgery, primary malignancies and skeletal metastases.

(iii) Renal Hypercalciuria (Fig. 2)

The clinical syndrome of renal hypercalciuria is said to be due to a disorder of distal tubular reabsorption, so-called calcium losing nephropathy. Studies by PAK (1975) revealed a decreased parathormone responsiveness of the distal tubule, resulting in decreased reabsorption of calcium from the glomerular filtrate. Under normal circumstances 5–10% of calcium passing the glomerulus is recovered in the loop of Henle and distal convoluted tubule (DIRKS et al. 1976; DIRKS 1984). This process is parathormone dependent.

In renal hypercalciuria distal tubular calcium recovery appears insufficient (PAK), despite raised serum parathormone levels and increased excretion of intracellular transmitter (cyclic AMP) (SCHWILLE and SEMBERGER 1975) (Fig. 3).

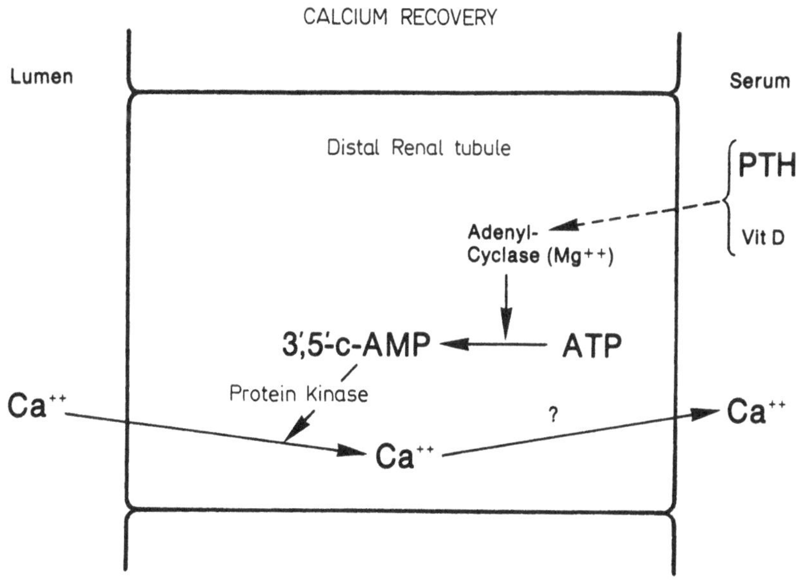

Fig. 3. Calcium recovery in the distal renal tubule

β) *Laboratory Differential Diagnosis of the Hypercalciurias*

A number of laboratory investigations are quoted as distinguishing between types of hypercalciuria (NORDIN 1976; PAK 1975; RITZ et al. 1975; YENDT and COHANIM 1973; HERING and LUTZEYER 1979). However much they may differ in detail, all these procedures have in common the measurement of calcium excretion following a period of starvation and after an oral calcium load. Patients with recurrent *calcium stones* who have on *one occasion* been *demonstrated* to be *hypercalciuric* are made to adhere to a low calcium diet for a period of three days before commencing the test (Table 3). At the end of this period they are starved for a minimum of twelve hours, during which an adequate diuresis is secured by the infusion of calcium-free solutions or by the administration of low calcium mineral waters or of distilled water. At the end of this period of starvation urine is collected over an interval of two to four hours, blood being taken at the midpoint of the collection period. Oral calcium loading can now be performed, either by the administration of a 1 g bolus or by the intake of 1 g evenly distributed over the day. This is followed by a defined urine collection period of 4 to 6 hours.

Urinary calcium, creatinine and, if possible, cyclic AMP are estimated, as well as *serum* calcium, creatinine and, where indicated, parathormone. The calcium-creatinine quotient is determined for the starving and post-calcium urines. Measurement of the serum calcium and parathormone levels and of urinary cAMP will then permit the three types of hypercalciuria to be distinguished (Tables 4, 5).

In the presence of *absorptive hpyercalciuria* both calcium excretion and urinary calcium-creatinine quotient will increase after an oral calcium load, the starving values having been normal. In both *renal* and *resorptive* hypercalciuria there will be raised calcium excretion and a correspondingly increased calcium-

Table 3. Protocol for the investigation of hypercalciuria

1. Low calcium diet for three full days prior to test period (restricted milk and dairy produce)
2. *Day 1*
   Starve from 8 pm (no food or oral fluids)
   From 8 pm to 6 am (day 2) 1500 ml levulose i/v
3. *Day 2*
   Accurate collection 6 am to 10 am under *starving* conditions of four hourly urines for laboratory estimation of calcium, phosphate, creatinine (plus cAMP). 8 am blood sample for calcium, phosphate, creatinine (ionised calcium, parathormone) estimation.
4. *Day 3*
   1 g calcium by mouth (e.g. 2 tabs. Calcium Sandoz forte, 1000 mg divided in 4 and dissolved in water, taken steadily throughout the day); simultaneously 24 hr urine collection for laboratory analysis as at 2. above.
5. *Day 4*
   Blood sample on concluding 24 hr urine collection, for estimation of calcium, phosphate and creatinine.

Table 4. Calcium/creatinine ratio under starving conditions and following an oral calcium load c-AMP in urine and serum parameters to distinguish the hypercalciurias

Type	Laboratory results: urine			Serum
	Calcium/creatinine ratio		cAMP	Ca^{++}, Ca, PTH
	4 hrly urines after 12 hour fast	24 hr urine and 1 g calcium by mouth		
Absorptive	<0.15	>0.30	No change	Normal
Resorptive or renal	>0.15	<0.30	Raised or No change	Normal or Raised
Mixed type	>0.15	>0.30	No change	Normal

Table 5. Measurement of cyclic AMP levels used to distinguish between renal and resorptive hypercalciuria

	Urinary calcium creatinine ratio		$\frac{\text{cAMP}}{\text{creatinine}}$	
	Starved period	Calcium loaded (oral)	Starved period	Calcium loaded (oral)
Resorptive (hyperparathyroidism)	Raised	Raised	Raised	Raised
Renal	Raised	Raised	Raised	Normal
Absorptive/ intestinal	Normal	Raised	Normal	Normal

creatinine ratio under both starving and calcium loaded conditions. Oral calcium loading will lead only to a small increase (Fig. 4, Table 4).

The method of Pak (1975, 1984) may then be used to distinguish between renal and resorptive hypercalciurias (Table 5). Urinary cyclic AMP should be determined. De Luca(1979) has identified this substance as the intracellular transmitter mediating the effects of parathormone in the distal tubule (Fig. 3). About half the urinary cAMP is filtered in the glomerulus and the remainder arises from tubular secretion (Schwille 1975). This tubular secretion is under parathormone control.

Whilst in renal hypercalciuria oral calcium will suppress cAMP excretion, this is not true of the resorptive picture. In other words, urinary cyclic AMP levels are continuously raised in resorptive hypercalciuria and cannot be suppressed by oral calcium loads. In renal hypercalciuria oral calcium loading will lead to a reduction in cAMP excretion.

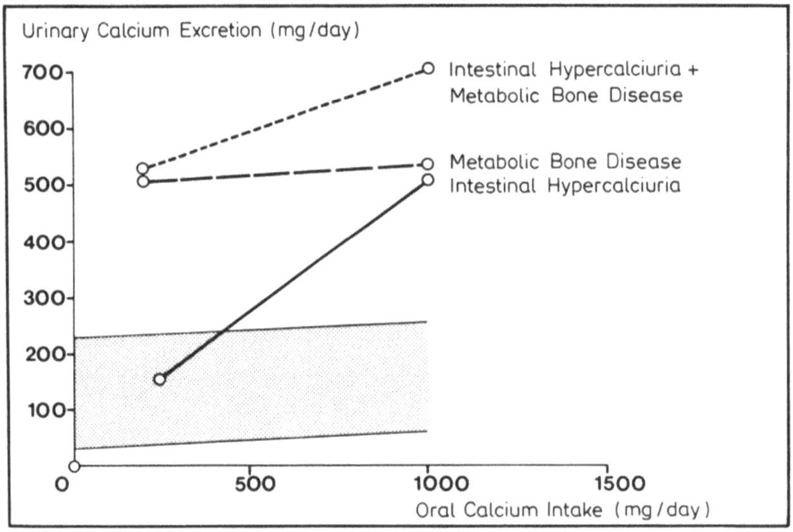

Fig. 4. The extent to which various types of hypercalciuria are related to oral calcium intake (modified after NORDIN 1976)

c) Calcium Oxalate Stones: Drug Therapy and Recurrence Prevention

α) Absorptive Hypercalciuria

The drug therapy of absorptive hypercalciuria is aimed at reducing dietary calcium intake and at inhibiting calcium uptake from the intestine. The daily calcium requirement of a healthy adult is of the order of 10 mg/kg body weight, so that individual calcium requirements may easily be calculated from dietetic tables (Table 1). The following is a rule of thumb, presenting the patient with a choice for his daily intake: 1–2 glasses of milk, 1 pot of yoghurt, 1 pack of cottage cheese or 100 g of cheese in addition to an otherwise balanced diet and mineral water. Drinks will need to be tested for their calcium content on an individual basis, since certain volcanic waters contain large quantities of calcium salts, occasionally in excess of 400 mg/l.

Where dietary measures alone prove inadequate, additional recourse may be taken to drug therapy.

The drug treatment of absorptive hypercalciuria usually centers on the administration of substances that act as ion exchangers within the intestinal lumen. To date two preparations are available:
1. Sodium cellulose phosphate
2. Sulphonated divinyl benzene copolymer (Campanyl)

Ion exchangers work by more or less selectively exchanging double charged cations for sodium or potassium. The exchange process is not specific for calcium, so that ions such as magnesium, iron or copper may also be bound, depending on the calcium content of the chyme. The sodium and potassium liberated during the exchange process are mostly eliminated in the feces, only a proportion being absorbed.

(i) Sodium Cellulose Phosphate

Principle: Sodium cellulose phosphate is the sodium salt of the phosphoric ester of cellulose. The substance has varying affinity for divalent cations, binding calcium and magnesium much more strongly than iron, copper or zinc. It is this property which renders it so effective as an ion exchanger.

The exchange process takes place throughout the gastrointestinal tract, mainly in the duodenum and upper jejunum. The exchanged sodium is absorbed with a corresponding quantity of water, as is the phosphorus liberated. The latter is excreted in the urine as orthophosphate. Approximately 10–20% of urinary orthophosphate arises from the hydrolysis of sodium and cellulose phosphate within the gastrointestinal tract, with the result that a daily dose of 15 g sodium cellulose phosphate would result in urinary excretion of 300 mg free orthophosphate (PAK 1974).

The work of PAK (1974) and of DELEN and BARTTER (1974) has shown this to result in a shift of the urinary solubility product for brushite (calcium hydrogenphosphate dihydrate) from a supersaturated to an unsaturated domain. At the same time, however, there is a slight but insignificant increase in the urinary brushite formation product.

HAYASHI et al. (1975) also demonstrated a slight and equally insignificant reduction in urinary calcium oxalate saturation. They explain these results as evidence of significantly reduced calcium excretion (50–70% of baseline), vitiated, importantly, by an increase in daily oxalate excretion of the order of 9–50 mg. Coupled as it is to a decrease in urinary magnesium loss, this rise in oxalate excretion does not result in any alteration of urinary calcium oxalate saturation. There was no evidence of any change in the formation product or rate of crystal growth for calcium oxalate.

The Development of Ion Exchanger Therapy: D. A. ADAMS and E. L. HOLMES discovered the ion exchanging properties of synthetic resins in 1935. The first industrial scale production of such resins was in 1938 (BURGHELE et al. 1967). Generally speaking ion exchange resins are high molecular weight condensation or addition polymers. As insoluble polyelectrolytes they bind dissociatable acid and alkali groups in a dense network over a large surface area (BURGHELE et al. 1967). These fixed "anchor" ions are able to exchange their electrostatically bound ionic partners for ions of like charge (DOSCH 1976). Ion exchange resins are themselves totally insoluble in water and are resistant to the common solvents. If administered by mouth they are duly passed in the feces without in any way entering the blood stream (GENOT 1956; DENT et al. 1964).

It was in 1958 that DEMPSEY et al. attempted to modify hypercalciuria by the administration of sodium phytate, which binds calcium as insoluble complexes within the intestinal lumen. This approach reduced the 24 hour urinary calcium loss of patients with idiopathic hypercalciuria by up to 100 mg, with evidence of increased urinary phosphate excretion (PARFITT et al. 1964). DENT et al. (1964) were first to report preliminary results of sodium cellulose phosphate treatment for idiopathic hypercalciuria.

Dosage: The usual daily dose is 3 × 5 g at main mealtimes. This regime may, however, be modified according to the amount of calcium excreted, drug compliance and the general and specific side effects experienced by an individual patient. In view of the side effects, a daily dosage of 15 g should not be exceeded.

Contraindications: In exchange for calcium, magnesium and other divalent cations every gram of sodium cellulose phosphate will liberate 90 mg of sodium within the lumen of the gut.

The result is a not inconsiderable uptake of sodium and water. Patients with latent or overt cardiac failure, hypertension or oliguric chronic renal failure with a tendency to idiopathic edema will need careful supervision and close monitoring during treatment. There is also a phosphate load which generally worsens the situation in cases of hyperphosphatemia and renal failure.

Clinical Experience: DENT et al. (1964) and PARFITT et al. (1964) reported the early results of clinical trials.

DENT et al. (1964) treated 8 patients (5 men and 3 women) suffering from idiopathic hypercalciuria with sodium cellulose phosphate for periods ranging from 4 to 14 months. In 4 patients calcium excretion returned to normal values, 1 patient suffered a recurrent calculus. It was not possible to evaluate the contribution due to a simultaneous low calcium diet.

Similar and comparable results were reported by PARFITT.

In 1970 RAPADO wrote up a therapeutic trial involving 15 patients with idiopathic hypercalciuria treated for periods of 1 to 8 months. He reports a significant decrease in calcium excretion and an increase in urinary phosphate. There was no effect on oxalate or uric acid excretion.

The group led by PAK et al. (1971) also found a calcium depressant effect of their treatment regime, with a shift of urinary brushite from the supersaturated to an unsaturated condition.

PAK et al. (1974) restricted their indications for treatment to "intestinal" or absorptive hypercalciuria. Furthermore PAK's patients were kept on a low calcium diet during treatment, their daily intake never exceeding 400 mg.

Numerous papers testify to an effect in reducing calcium excretion and in altering urinary brushite saturation (KALLISTRATOS 1972; PIETREK and KOKOT 1973; BLACKLOCK and MACLEOD 1974; FINLAYSON 1974; ROSE and HARRISON 1974; KAPLAN and PAK 1975; COOK 1975; ETTINGER 1976; HAUTMANN et al. 1978; HERING and LUTZEYER 1979; HERING et al. 1979). SMITH (1984) reported a recurrence free rate of only 47 p.c. in comparison to thiazides of about 85 p.c. Observation time was 2 years.

Side Effects: Precautions should be taken when treating patients with hypertension, renal or cardiac failure or any tendency to edema. The binding of other divalent ions such as magnesium, iron, copper and zinc must also be born in mind (PAK et al. 1971; PIETREK and KOKOT 1973; COOK 1975). A fall in serum magnesium and urinary magnesium excretion has also been documented during sodium cellulose phosphate treatment. However, the reduction in magnesium excretion was without effect on the products of activity or formation for urinary brushite. Administration of sodium cellulose phosphate also leads to a fall in serum levels of the divalent cations iron, copper and zinc, apparently without any clinical effect.

Continuous ion exchanger therapy might be expected to lead to increased parathyroid activity and consequent secondary or tertiary hyperparathyroidism. A long term study was unable to confirm any such effect in the laboratory over a two year period (HERING and LUTZEYER 1979). Bone biopsies did indeed reveal a reduced calcium content per unit volume, yet serum calcium and parathormone levels remained within the normal range (MALLUCHE et al. 1981). Animal experiments confirmed the occurence of bone demineralization (HAGMAIER et al. 1978).

The development of *hyperoxaluria* during such treatment is of far greater import (HAUTMANN et al. 1978; PAK 1973), for it will lead to an increase of relative urinary calcium oxalate saturation. Note that a rise in oxalate excretion has a more powerful effect than the same percentage increase in calcium excretion (ROBERTSON 1976). The explanation of this mechanism is as follows: Normally about 3–12% of dietary oxalate is absorbed by the intestine (BINDER 1974; CASPARY 1979; HODGKINSON 1968, 1977; WILLIAMS 1976; HAUTMANN et al. 1978). Thus the majority of dietary oxalate exists as calcium oxalate, poorly soluble and barely crossing the intestinal lipoprotein barrier. This oxalate is therefore eliminated in the feces.

If the bulk of dietary calcium were to be bound to sodium cellulose phosphate, the corresponding oxalate will be robbed of its usual ionic partner. Sodium, potassium and magnesium salts are therefore formed, all of which have higher solubility. Alternatively there may be no such binding and free ionised oxalic acid will persist (Fig. 5).

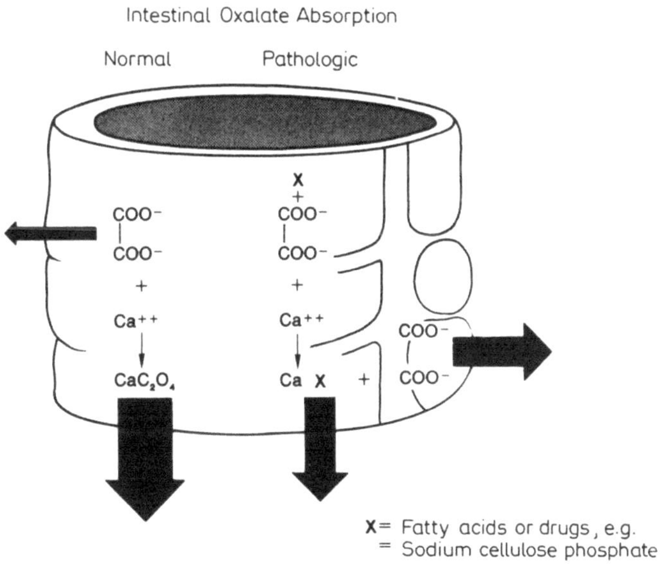

Fig. 5. The physiology and pathophysiology of intestinal oxalate absorption (modified after HAUTMANN 1978)

In other words, if intestinal formation of calcium oxalate is blocked by ion exchanger therapy, as much as 30–50% of dietary oxalate may be absorbed (KNAPPWORST 1978). *The pathophysiology is therefore identical to that of secondary intestinal hyperoxaluria,* a metabolic disorder occuring in fat malabsorption states, such as tropical sprue, Whipple's disease or disturbed bile acid turnover and furthermore in extensive inflammatory bowel disease (regional ileitis, ulcerative colitis), after small bowel resections and following bypass surgery for morbid obesity (HAGMAIER et al. 1984).

A computer program written in FORTRAN IV and modified after FINLAYSON has been used to evaluate data from measurements of relative urinary calcium oxalate saturation. It emerges that in those patients in whom hyperoxaluria occurs as a side effect of sodium cellulose phosphate there is a tendency to steadily increasing urinary saturation. Despite the reduction of calcium excretion to normal values, rising oxalate levels increase the degree of urinary calcium oxalate saturation in these patients, who are therefore at risk of crystal precipitation and further calculus formation (HERING et al. 1980).

Discussion: Sodium cellulose phosphate is an excellent blocking agent for calcium excretion. At the same time, however, it worsens the degree of oxaluria and reduces urinary magnesium excretion. Its therapeutic use is therefore only appropriate in proven cases of pure absorptive hypercalciuria and in the presence of a low calcium, low oxalate diet.

(ii) Synthetic Resin

Principle: Sulphonated styrene divinyl benzene copolymer is cross linked with 8% divinyl benzene to provide a preparation that acts in a similar way to sodium cellulose phosphate. Sorbitol and sodium carboxymethyl cellulose are also added and the potassium content is 120 mg/g. It differs from sodium cellulose phosphate in that calcium is absorbed in exchange for potassium.

Such an ion exchange resin will be in a state of dynamic equilibrium with exchangeable ions. Although exchange can therefore take place anywhere along the alimentary canal, there will be variations in exchange rate, generally a decrease from the stomach towards the rectum.

Synthetic ion exchange resins are also not perfectly selective for calcium ions. As with sodium cellulose phosphate, iron, magnesium, zinc and copper may also be bound. Measurable iron-, zinc- or magnesium deficiency has not, however, been recorded during prolonged ion exchange resin therapy (WOLF 1969). The exchange mechanism is based on substituting potassium, of which the body receives a load of 984 mg/24 hrs at a daily dose of 15 g resin. Prolonged treatment did not give rise to detectable hyperkalemia (RUGENDORFF et al. 1981). It is theoretically possible for water soluble organic cations, vitamin precursors and drugs to be bound. Such effects have never been documented, either in animal experiments or in clinical practice (BECKER and SWIFT 1959; DOCK and FRANK 1950; WOLFF 1954). Care should be taken with digitalized patients, to whom the daily intake of 984 mg potassium may be a hazard.

Toxicologic studies and teratogenicity tests have failed to show any adverse effect of synthetic ion exchange resins on reproduction, growth, bone marrow maturation, endocrine histology or major organ function (BECKER and SWIFT 1959; FLANAGAN et al. 1951; McCHESNEY and McAULIFF 1950).

Dosage: Synthetic ion exchange resin therapy is indicated in proven cases of absorptive (= intestinal) hypercalciuria. The usual daily dose is 15 g of granules in two divided doses. The granules are made up into an aqueous slurry and should normally be taken at standard mealtimes. A daily dose of 15 g granules corresponds to approx 4–8 g of active resin moieties and thus to a total in vitro calcium exchange capacity of 16–32 mg (according to the manufacturer, Temmler-Werke, Marburg). The standard daily dose may be modified according to the therapeutic response.

Contraindications: No absolute contraindications have been established. Primary hyperparathyroidism, resorptive or renal hypercalciuria and distal renal tubular acidosis represent relative contraindications.

Beware: Patients with chronic renal failure or hyperkalemia should be treated only if the serum potassium can be carefully monitored!

Note also the hazard to digitalized patients of an increased potassium load.

Clinical Experience: RUGENDORFF et al. (1981) have reported reduction of calcium excretion to normal levels in previously hypercalciuric patients. Medication was generally well tolerated and there were no notable abnormalities of clinical chemistry, such as changes in serum phosphate, sodium, calcium, magnesium or iron levels. A long term study has confirmed this evidence (HERING et al. 1979). It was of some interest that relative calcium excretion, as defined by the calcium-creatinine ratio, remained remarkably constant throughout the trial period.

Side Effects: No general side effects or hypersensitivity reactions are on record. Digitalized patients have been discussed above. Vitamins of the B group would need to be taken at times well separated from doses of resin, since binding of vitamins is theoretically possible.

One serious side effect of prolonged treatment is the occurence of hyperoxaluria. The etiology and consequences of this effect are similar to those discussed above for sodium cellulose phosphate (HERING et al. 1979).

Discussion: In the presence of appropriate indications synthetic ion exchange resins may be used to lower urinary calcium excretion. Prolonged resin therapy of absorptive hypercalciuria should only be undertaken where there are facilities for monitoring urinary oxalate.

β) Resorptive and Renal Hypercalciuria

Both resorptive and renal hypercalciuria are only slightly influenced by daily calcium intake. Restricting dietary intake is therefore of little avail. Although, where primary hyperparathyroidism is the cause of resorptive hypercalciuria, there is increased intestinal calcium uptake, the latter is not sensitive to dietary or drug therapy. In such a case surgical exploration of the parathyroids and removal of the autonomous focus will be the treatment of choice.

All other forms of resorptive hypercalciuria (e.g. osteoporosis, osteomalacia, Paget's disease of bone, prolonged immobilization, primary or secondary malignancy of the skeleton) will require treatment both of the underlying condition and of its manifestation as hypercalciuria. With the sole exception of primary hyperparathyroidism, *all forms of hypercalciuria are amenable to thiazide treatment.*

(i) Thiazides

Principle: Hydrochlorothiazide is a loop diuretic acting on cortical segments of the proximal convoluted tubule, where it inhibits the reabsorption of sodium chloride and water. This results in increased exchange of sodium for potassium in the distal tubule, with a consequent marked kaliuretic effect, – the cause of the hypokalemia seen after prolonged thiazide treatment. The sodium-potassium exchange mechanism of the distal tubule is unable to completely compensate for the proximal tubular inhibition of sodium reabsorption, so that a considerable natriuresis and passive water loss develop. This usually results in contraction of the extracellular volume and loss of weight. Increasing solute concentration in the extracellular space in turn leads to increased equimolar reabsorption of salt and water from the proximal tubule in an attempt to conserve sodium. Parallel to this sodium recovery there is proportionally equal reabsorption of calcium from the proximal tubule. The latter effect is most marked when there is mild sodium depletion of the extracellular space. If thiazides are to be given as a treatment of hypercalciuria they will therefore exert their optimal effect in the presence of a sodium restricted diet (DEETJEN et al. 1975; RITZ et al. 1975).

A further site of action for thiazide diuretics is suspected in the distal tubule, where a parathormone dependent activation of intracellular adenyl cyclase is said to lead to the isolated reabsorption of calcium. The thiazides constitute the only group of diuretics with a hypocalciuric action. All other diuretics have a calciuric effect.

Dosage: Depending on the severity of hypercalciuria the usual daily dose will be 50–100 mg by mouth. In view of the mode of action, it will be clear that all forms of hypercalciuria are suitable for thiazide treatment, including the absorptive group.

Contraindications: Primary, secondary and tertiary *hyperparathyroidism* constitute absolute contraindications, since in these conditions thiazides may provoke dangerous hypercalcemic crises.

Any syndrome embracing *hypokalemia* represents a relative contraindication. Regular serum potassium estimations will then be required, since the duration of thiazide therapy needed for the effective treatment of recurrent urolithiasis may lead to hypokalemia so profound as to endanger the patient. This is especially true of digitalized patients.

Beware: *Hypotension* – thiazides have a hypotensive action!

In hypertensive patients this effect is beneficial, and the dose should then be adapted to preexisting hypotensive needs.

Initially, patients with mild or latent *hyperuricemia* must have regular serum uric acid estimations performed, since thiazides may, above a certain dose, give rise to hyperuricemia. If necessary, allopurinol can be added to the medication of such patients.

Similar considerations apply to latent *diabetics*, who may develop overt disease on thiazide treatment.

Clinical Experience: YENDT and COHANIM (1973) reported on 197 patients treated with thiazides over periods up to eleven years at an oral daily dose of 100 mg. All patients had previously elevated 24 hour urinary calciums, and in all of them the values became normal on treatment. Over 90% of patients reported cessation of stone formation. No new stones occurred and existing stones ceased to enlarge. Within this group YENDT and COHANIM (1973) observed the best effect in patients with non-infective calcium calculi, whereas those with calcium calculi of infective etiology had an increased tendency to recurrence. Since the effect of thiazides depends on extracellular sodium levels (PAK 1973, RITZ et al. 1975). PAK has instituted additional dietary sodium restriction to enhance the response.

Effective control and reduction of urinary calcium excretion to normal levels was first reported by LAMBERG and KUHLBAECH (1959), LICHTWITZ et al. (1961), PARFITT et al. (1964), DUARTE and BLAND (1965) and by YENDT et al. (1966). More recent publications by ROSE and HARRISON (1974), RAPADO et al. (1976), PAK et al. (1978) and by HERING et al. (1979), JACOBSON et al. (1979), LJUNGHALL et al. (1981), and SCHOLZ et al. (1981) have tended to confirm the effectiveness of thiazides in the treatment of hypercalciuria and their influence on the frequency of stone recurrence, whilst stressing the need to appreciate their side effects.

Side Effects: Hypercalciuria is only *one* aspect of the multifactorial etiology of calcium oxalate lithiasis. The possible effects of thiazides on urinary levels of other electrolytes and stone forming or -preventing substances should not be forgotten!

Oxalate: GLAZENBURG (1972), COHANIM and YENDT (1981), PAK et al. (1978), YENDT and COHANIM (1973), SCHOLZ et al. (1981), and YENDT (1984) have all documented reduction of both calcium and oxalate excretion to normal levels on thiazide treatment. Yet other authors have reported a deterioration in oxalate excretion (HERING et al. 1979; ROSE et al. 1974). The chief difficulty in assessing these conflicting reports lies in technical variations in oxalate estimation. Different methods tend not to yield comparable results, and at the time of writing a definite opinion on the effects of thiazide therapy on oxalate excretion cannot therefore be given.

Magnesium: YENDT and COHANIM (1973) report a mild increase in magnesium excretion. Magnesium is said to form complexes with oxalate and thus to have a degree of calculus inhibiting effect. There is no further evidence for a hypermagnesiuric effect of thiazides. Both SCHOLZ et al. (1981) and LJUNGHALL et al. (1981) report a mild decrease in magnesium excretion.

Zinc: In separate papers YENDT and COHANIM (1973) and PAK et al. (1978) report thiazide-promoted zinc excretion. Zinc is considered to inhibit crystal deposition in organic matrix. In the context of urolithogenesis zinc helps inhibit crystallisation in organic substances, the latter making up 3–5% of urolith material.

Pyrophosphate: Increased pyrophosphate excretion is likewise reported by both PAK and YENDT. Pyrophosphate is an effective inhibitor of calcium oxalate crystal aggregation.

Uric Acid: Hyperuricemia developing during thiazide therapy has been recorded by ROSE and HARRISON (1974), YENDT and COHANIM (1973) and PAK et al. (1978). PAK, furthermore, describes hyperuricosuria as occuring in not quite 50% of his patients. This phenomenon has been ascribed to an increase in uric acid clearance, considered by PAK to be due either to an increase in uric acid production or to a decrease in extrarenal metabolism. In any event, an increase in uric acid excretion must be looked on as undesirable in a patient with calcium oxalate lithiasis. Uric acid blocks the usual inhibitory effects of acidic mucopolysaccharides on crystal aggregation (ROBERTSON et al. 1976).

Recent work by LJUNGHALL et al. (1981) failed to reveal any increase in uricosuria, whilst SCHOLZ et al. (1981) actually observed a decrease in urinary uric acid.

Citrate: According to reports by the group of SCHOLZ and SCHWILLE (1981) and by LJUNGHALL and his colleagues (1981) thiazide therapy is without effect on citrate excretion.

Discussion: Thiazide therapy will be effective in the treatment of any type of hypercalciuria. The effects of treatment will be potentiated by sodium restriction. There are no known side effects liable to precipitate further stone formation. On the contrary, those substances whose excretion is increased tend to be stone inhibitors, such as magnesium, zinc or pyrophosphate.

General side effects and intolerance symptoms may arise through hypokalemia, hyperuricemia or exacerbation of diabetes mellitus. Hypotension may also be a problem. Therefore any patient on long term thiazide therapy for stone disease requires regular laboratory investigation!

γ) Drug Therapy of Hyperoxaluria

Because the disease is due to an inherited hepatic enzyme defect, only limited causally directed drug treatment is available for primary hyperoxaluria. GERSHOFF (1964), ROSE (1981), and ROSE et al. (1982) have all reported isolated successes with vitamin B_6 administration. Attempts to influence the quantities of oxalate formed in normal intermediate metabolism or to control renal excretion and diffusion processes have also met with little success. Yet only 5–40% of renally excreted oxalate can have been taken up by the gut (BINDER 1974; CASPARY 1979; KNAPPWORST et al. 1967). The so-called secondary hyperoxaluria occurring in a variety of conditions arises from abnormal intestinal absorption (Fig. 5). Many diseases may be responsible: recurrent gastroenteritis, Whipple's disease, sprue, the enterocolitides, pancreatitis, regional ileitis, ulcerative colitis, enterocolic bypass procedures for morbid obesity, fat malabsorption, viral enteritides and, furthermore, iatrogenic states brought about by misconceived hypocalciuric therapy with intestinally active ion exchangers or by overzealous calcium restriction.

Apart from the few case reports on vitamin B_6 therapy for the primary form, it is only secondary "intestinal" hyperoxaluria that offers any quarter to pharmacologic attack. Drug and dietary therapy will both depend on the underlying condition.

The enzyme defect of fat malabsorption leaves long chain fatty acids inadequately cleaved. The latter then combine with dietary calcium to form insoluble calcium soaps with a consequent fall in calcium concentration in the chyme. Calcium normally combines with oxalate to form poorly soluble and barely diffusible salts. For this reason only 3–12% of dietary oxalate is normally absorbed from the gut (ZAREMBSKI and HODGKINSON 1969). In the absence of its usual partner, calcium, oxalate will persist either in the ionised, freely diffusible form or as more soluble sodium-, potassium- or magnesium salts. Depending on the concentration gradient, such oxalate can be absorbed throughout the gastrointestinal tract preferentially in the colon. In this way up to 40% of renally cleared oxalate may originate from the gut lumen.

(i) Cholestyramine

The treatment of secondary intestinal hyperoxaluria will require dietary restriction of long chain fatty acids and their replacement by medium chain species. A trial of drug therapy may also be undertaken, using cholestyramine (commerically available as Questran or Quantalan). This substance is reputed to be beneficial in steatorrhea of biliary origin, in regional ileitis and after extensive resections, both in terms of its effect on the diarrhea and as a hypooxaluric agent (CASPARY 1979; KNAPPWORST 1978).

Side Effects: The administration of cholestyramine may initially exacerbate fat malabsorption and thus further impair the absorption of fat soluble vitamins. Concomitant vitamin replacement therapy is therefore recommended.

(ii) Diethyl Cellulose

Diethyl cellulose is not yet on the market. It acts as an ion exchanger, binding oxalic acid within the lumen of the gut. At a dose of 3 × 5 g after meals each gram of diethyl cellulose is capable of binding 700 μmol of oxalate within the intestine, whence it is removed in the feces. There is no evidence of absorption from the intestinal lumen.

PINTO and BERNSHTAM (1978) tested the drug in a clinical trial on a small number of patients. The duration of treatment was too brief to allow any firm conclusions about the effectiveness or side effects of this substance.

(iii) Succinimide

In 1972, THOMAS et al. described an effective reduction in hyperoxaluria after administration of the succinic acid derivative succinimide. During the follow-up period these authors recorded a decrease in recurrence rates for calcium oxalate calculi, coinciding with a return of urinary oxalic acid levels to the normal range. Other authors were not, however, able to completely reproduce these findings (HAUTMANN et al. 1978; HODGKINSON et al. 1975; ROHDE et al. 1978).

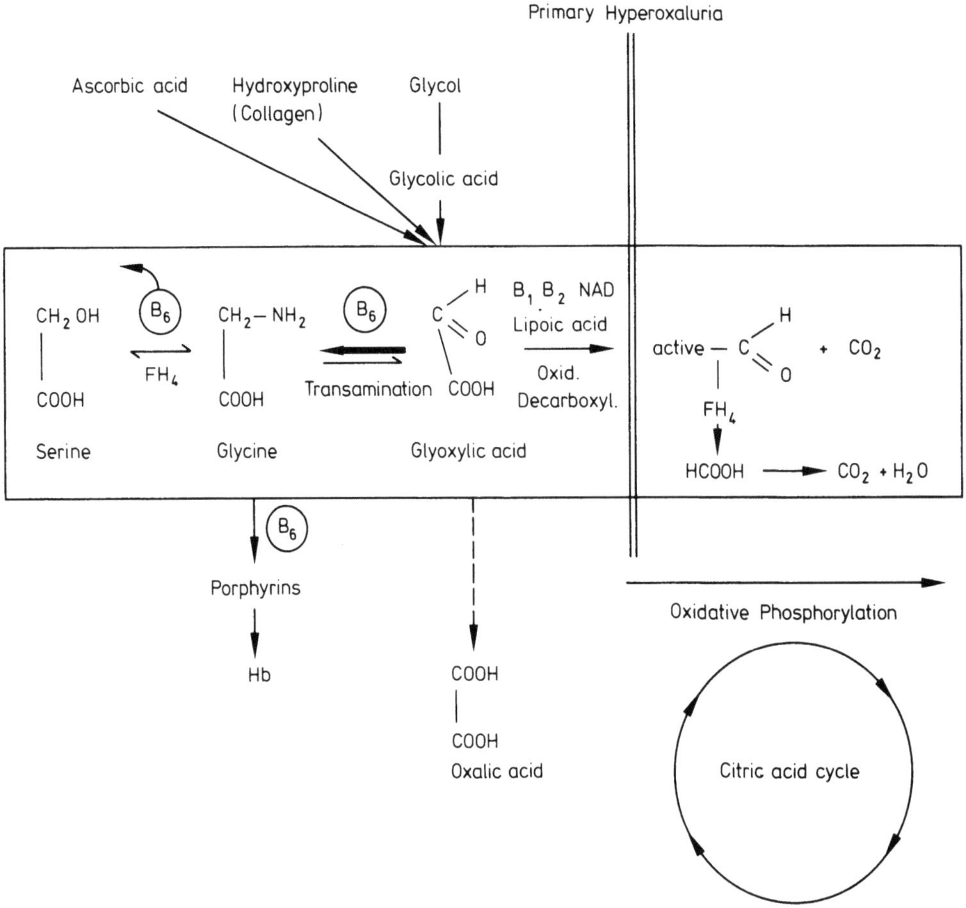

Fig. 6. Oxalic and glyoxylic acids in intermediate metabolism (after HAUTMANN 1980)

Principle: To date it has been impossible to elucidate the exact role of succinimide in intermediate metabolism or within the kidney, either in vivo or in vitro. The site of action on intermediary metabolism is assumed to be the liver (ZILLEKEN 1975), although other authorities prefer the kidney. It is at this site that there is said to be an effect on calcium-oxalate aggregation (SCHULTE et al. 1979). The effect on hepatic metabolism is thought to be associated with the insertion of succinimide into the Krebs cycle (Fig. 6). Succinate is generated by deamination in the intestinal wall and would accelerate oxidative phosphorylation. Such a rise in redox potential would in turn stimulate oxidative degradation of the oxalate precursor glyoxalate via the tricarboxylic acid cycle. The result should then be reduced oxalate production.

A second possible metabolic pathway would be introduction of succinate into the Shemin cycle. That would result in activation of glycine metabolism, leading to increased hemoglobin synthesis and consequent improved tissue oxygenation. This in turn could lead to a reduction in the formation of oxalate from glyoxalate.

Dosage: The dose is set at 3 × 3 g by mouth at mealtimes.

Contraindications: No absolute contraindications are known. In view of the unknown mechanism of action, one should refrain from prescribing succinimide during pregnancy and lactation.

Clinical Experience: In 1972, THOMAS et al. reported effective control of hyperoxaluria and cessation of stone recurrences. HODGKINSON and his colleagues, however, were unable to detect any effect at all of succinimide administration on oxalate excretion in their animal system (HODGKINSON et al. 1973). ROHDE and coworkers also failed to find any change in oxalate excretion (ROHDE et al. 1978). Studies by HAUTMANN et al. (1978), involving 19 patients with recurrent calcium oxalate lithiasis and proven pretherapeutic hyperoxaluria, demonstrated a significant decrease in urinary oxalate excretion during the 19-month trial period. 57% of patients had an initial fall in oxalate excretion, followed by a drift back up into the pretherapeutic range. Succinimide therapy brought about a significant decrease in recurrence rate.

Side Effects: No untoward effects on the excretion of lithogenic material or in terms of general acceptability could be demonstrated in the laboratory. There were, however, subjective complaints of gastrointestinal upset, occasionally leading to the abandonment of treatment.

Discussion: The exact mechanism of action of succinimide remains obscure. The results of its clinical application are less than uniform, and a definitive opinion cannot at present be given. In cases of extreme hyperoxaluria, however, a trial of therapy could always be justified, particularly in the absence of any evidence of serious side effects. The exceptional contraindications remain pregnancy and lactation.

(iv) Pyridoxine (Vitamin B_6 Complex): (Primary Hyperoxaluria)

Pyridoxine is a coenzyme in transamination reactions between glyoxylic acid and glycine and between glyoxylic acid and activated formaldehyde. This glyoxylic acid–glycine–glyoxylic acid-activated formaldehyd pathway provides the organism with a route of degradation for (toxic) oxalic acid at the glyoxylic precursor stage, thus preventing further formation of the toxic end product oxalic acid (Fig. 6).

Dosage: The dose will depend on the level of oxaluria, 200 mg/day being suitable for severe cases (ROSE et al. 1981).

Contraindications: No symptoms of intolerance, clinical side effects or laboratory abnormalities are known.

Clinical Experience: GERSHOFF (1964) reported positive results for the control of hyperoxaluria, a finding at odds with that of WILLIAMS (1968), the latter failing to detect any very satisfactory effect of vitamin B_6. Nevertheless, in the absence of any other available treatment he recommends the administration of up to 200 mg/day for cases of proven primary hyperoxaluria. This recommendation is shared by KALLISTRATOS (1972), TERHORST and LUTZEYER (1973), and by BUELOW and FROHMUELLER (1976).

In 1981 a report came from ROSE et al. on the successful treatment of extreme hyperoxaluria with vitamin B_6. Indeed these authors suspect vitamin B_6

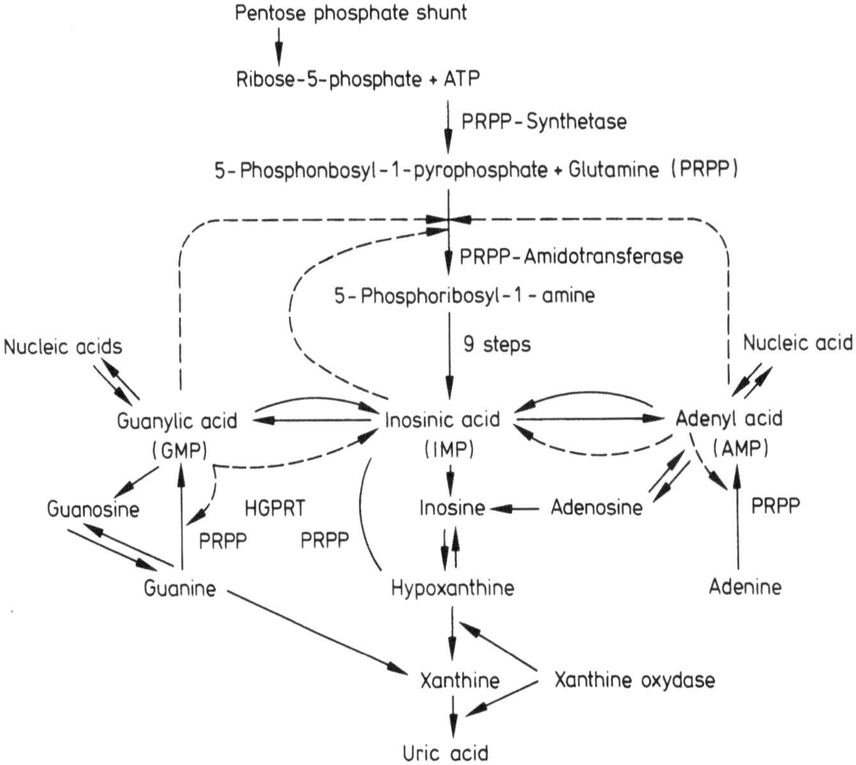

Fig. 7. Degradation pathways for purine nucleotides and the reutilization of xanthine and hypoxanthine

deficiency to be a cause of hyperoxaluria, the mechanism being impaired degradation of glyoxalate to activated formaldehyde. Longer term and more extensive clinical trials are needed to confirm the effectiveness of this treatment.

Side Effects: Despite the high dosage, no side effects are reported. In the absence of any other effective treatment a trial of vitamin B_6 therapy is probably justified, particularly in view of the lack of side effects. Individual case reports tend to encourage such an approach.

δ) Hyperuricemia and Hyperuricosuria

Hyperuricemia and hyperuricosuria may be primary or secondary. In primary gout and in the clinical syndromes of hypoxanthine-guanine phosphoribosyl transferase (HGPRT) deficiency or of phosphoribosyl pyrophosphate (PRPP) deficiency the clinical effects are due to disordered uric acid metabolism. The enzyme defects cause disorganisation of purine and nucleic acid degradation with a rise in level of the endogenous uric acid pool. In man uric acid represents the end product of nucleic acid degradation, although there are many mammals in which this is not the case (Fig. 7). The serum uric acid lies between 3.5 and

6.5 mg in normal men and between 3.3 and 5.7 mg in women. Normal daily excretion (off a high purine diet) amounts to less than 800 mg/day of uric acid.

According to BOSS and SEEGMILLER (1979) uric acid is 100% filtered by the glomerulus, 98–100% being reabsorbed in the proximal tubule and 50% being actively secreted in the descending limb of the loop of Henle. Finally 40–44% are reabsorbed in the distal tubule. The net excretion is thus of the order of 6–12% of glomerular filtrate uric acid. In primary renal failure or secondary tubular impairment due to interstitial nephritis or pyelonephritis the uric acid secreting mechanism may be embarassed. The result will be a rise in the endogenous uric acid pool and hyperuricemia. That, in essence, is the renal gout theory of GARROD (1853). THANNHAUSER (1952, 1956) and ZOELLNER (1960) gave the renal theory its resurrection and some experimental support.

According to BENEDICT et al. (1949) primary gout can be explained on the basis of excess uric acid production. This theory derives from the existence of HGPRT and PRPP deficiencies. Lack of the enzyme HGPRT or of the substrate PRPP results in incomplete reassembly of the purine derivatives xanthine and hypoxanthine into new nucleotides. Xanthine and hypoxanthine are degraded by xanthine oxidase to uric acid.

ε) *Secondary Hyperuricemia*

This syndrome may arise wherever there is pathologically increased cell turnover or cell breakdown (myeloproliferative disease, leucoses, malignancy, cytotoxic therapy, radiotherapy or substantial weight loss) as well as in obesity or in response to increased dietary purine intake.

(i) Clinical Significance of Disorders of Purine Metabolism in Relation to Calcium Oxalate Calculi

It was BERGER and YÜ (1975) who drew attention to the pathogenetic significance of uric acid for calcium oxalate stone formation. They were able to demonstrate that 15.8% of patients with primary gout had uroliths, whilst in turn 27% of their patients with oxalate stones had a demonstrable abnormality of purine metabolism. The FRAMINGHAM study (described in M. J. V. SMITH and W. H. BOYCE: "Allopurinol and Urolithiasis", 1969) also uncovered an increased incidence of urolithiasis in patients with elevated serum uric acid levels.

Two possible mechanisms have been suggested to account for this link:

1. MANDEL and MANDEL (1981) were able to demonstrate by X-ray diffractometry that uric acid and calcium oxalate possess similar crystal lattice structure and lattice angles. Uric acid crystals might thus act as seeds for heterologous nucleation and so trigger calcium oxalate aggregation.
2. Studies by ROBERTSON et al. (1976) suggest that, among other substances, acidic mucopolysaccharides exert an inhibitory influence on calculus formation. Uric acid in turn blocks this effect.

The mechanism suggested by ROBERTSON consists of surface coating of crystals by mucopolysaccharide, so inhibiting the attachment of further crystals. Increased urinary uric acid concentrations will occupy positive binding sites on the mucopolysaccharide molecules, preventing these from proper attachment to crystal complexes. The inhibitory effect of mucopolysaccharides on crystal aggregation is thus lost. Drug therapy is aimed at correcting excessive uric acid excretion, and it is therefore the renal and postrenal aspects of uric acid metabolism that are most relevant to the treatment of urolithiasis.

ζ) Allopurinol

Principle (Fig. 8): This drug acts at two points in intermediate metabolism:

1. It blocks nucleotide synthesis by forming the false substrate allopurinolribonucleotide. This blockade is only partial.
2. Competitive inhibition of xanthine oxidase.

As a hypoxanthine analogue allopurinol is converted by hypoxanthine-guanine-phosphoribosyltransferase (HGPRT) to a "false" allopurinolribonucleotide. This process consumes phosphoribosyl pyrophosphate. The false nucleotide acts via a feedback mechanism to inhibit de novo purine synthesis and thus the formation of uric acid. The inhibition of xanthine oxidase is specific and arrests nucleotide degradation at the hypoxanthine-xanthine step.

Unlike uric acid, xanthine and hypoxanthine are soluble in an acid milieu and can be excreted without crystallising.

Allopurinol is a xanthine oxidase inhibitor. Although one might expect deleterious consequences of long term allopurinol therapy in the form of whole body xanthine- or hypoxanthine depletion, no such effect has been documented with any certainty (SIMMONDS 1979).

Dosage: The daily dose is 300 mg by mouth. Depending on the actual serum uric acid level and the degree of hyperuricosuria, this value may be raised or lowered on an individual basis. Allopurinol is rapidly absorbed following in-

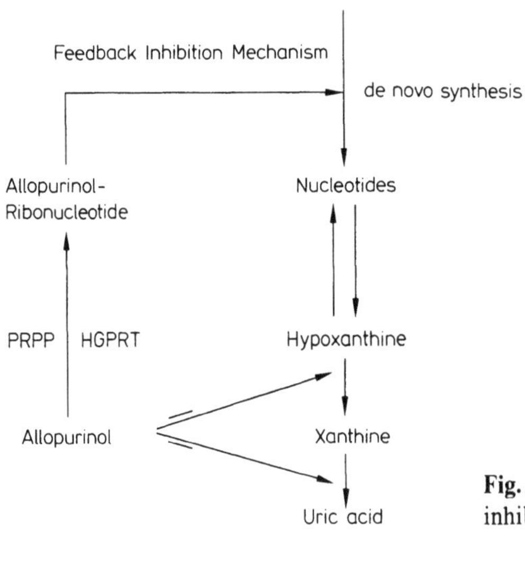

Fig. 8. Mode of action of the xanthine oxidase inhibitor allopurinol

gestion, two thirds being oxidised in the liver and excreted by the kidneys (WELLHOENER 1976).

Contraindications: Pregnancy and lactation.

Clinical Experience: Allopurinol was introduced in 1963 by RUNDLES et al. for the treatment of primary gout and of the hyperuricemia of leukemics. First reports of successful treatment of uric acid metabolism disorders were by YÜ and GUTMAN (1964). In the meantime numerous papers have appeared, all testifying to the efficacy of allopurinol (SCOTT 1966; SCOTT et al. 1969; ANDERSON et al. 1967; SEEGMILLER et al. 1967; SILBERMANN 1967; ZOELLNER and SCHATTENKIRCHNER 1967; KOLLWITZ and BRAUER 1968; GODFREY and RANKIN 1969; HOLLÄNDER and SCHWARCZMANN 1969; SMITH and BOYCE 1969; BAND 1970; HELBIG and FINDEISEN 1971; MILLIS 1971; COE and RAISEN 1973; COE and KAVALACH 1974; YÜ 1974; HARTUNG 1975; VABUSEK 1976; DE VRIES and SPERLING 1976; BRAUN et al. 1977; MIANO et al. 1979). All these publications report a lowering of previously raised serum uric acid and/or of elevated urinary uric acid values. Attention has been drawn to the risk, early on in treatment, of a transient rise in uric acid excretion and possible intratubular precipitation. TERHORST and MELCHIOR (1972) and KALLISTRATOS (1972) have both documented an effective reduction in the recurrence rate of calcium oxalate calculi during allopurinol therapy. These observations are confirmed by the work of GUTMAN and YÜ (1968), of SCHNEIDER (1969), of SCULTETY and BALOGH (1967) and of SMITH and BOYCE (1969).

Side Effects: None of the above papers mention any serious objective problems. At the beginning of treatment complaints of fever, rigors and dermatologic symptoms may arise. Overt allergy is rare, but there are not infrequently such symptoms as gastritis, anorexia and lassitude. Generally these complaints all settle as treatment progresses, and it rarely becomes necessary to discontinue the drug.

Discussion: Allopurinol is the treatment of choice for uric acid lithiasis and proven disorders of uric acid metabolism. The mode of action is such that no permanent increase in uric acid excretion will develop.

η) Probenecid

Probenecid is also used to treat disorders of uric acid metabolism.

Principle: Probenecid lowers the serum uric acid by a uricosuric action.

The mechanism is inhibition of tubular reabsorption. Therein lies the explanation for the undesirable side effects of probenecid, which may be a serious hazard to patients with uric acid stones. Depending on the state of the endogenous uric acid pool there may be so marked a rise in urinary uric acid excretion as to cause intrarenal precipitation of uric acid crystals, particularly when the saturation limit of 6.4 mg% at pH 7 is exceeded. Note that it is specifically in acid urine that precipitation may occur at lower concentrations.

If for some reason probenecid has to be given in place of allopurinol, the following requirements must always be met:

1. The daily diuresis must be at least 2–3 liters
2. The urinary pH should be adjusted to lie between 6.8 and 7.2.

If either of these demands is unsatisfied, the kidney may become completely blocked with uric acid crystals. This risk pertains whenever the saturation limit of uric acid is exceeded (SAMBERGER, BRAUN, LUX and MAY 1979).

Another hazard is triggering an acute attack of gout, usually at the beginning of treatment when the endogenous pool is being mobilised.

Contraindications: Renal failure and pregnancy.

Discussion: Wherever and for whatever reason urolithiasis has to be treated without increasing the daily diuresis or neutralising the urine one should take the hazards of probenecid very seriously. The risk of inducing acute renal failure is considerable (SAMBERGER et al. 1979).

ϑ) *Hyperphosphaturia*

Hyperphosphaturia is important not only in relation to phosphatic calculi (nucleation by phosphates), but also because of its effect on calcium oxalate stones and its role in the formation of mixed calcium oxalate-calcium phosphate calculi. Phosphatic "microliths" appear in phosphate saturated urine and may serve as seedlings for the formation of calcium oxalate calculi. This concept is substantiated by electron microscopy of urine sediment (BLASCHKE and MAAR 1979; HERING et al. 1981).

Aluminium hydroxide preparations offer one method of treating hyperphosphaturia. Indeed they are often used in patients with end stage renal failure to prevent the advent of hyperphosphatemia. Aluminium hydroxide binds phosphate and thus prevents its intestinal uptake.

(i) *Aluminium Hydroxide*

Principle: Aluminium hydroxide is a weak base often employed as a neutralising agent in the treatment of hyperacidic gastritis. There is up to date no evidence for systemic uptake from the gut. Aluminium hydroxide exhibits relatively non-specific binding of phosphate as phosphates of aluminium. Tetracyclines, alkaloids and phosphate containing enzymes are also bound in a concentration dependent way (WELLHOENER 1976).

Dosage: The daily dose consists of 440 mg three times daily, by mouth.

Contraindications: None known. Intestinal disorders causing decreased motility are a relative contraindication, since aluminium hydroxide may itself reduce gut motility.

Clinical Experience: The role of this agent is well known and long established in the treatment of end stage chronic renal failure, where it is intended to prevent the occurrence of renal hyperphosphaturia.

A reduction in urinary phosphate levels is important in the treatment of calcium oxalate lithiasis whenever the urine tends to become alkalinised – the most usual cause being infection. Calcium phosphate may precipitate from an alkaline urine, and according to the heterologous nucleation hypothesis calcium oxalate deposits may form on the surface of calcium phosphate crystals. The result is a mixed calcium oxalate-calcium phosphate stone.

Side Effects: No serious or obvious side effects are on record. Prolonged treatment may so reduce intestinal motility as to lead to constipation and fecal impaction. This effect is fully reversible on discontinuing the drug. An increase in parathormone secretion due to transitory hyperphosphatemia and a rise in intrarenal 1-hydroxyhydrolase activity, raising 1,25-dihydroxycholecalciferol levels, may occur but are without clinical significance (TSCHOEPE et al. 1979).

Discussion: Long term aluminium hydroxide therapy is only of use in cases of calcium oxalate or calcium oxalate–calcium phosphate lithiasis simultaneously characterised by marked hyperphosphaturia. The treatment is usually entirely safe.

i) Inhibitors of Calcium Oxalate Stone Formation and Treatment with So-called Inhibitors

General Considerations: Numerous experiments in vitro and in vivo confirm that urine contains a number of substances acting in different ways to inhibit crystal nucleation or aggregation. The following are said to be inhibitors of crystal aggregation: acidic mucopolysaccharides, pyrophosphate, phosphocitrate, citrate, magnesium, diphosphonate, methylene blue and various glycosaminoglycans. Their effectiveness is variable (1. Phosphocitrates: TEW et al. 1981; WILLIAMS and SALLIS 1981; 2. RNA and RNA-like substances, glycosaminoglycans, "GAGS": SCHRIER et al. 1981; 3. Diphosphonate EHDP, chondroitin sulphate, glycosaminoglycans "GAGS", methylene blue, pyrophosphate, urate and xanthine: HALLSON et al. 1981; SCURR et al. 1981; 4. Magnesium, sodium chloride, pyrophosphates, vitamin B_6, glucuronic acid, citrate: SUR and PANDEY 1981; RYALL and MARSHALL 1981; SALLIS et al. 1981; TISELIUS and LARSON 1981; PINTO and PUJOL 1981; RODGERS and GARSIDE 1981; HARTUNG et al. 1981; VAN'T RIET and O'REAR 1981). It has not yet been possible to critically evaluate these communications in clinical practice. The results given are not strictly comparable between papers, the activities quoted vary from author to author and the measuring systems differ. Suitable among these for oral administration are: Orthophosphate, excreted in the urine as pyrophosphate, diphosphonate, which exerts a pyrophosphate-like action, magnesium and methylene blue. The degree of absorption from the gut is variable and in some cases unknown. Treatment with any inhibitor presupposes proven inhibitor deficiency. Treatment instituted on false premises is not only useless but, as in the case of inappropriate magnesium therapy, often vitiated by the opposite of the intended effect. In the presence of urinary tract infection and an alkaline urine magnesium therapy may simply lead to the formation of magnesium ammonium phosphate calculi. It is precisely in cases of calcium oxalate lithiasis, which are so common and represent such a therapeutic challenge, that we have no idea of the quantity of inhibitor to give, if we are to slow down or abolish calcium oxalate crystal nucleation or aggregation. The available data are derived from measurements in vitro and are intrinsically inapplicable to real patients.

(i) Orthophosphate

Principle: Pyrophosphate inhibits the precipitation of calcium oxalate and the formation of calcium carbonate crystals (FLEISCH and BISAZ 1961). According to FLEISCH and his colleagues condensed phosphates block crystal growth by attaching to the crystal surface. This is particularly true of the hydroxyapatite group, which has a high affinity for pyrophosphate. Pyrophosphate excretion rises in the wake of orthophosphate ingestion (EDWARDS et al. 1965). A generally valid explanation for this phenomenon is still not available. There are three working hypotheses:

1. Inhibition of pyrophosphate synthetase by orthophosphate.
2. Downmodulation of pyrophosphatase activity.
3. Inhibition of renal tubular pyrophosphate reabsorption by orthophosphate (RUSSEL et al. 1964).

FLEISCH and his colleagues consider the kidney the principal site of action, pointing out that orthophosphate administration is followed by a simultaneous rise in orthophosphate- and pyrophosphate clearances, although there is no change of plasma pyrophosphate concentration.

Dosage: The maximum daily dose is 1–1.5 g, which should never be exceeded because of the risk of inducing secondary hyperparathyroidism (FLEISCH). The indications for this therapy are limited to sterile calcium oxalate lithiasis, since orthophosphate treatment of magnesium ammonium phosphate-, brushite- and apatite calculi is hazardous. In animal experiments orthophosphate has been given to induce calculi of this type.

Covert urinary tract infections are also a potential hazard, since the associated urine is frequently alkaline in reaction. Once again, orthophosphate may cause the formation of phosphate calculi.

Rule of Thumb: Orthophosphate treatment requires continuous monitoring of urinary pH and should be interrupted if this enters the alkaline range.

Contraindications: Orthophosphate is absolutely contraindicated in the presence of Gram-negative urinary tract infection, especially when associated with organisms of the Proteus- or Pseudomonas group. These bacteria are urease positive and split urinary urea into ammonia, alkalinising the urine. For the same reason, orthophosphate should not be used to treat "infectious" calculi.

Other contraindications would include chronic renal failure with hyperphosphatemia and primary, secondary or tertiary hyperparathyroidism.

Clinical Experience: FLEISCH and BISAZ (1961) were the first to report useful results of orthophosphate treatment for calcium oxalate stones. Their results were confirmed in 1969 by SUTOR and a reduction in recurrence rates for calcium oxalate calculi has also been reported by DULCE (1965), by HORN (1971), by TERHORST and LUTZEYER (1973). TERHORST reports not only increased pyrophosphate excretion but also a drop in urinary calcium levels. WILLIAMS (1977) has recommended an oral daily phosphate intake in the region of 1.5–2 g, claiming this to be as effective as orthophosphate.

Orthophosphate therapy is further recommended for calcium oxalate lithiasis by HOWARD and THOMAS (1968), FINLAYSON (1974) and by ETTINGER (1976) on the grounds that crystalluria will cease instantaneously when treatment starts. At the same time FINLAYSON expresses some doubt about the effectiveness of this treatment, since oral orthophosphate, for all it produces a palpable increase in pyrophosphate excretion, only raises it to the levels found in healthy subjects. Either this weak effect is itself sufficient, or it merely affects one component in a multifactorial pathogenetic mechanism.

All the literature on oral orthophosphate therapy has in common that either the patient cohorts are too small or the trial period is too short to permit any objective conclusions. SMITH (1984) reported about 37 patients ten years on this trial. The stone recurrence rate was reduced from 6 stones/year before treatment to 2.6 stones/year after onset of treatment. Treatment was started for patients with idiopathic stone disease, primary hyperoxaluric, renal tubular acidosis type I and mild form of primary hyperparathyroidism.

Side Effects: No serious side effects are known. Gastrointestinal intolerance in the form of gastritis or fecal impaction have been reported for long term treatment, but these complaints appear reversible by discontinuing medication. A hypertension may develop in patients with prestanding hypertension (SMITH 1984). In case of impaired renal function creatinine clearance should be higher than 50 ml/min (SMITH 1984).

Discussion: No definite statement can be made on the subject of recurrence prevention, since the clinical data is simply inadequate.

(ii) Magnesium

Following early studies by HAMMARSTEN in 1928 and 1929, PRIEN and GERSHOFF (1974) have reported relatively successful treatment of calcium oxalate lithiasis with magnesium oxide.

Other papers on the effects of magnesium on oxalate solubility are by SUTOR (1969), ELLIOT and RIBEIRO (1970), WILLIAMS (1977), and by DANIELSON (1985).

Principle: Magnesium administration leads to the formation of a magnesium oxalate salt in the urine. Calcium is thus displaced from oxalate binding, depending on the exact concentrations. Magnesium oxalate is very substantially more water soluble than the calcium salt. Following oral intake of magnesium there is a rise in urinary magnesium excretion. The mechanism of absorption, the site and the proportion absorbed are all unknown. According to TERHORST and MELCHIOR (1972) there is no effect on urinary calcium-, phosphate-, pyrophosphate-, uric acid- or citrate excretion, FLEISCH and BISAZ (1966) state that around 30% of dietary magnesium appears in the urine.

Dosage: MELNICK et al. (1971) recommend 600 mg twice daily. Magnesium therapy should only be instituted *when* there is proven urinary magnesium deficiency. The administration of magnesium oxide is thus indicated for cases of sterile calcium oxalate calculus.

Contraindications: The danger of magnesium therapy actually generating calculi is similar to that in orthophosphate treatment. This hazard is increased in alkaline urine or in the presence of Gram-negative urinary tract infection. Magnesium ammonium phosphate calculi may then form. Where urinary tract infection occurs treatment should therefore be interrupted.

Clinical Experience: From the point of view of the patient cohort and the duration of the study the best report on magnesium oxide as a treatment of calcium oxalate lithiasis is by MELNICK et al. (1971). Over a period of 4 years these workers were able to reduce the recurrence rate by a factor of ten. This degree of success was only achieved in a group of patients with obvious urinary magnesium deficiency at the outset. In the absence of such magnesium deficiency there was little definite benefit. KING (1971), on the other hand, found no increase in the incidence of stones among alcoholics, a group who may present with considerable magnesium deficiency. It is not known to what extent increased diuresis might be a factor among alcoholics.

JOHANSSON et al. (1981) have reported some success among their patients with calcium calculi, even though magnesium therapy did nothing to alter urinary calcium excretion. Over the three-year period of their study about 90% of patients on treatment remained recurrence free, compared to only 40% in the control group. DANIELSON (1985) reported a five-year recurrence-free rate of about 80%.

Side Effects: No serious subjective or objective effects have been met with. Less than 5% of patients complained of gastrointestinal symptoms; all the latter resolved after stopping magnesium oxide (JOHANSSON et al. 1981).

Discussion: Magnesium oxide treatment is frequently combined with vitamin B_6 therapy and appears to represent an effective means of preventing recurrence. The prerequisite for avoiding serious side effects is sterility and neutral pH of the urine. Magnesium oxide therapy is contraindicated for any so-called infectious stone.

(iii) Ethanehydroxydiphosphonate (EHDP)

In 1970 FLEISCH et al. reported in vitro inhibition of calcium phosphate precipitation by a 10^{-7} molar EHDP solution. EHDP is an artificial crytallisation inhibitor of similar structure to pyrophosphate. Since EHDP is not broken down by naturally occurring phosphatases, it is both incorporated into the skeleton and excreted unchanged in the urine (BAUMANN et al. 1975).

EHDP was originally introduced for the treatment of Paget's disease (ALTMANN et al. 1973), myositis ossificans (BASSET et al. 1969) and generalized calcinosis (CRAM et al. 1971). In 1975 BAUMANN and his colleagues published their experience in the treatment of 9 patients. The recommended daily dose was 1.100 mg divided into four. 8 out of 9 patients remained free of recurrences over a twelve month period. Urinary pyrophosphate excretion increased by 14%. The side effects included a rise of urinary uric acid by 90% and of oxalic acid by 70%.

The fact that EHDP accumulates in the skeleton, where its long term effects remain unknown, has prevented this treatment from gaining general acceptance.

At the time of writing nothing further can be said of its effectiveness, side effects or hazards in clinical use.

(iv) Oxalyt-C

Studies with the sodium-potassium citrate preparation Oxalyt-C have been carried out at various centers (HESSE et al. 1985; DULCE et al. 1985; HAUSER and FRICK 1985; MAY and BRAUN 1985; SCHWILLE 1985) over relatively short periods of time with small numbers of subjects (stone patients and stone-free controls), and have shown an influence of this agent on various urinary parameters

Effects: There is a dose dependent increase in urinary citrate excretion and thus a rise in urinary pH, the final values varying between 6.2 and 6.6

In addition, there is a dose-dependent decrease in calcium excretion, the reason for which has not yet been explained, but which is possibly due to intestinal complex formation with citrate or to temporary systemic alkalosis, although no systemic alkalosis could be achieved by oral citrate administration.

Further effects are a decrease in ammonia excretion and a temporary fall in serum parathormone values.

Dosage: The normal dose is 3 × 3 g daily. In the case of therapy-resistant aciduria, 4 × 3 g daily can be administered.

Side Effects: The side effects described are dose dependent and disappear on discontinuation of therapy. They include loose stools and urinary infections. Existing urinary infections can also be exacerbated.

Contraindications: Contraindications are manifest urinary infections, infected calculi, and calculi formed predominantly of phosphate, as in neutral or alkaline urine there is a danger that the phosphate will crystallize out. Caution is advisable when the spontaneous urinary pH value is above 6, since additional alkalizing therapy can provoke urinary infection or formation of an infected calculus.

Evaluation: No conclusive assessment of the efficacy of Oxalyt-C is possible at this point, as the duration of administration has been too short and the number of patients too low.

(v) Urinary pH

The solubility of calcium oxalate is essentially constant over a wide range of urinary pH. The consequence is that pharmacologic manipulation of urinary pH is of little benefit in the treatment of calcium oxalate lithiasis per se. Only in cases of mixed calcium oxalate calculi, of so-called infectious stones and also of mixed calcium oxalate–uric acid stones are such maneuvers helpful. The necessary pH change will depend both on the nature of the stone components and on their actual concentrations, since the exact mineral formed will be of some importance. The details are to be found in the relevant chapters.

(vi) Urinary Tract Infection

Urinary tract infection is not a frequent feature of calcium oxalate lithiasis, and this type of calculus is usually classified among the sterile group. Should infection supervene it must receive specific treatment, since there is otherwise a danger of phosphate deposition on oxalate calculi. The addition of infectious components to such mixed calculi worsens the recurrence rate of calcium oxalate lithiasis. Specific antibacterial chemotherapy is therefore always indicated in cases of proven infection.

(vii) Treatment of Mixed Calcium Oxalate Calculi

The basic principle is to treat each component on its own merits. Consideration should also be given to the underlying metabolic cause of increased urinary lithogen excretion.

The choice of drug treatment and diet should be independent of the proportions of individual components. Mixed stones tend to recur more often, and every lithogenic abnormality should therefore be treated.

2. Infective Calculi

This term embraces all types of calculus arising in infected or alkaline urine. The commonest pathogens are Gram-negative organisms such as Proteus, Pseudomonas and Klebsiella. Their possession of the enzyme urease enables them to produce ammonia, thus alkalinising the urine. Phosphate salts are poorly soluble in an alkaline urine and the consequence is therefore stone formation, with an incidence according to GRIFFITH (1978) and HERRING (1962) of the order of 15–20%.

The following types of stone may be infective: Any calcium phosphate calculus (hydroxyapatite, carbonate apatite, brushite, octacalcium phosphate and whitlockite); any magnesium phosphate calculus (struvite and rarer magnesium phosphate minerals such as newberyite and bobierite).

The main aim of pharmacologic and dietary recurrence prevention is to improve the solubility of the calcium phosphates. It is with this in mind that the urine should be acidified and infection eradicated as far as possible. In the presence of preexisting calculi it remains desirable to maintain a sterile urine, since bacteria will bind to the surface of the calculus (GRIFFITH et al. 1976). If urinary infection is longstanding and where renal calculi have arisen, there is a risk of intrarenal reflux giving rise to interstitial nephritis and pyelonephritis. Classical treatment of the calculi will fail to eradicate them, even if powerful and specific antibiotics are exhibited.

Diet: The basic requirement to restrict food of a high calcium content is as for the treatment of calcium oxalate lithiasis, but oxalate need only be limited where mixed calculi occur. Any food or drink likely to alkalinise the urine should be strictly avoided. Citrus fruits and their juice are important culprits, alkalinising the urine with the salts of weak acids. Beer, coca cola and acidifying mineral water are permitted. The urine should be diluted by an increased fluid intake and metabolic disorders require treatment on their own merits. Brassicas have an alkalinising effect and should be avoided.

Ammonium urate lithiasis imposes special dietary requirements, since there is both an infective and a metabolic uric acid component. The urine should still be acidified, but only down to a pH of 6.5 Overzealous acidification carries a risk of urate precipitation. A steady fluid intake of 1.5–2 liters or more (if possible) is fundamental to therapeutic success.

Drug Treatment of Urinary Tract Infection: A rational strategy for preventing recurrent infective stones must first aim to completely eradicate existing stones (SCHNEIDER 1980). Antibacterial therapy is unlikely to be successful where pseudorecurrences or organic material were left behind. As a rule any remaining debris is contaminated and will give rise to a recrudescence of infection with a renewed rise in urinary pH and the seeding of recurrences around such infected nuclei.

BUDEVSKI (1975) quotes a recurrence rate of 14% where there was previous complete clearance. This figure rose to 52% for cases with residual stones and attained a peak of 75% if calculi remained in the presence of infection. According to WILLIAMS (1977) the spontaneous recurrence rate may reach 80% over a 20 year period. It is misguided to expect spontaneous regression of residual calculi (GRIFFITH 1978), hence the requirement for complete surgical clearance of all calculous material and infected matrix.

Stone clearance should be followed by specific antibiotic treatment, achieving adequate tissue levels within the renal parenchyma, as well as adequate urine levels. Even after successful removal of e.g. struvite calculi there is likely to be persistent soft tissue infection (interstitial nephritis and pyelonephritis) demanding prolonged and aggressive chemotherapy. GRIFFITH suspects intrarenal reflux as the cause of persistent infection following stone clearance and quotes an incidence of 40%. The proper duration of antibiotic therapy is controversial, opinion ranging from denial of any need in cases of struvite calculi to a lifelong sentence to prophylaxis. Since the protagonists of aggressive antibiotic treatment quote lower recurrence rates, in the region of 4–10%, their point of view seems not without merit (BRUCE and GRIFFITH 1981; SEGURA et al. 1981; GRIFFITH et al. 1981). By contrast BOYCE (1974) quotes a figure of 18%.

The choice of antibiotic must take account of nephrotoxicity. The aminoglycosides (gentamicin, tobramycin and amikacin) are markedly nephrotoxic, a property amplified by renal damage of any cause. The dose may depend on the creatinine clearance.

Recurrent or persistent infection may reflect anatomical tract abnormality, congenital or acquired (obstructive uropathy, stricture, stenosis, megaureter, vesicoureteric reflux, infravesical obstacles). These conditions require surgical correction to eradicate infection.

Treatment of Urinary Tract Infection in the Presence of Calculi: If for some reason surgical stone clearance cannot be contemplated (age, previous surgery, anaesthetic objections), conservative management by urinary antiseptic treatment may be appropriate, if adequate urinary acidification (pH 6.5) can be achieved. On the other hand, as long as the stone remains in situ it will always prove impossible to eradicate interstitial nephritis or pyelonephritis as a source of persistant sepsis. Every acute exacerbation of symptomatic urinary tract infection will require high dose antibiotic treatment. Regular examination of urinary sediment and a strict watch on urinary pH are an integral part of this form of management.

(i) Acetohydraxamic Acid

In 1973, GRIFFITH et al. published the first report of successful urease inhibition by acetohydraxamic acid. The enzyme urease is produced by all groups of Proteus and by certain Pseudomonas-, E. coli-, Klebsiella- and staphylococcal species. Urea is split in the following reaction:

$$NH_2CONH_2 + H_2O \xrightarrow[\text{urease}]{} 2NH_2 + H_2CO_3$$

$$2NH_2 + H_2O \rightarrow NH_4 + OH$$

The resultant hyperammonuria alkalinises the urine, promoting the formation of phosphatic calculi, particularly of struvite.

In animal experiments hydraxamate was shown to be a highly effective inhibitor of bacterial urease. GRIFFITH et al. (1973) demonstrated neutralization of the urine, inhibition of struvite calculus formation and a bacteriostatic action on Proteus organisms. The intermediate metabolism of hydraxamix acid is unknown, yet clinical trials so far suggest low toxicity and good therapeutic effect. Animal experimentation has also suggested a protective effect against hyperammonuric renal damage. Acetohydraxamic acid is not yet on the market in Germany (FRG) and in the USA the clinical use is still under control by the FDA.

Mode of Action: AHA is rapidly and completely absorbed from the gut. Peak blood levels occur after half an hour and 40–60% of oral intake appear unchanged in the urine. Approximately 50% is metabolised by an unknown pathway and at an unknown rate, the latter apparently more rapid at lower than at higher doses. It appears, therefore, that the metabolic pathway becomes saturated by high quantities of AHA. According to GRIFFITH et al. (1976) 25–30% of ingested AHA is broken down to carbondioxide and blown off by the lungs. For normal renal function the half life is 5–10 hrs, more in patients with renal impairment.

Clinical Experience: In a trial involving 76 patients GRIFFITH et al. (1981) gave AHA for periods in excess of 3 months. Despite preexisting urinary tract infection and anatomical tract abnormalities (trabeculated bladder, indwelling catheter, nephrostomy, paraplegia or quadriplegia) they found a reduction in urine alkalinity and in urinary ammonia concentrations. In only four cases did preexisting stones regress, but further growth or recurrence of stones occurred in none of their patients. RODMAN (1985) reported a double blind trial of 31 patients. Patients on AHA treatment showed no stone growth or new formation.

Side Effects: The side effects and toxicity of AHA are dose dependent and fully reversible by stopping medication. Approximately 50% of patients complained of headache and a further 50% of gastritic symptoms, diarrhea or constipation – a spectrum of gastrointestinal effects. 4% reported somnolence or lassitude and 8% noted flushing in combination with alcohol. The latter phenomenon would persist approximately 30 minutes and then suddenly cease. More serious side effects occurred with the following frequency: Mild anemia, 17%; severe anemia, 13%; phlebitis, 13%; pulmonary embolus, 1.4% and tremolousness 30%.

Comment: Further discussion should await the outcome of more extensive controlled clinical trials.

Instrumental Chemolysis of Infective Stones: Instrumental chemolysis via a nephrostomy or indwelling catheter is not only – in the final analysis – impossible, the attempt may even be life-threateningly dangerous. Despite sporadic reports in the literature of the 60s and 70s (TIMMERMAN and KALLISTRATOS 1973; SUBY and ALBRIGHT 1943) of successful dissolution of infective calculi using EDTA (TIMMERMANN), Renacidin (MULVANEY 1960; RIES and MALAMENT 1962; KOHLER 1962) or Suby's solution (SUBY 1943), large scale trials have been unable to prove any benefit. Fatal accidents were not infrequent, and in the USA intrarenal perfusion with Renacidin is now prohibited. Indeed the stipulation that Renacidin therapy only be undertaken in the absence of infection and at pressures below the intrapelvic pressure limits its application to the point of extinction. In view of the complication rate and very doubtful benefit, such treatment should be regarded with suspicion.

In a similar way, occasional reports of successful stone dissolution by *hemiacridine* should not lead one to hope for any widespread applicability of this treatment, since successes were occasional and related only to individual problem cases. None of the authors mentioned reports a large series (FAM et al. 1976; JACOBS and GITTES 1976; NEMOY and STAMEY 1976; BROCK et al. 1980). Chemical dissolution of stones via percutaneous nephrostomy has generally only met with success in cystinurics (SMITH et al. 1979; STARK and SAVIR 1980; DRETZLER et al. 1979).

Drug Treatment of Metabolic Disorders: For the drug treatment of hypercalciuria, hyperuricosuria and hyperphosphaturia, see the above sections on the treatment of calcium oxalate lithiasis.

(ii) Urine Acidification

Principle: Acidifying the urine is intended to improve the solubility of phosphates. Nucleation of phosphate and carbonate crystals is inhibited in neutral or acid urine. The technique of urine acidification depends on the administration of salts of strong acids and weak bases. Following absorption from the gut there is transient metabolic acidemia, for which the kidney will compensate by substituting hydrogen ion for potassium ion exchange with sodium. Intracellular carbonic anhydrase splits carbonic acid into bicarbonate and hydrogen ion. The bicarbonate returns to the bloodstream by diffusion, whilst the hydrogen ion is entered into distal tubular active transport and exchange mechanisms. This hydrogen ion secretion acidifies the urine. It is thus clear that such a strategy will only be effective where renal function is preserved. Interstitial nephritis of calculous or infective origin may cause a secondary distal renal tubular acidosis and therefore block any therapeutic benefit.

Dosage: The exact dose of a given drug will depend on the starting pH of the urine, on renal function and on the severity of possible side effects. A variety of preparations is commercially available. In Europe these include "Acidol pepsin", "Extin", "mixt. solvens" and, more recently, "Uralyt-acid". Nearly all these formulations contain a wide variety of compounds, but the active principle is consistently ammonium chloride or a similar hydrogen ion donor and they are all suitable.

Contraindications: Urine acidification is contraindicated in all forms of acidosis, especially in distal renal tubular acidosis. In cases of ammonium urate calculus the urine pH should not be allowed to fall below 5.8–6, since further acidification risks precipitating urates.

Clinical Experience: Effective urine acidification can only be achieved with concomitant antibacterial attack on the causative organism. Otherwise excessive doses of acidifying agents may be necessary with an inherent risk of iatrogenic metabolic acidosis.

Side Effects: Gastrointestinal intolerance is dose dependent and fully reversible by stopping medication. Nausea and retching without histologically proven gastritis or ulcer is the chief symptom.

Discussion: If urinary tract infection is treated at the same time, good dose dependent urine acidification can be achieved. Patient cooperation is necessary for proper control of urinary pH by daily testing. The fundamental requirements for successful treatment are complete stone clearance and rigorous, perhaps long term, antibacterial chemotherapy.

Problems of Conservative Treatment for Infective Calculi: The initial decision to treat conservatively and the subsequent therapeutic strategy are both vitiated by a variety of problems. Conservative treatment may be necessary in circumstances such as the preoperative assessment period, episodes of pseudorecurrence, unilateral or bilateral staghorn calculus and cases of staghorn- or infective calculus unsuitable for surgical removal on anaesthetic grounds. Established or incipient renal sepsis, fever and rigors related to infective calculi, the threat of peri- or paranephric abscess and outflow obstruction to infected kidneys all present a hazard to the patient which may demand a period of conservative management. Any decision between conservative treatment and surgical intervention will have to take a balanced view of renal function, potential nephron loss following an attack on the parenchyma and the fate of renal function following interstitial nephritis or pyelonephritis, if the stone is left in situ. Such sequelae as hypertension and the emergence of a potential source for recurrent metastatic infection should also be considered.

The final decision, which course to adopt will have to be made on the merits of each individual case.

The decision to treat conservatively may avoid all the hazards associated with surgery, but the stone will remain as a continuing source of future infection. As already stated, this factor cannot be influenced by high dose antibiotics or by urine acidification. Renal function will slowly but surely be eroded by infection, by interstitial nephritis and by pyelonephritis. Because of the creatinine excretion reserve, such events will only become apparent at a relatively late stage, unless the function of both kidneys is reassessed individually on a regular basis (iodohippuran clearance, radiology, ultrasonographic renal outline) so as to detect the extent and progression of renal damage at an early stage.

Apart from bacterial insult Lipid A, an E. coli cell wall component, may engender chronic renal destruction, apparently by some shared antigen mechanism (WESTENFELDER et al. 1975).

Superadded metabolic disease, such as hyperparathyroidism, hyperuricemia or hypokalemia may exacerbate tubular damage. Further stone enlargement and outflow obstruction, the development of a septic kidney or the spread of infection to the peri- and paranephric tissues with abscess formation are ever present hazards. Infected renal calculi are a well established source of such unpleasant sequelae as endocarditis, iridocyclitis and rheumatic disorders. *In view of their overall life expectancy, young and middle-aged patients are best protected from these complications by surgical clearance of their stones.*

Operative removal of renal stones may be problematic where a staghorn is confined within narrow calyceal necks, preventing a simple approach from the renal pelvis or pelvicalyceal junction. In such cases a *transparenchymal* approach will require formal nephrotomy. These kidneys have frequently been operated on in the past and the ensuing scar tissue presents both a source of operative bleeding and a cause of reduced renal function. Without any doubt nephrolithotomy with surface cooling (BOYCE and ELKINS 1974) or with perfusion hypothermia (EISENBERGER et al. 1973; MARBERGER and EISENBERGER 1980; MARBERGER and STACKL 1981), with or without inosine infusion (MARBERGER et al. 1976) represents a real advance. Nevertheless, a 10–20% loss of renal function due to scar formation is to be expected. Radial nephrolithotomy along "avascular" planes identified by methylene blue injection (BOYCE and ELKINS 1974) or by Doppler flow studies (RIEDMILLER et al. 1981) has allowed some improvement by reducing tissue damage. The feasibility of workbench surgery (GIL-VERNET 1965) does not in itself represent an indication to employ the technique, particularly since it brings no further advantages in terms of renal function. Nevertheless it does allow the surgeon to achieve improved clearance without being subject to the pressure of time limits. It should perhaps be reserved for surgery to solitary kidneys.

Quite apart from the difficulties of preserving renal function, the completeness of stone clearance remains a problem, despite improved intraoperative stone localization techniques (ALBRECHT and MONCADA 1981; MELCHIOR and LANG 1981; DE SY and OOSTERLINCK 1981; LYTTON 1979). Intraoperative stone localization by ultrasound has no advantages over radiology for fragments smaller than 2 mm, chiefly because of masking by air entering the renal pelvis once the kidney is opened (HUTSCHENREITER et al. 1981). Pseudorecurrence rates of the order of 20–40% are frequently quoted (GRIFFITH 1978). Residual material, be it crystalline or not, has to be regarded as a nucleus for recurrences, however energetic antibiotic and acidification therapy may be. For the true recurrence rate following surgery for staghorn calculi figures of 40–60% are mentioned (GRIFFITH 1978).

Therefore the best strategy will have to be decided on from case to case: If surgery is to be embarked on it must be followed by energetic postoperative recurrence prevention, for the recurrence rate of infective calculi is inherently high!

New developments in the field of percutaneous litholapaxy (ALKEN et al. 1981; MARBERGER et al. 1982) and of remote extracorporeal shockwave litholapaxy (CHAUSSY et al. 1982) promise some progress in the treatment of problem cases.

(iii) Renal Tubular Acidosis

The etiology and pathogenesis of this condition are discussed in ROBERTSON and PEACOCK (1985).

With an overall frequency of 1% renal tubular acidosis is a rare feature of urolithiasis. Among cases of infective stones, however, the frequency reaches 10–40% (BACKMANN et al. 1981; SOMMERKAMP 1977).

Rule of thumb: recurrence of calcium stones, medullary sponge kidney, nephrocalcinosis or urinary pH fixed at 6–7 carry a high index of suspicion for renal tubular acidosis.

Principle: The mechanism of this disorder consists in partial impairment of distal tubular hydrogen ion secretion. The result is inadequate urine acidification, the pH usually being above 6. Blood chemistry reveals a hypokalemic hyperchloremic metabolic acidosis. This acidosis in turn acts on the skeleton to provoke increased osteoclastic breakdown of apatite and so leads to temporary hypercalcemia and hyperphosphatemia. Both ions undergo glomerular filtration.

Since the increased calcium and phosphate loads cannot be completely reabsorbed by the proximal tubule, distal segments will be overloaded with these substances. Poorly soluble in alkaline or neutral urine, calcium and phosphate will precipitate, giving rise to nephrocalcinosis or recurrent urolithiasis.

(iv) Treatment

Diet: No specific dietary treatment is available for renal tubular acidosis.

Drug Treatment: Drug treatment must take account of *five important factors:*

1. The extent of the *metabolic acidosis* must be determined by blood gas analysis and calculation of the base excess. Acidosis may be corrected by giving bicarbonate or so-called "Shohl's solution". In either case the dose should be tailored to the extent of the metabolic acidosis and the base excess, using to the formula: *base excess* × *body weight in kg* × *0.3* to arrive at the required quantity of bicarbonate in mmol. Bicarbonate treatment requires continuous blood gas monitoring to avoid the danger of alkalosis. This treatment will not result in any change in urinary pH, particularly not in acidification.
2. The extent of *hypokalemia* will determine the necessary potassium replacement. Depending on the severity of the syndrome (complete or incomplete renal tubular acidosis) considerable quantities may need to be taken. Since potassium preparations are not always well tolerated, slow release formulations liberating their potassium in the small intestine may be preferred.
3. The extent of *bone demineralization* may be quite considerable and require the administration of calcium and vitamin D preparations. The exact degree

of demineralization is best measured by iliac crest biopsy or by skeletal densimetry of the hand or forearm. The clinical presentation of demineralisation is often a complaint of backache. Giving vitamin D (1,25-dihydroxycholecalciferol) should improve skeletal calcium uptake. The calcium requirement will depend on the skeletal deficit. The additional intake during the replacement phase should never exceed the daily requirement of a 70 kg man (10 mg/kg). This replacement therapy should be supplemented with physiotherapy. Occasionally a support corset may be needed.

4. *Hypercalciuria* should be treated with thiazides: Attempts must be made to reduce the renal clearance of calcium, as in the treatment of renal and resorptive hypercalciuria. A sodium restricted diet enhances the effect of thiazides. Sodium depletion of the extracellular space enhances proximal tubular calcium recovery and the effect of thiazides on the distal tubule is also amplified. Preexisting hypokalemia will require adequate replacement therapy, since thiazides potentiate hypokalemia.
5. *Distal Tubular Hydrogen Ion Excretion may be Promoted by Ethacrynic Acid:* In 1972, HEIDBREDER described ethacrynic acid treatment of renal tubular acidosis, stating the substance to increase distal renal tubular hydrogen ion excretion. SOMMERKAMP (1981) reported on 8 patients with proven renal tubular acidosis treated with 50 mg by mouth daily. The therapeutic effect consisted of urine acidification and increased renal acid production. Because of the hazard of hypokalemia SOMMERKAMP recommends the drug be given alternate days only.

The usual form of urine acidification therapy is contraindicated, as it would generally only worsen the existing metabolic acidosis. In fact, the hydrogen ion secretion defect in itself renders urine acidification impossible. Recurrent stone formation and the advent of nephrocalcinosis or medullary sponge kidney can only be prevented by correcting the acidosis.

Laboratory Investigations: The course of the illness and the effect of drug therapy should be checked and monitored by laboratory investigations, repeated as often as necessary:

1. Serum electrolytes, particularly potassium
2. Urinary excretion products
3. Blood gas analysis
4. 24 hr urinary calcium and phosphate excretion.
5. Screening for bacterial urinary tract infection, followed by antibiotic therapy as indicated.
6. Intravenous urography at yearly intervals.

3. Uric Acid Stones: Treatment, Recurrence Prevention, Oral Chemolysis

Pure uric acid stones represent the sole type of urinary calculus amenable to dissolution by drugs. Where the pathogenesis is fully understood, oral litholysis is feasible.

With a frequency of 5–20% uric acid stones take third place in Western Europe and the United States, after only calcium oxalate and infective calculi (HERRING 1962; GEBHARDT and BASTIAN 1976). Dietary changes appear to have brought about a steady rise in frequency since the last war. Furthermore there is a definite north-south socioeconomic distribution, the incidence of uric acid lithiasis appearing correlated to dietary protein content. Increasing consumption of purine rich foodstuffs has not only led to an overall rise in serum- and urinary uric acid levels but also to an increase in the actual incidence of gout. The same group of patients is also likely to have calcium and oxalate stones (ZOELLNER 1960).

The *pathogenesis* of uric acid stones lies in increased urinary uric acid excretion with an inappropriately high urinary hydrogen ion concentration. This latter is due to abnormal ammonia excretion, but the former arises from an *external causative* factor such as increased dietary purine intake (meat, offal, various brassicas) or from an endogenous increase in uric acid production (primary gout, increased cell turnover in the myeloproliferative disorders or during cytotoxic therapy for malignancy).

The urinary pH is often below 5.4. Uric acid is a weak acid with a pK of 5.5 and is therefore neither much dissociated nor noticeably soluble at this pH. The combination of an acid urine with hyperuricuria therefore predisposes to uric acid stone formation, but at the same time it is easy to see how dietary and pharmacologic measures can break the pathogenetic chain.

a) Diet, Fluid Intake and Choice of Drinks in Uric Acid Lithiasis

The dietary purine content must be held at a low level. Offal such as liver, kidney or sweatbreads, as well as excessive overall meat and fish intake (especially marine fish like sardines or herrings) should be strictly limited. Brassica and nut consumption should also be reduced.

Strong alcoholic drinks are prohibited, as they may precipitate hyperuricemia. Drinks likely to acidify the urine (Coca Cola, beer) should be restricted and citrus fruit and its juice recommended in their place. The latter contribute by neutralising the urine. The total fluid intake must be adequate; the usual 1.5–2 liters is quite insufficient and should be increased to at least 2–3 l/day.

b) Preventive Drug Treatment of Uric Acid Lithiasis

There are two possible points of pharmacologic attack:
1. Reduction of excessive uric acid excretion
2. Solubilising urinary uric acid by raising a low urine pH

(i) Allopurinol Treatment of Hyperuricemia and Hyperuricosuria

Principle: Allopurinol acts on uric acid metabolism at two sites (Fig. 8):
1. Its property as a xanthine oxidase inhibitor blocks the conversion of hypoxanthine to xanthine and of xanthine to uric acid. Both these reactions are

normally controlled by xanthine oxidase. Purine degradation is thus blocked by allopurinol at the hypoxanthine-xanthine stage. In contrast to uric acid, both these substances are soluble in urine and rarely give rise to stones. Some qualification should be added in respect of xanthine, which is also apt to crystallise out if excreted in vast quantities – see the chapter on xanthine stones.

2. The second mode of action of allopurinol consists of inhibiting nucleotide synthesis. Allopurinol is a hypoxanthine analogue and is thus converted by the enzyme hypoxanthine guanine phosphoribosyltransferase (HGPRT) and the addition of phosphoribosyl pyrophosphate to allopurinolribonucleotide, a false purine base. The false base blocks uric acid synthesis by product inhibition. What is more, the phosphoribosyl pyrophosphate used to synthesize allopurinolribonucleotide is then unavailable for further de novo synthesis (conversion of hypoxanthine and xanthine to ribonucleotides). The false base allopurinolribonucleotide also inhibits glutaminephosphoribosyltransferase, another enzyme involved in nucleotide precursor synthesis. In addition, allopurinolribonucleotide inhibits phosphoribosyl transferase.

The reactions described above result in suppression by allopurinol of uric acid production. Allopurinol has no effect on renal uric acid clearance and treatment thus results in reduced uric acid excretion, the very reverse of the effect achieved by agents such as probenecid and other uricosurics.

Allopurinol is rapidly absorbed following oral ingestion. Two thirds are metabolised in the liver by the enzyme xanthine oxygenase to oxypurinol, which is subsequently eliminated by the kidney (WELLHOENER 1976). Its half life is two to three hours and allopurinol is fully effective in patients with reduced renal function.

Dosage: The dose should be varied according to the serum uric acid and the 24 hr urinary uric acid excretion. A normal starting dose is 300 mg daily by mouth, but this will have to be modified in the light of subsequent changes in uric acid levels.

Contraindications: Because of possible teratogenicity allopurinol should not be taken in pregnancy or during lactation.

Clinical Experience: The uric acid depressant effect of allopurinol is well established in the treatment of primary and secondary gout (GUTMAN and YÜ 1968; KRAKOFF and MEYER 1965; RUNDLES et al. 1963; SEEGMILLER et al. 1967; WATTS et al. 1966). The substance was introduced by RUNDLES and his colleagues in 1963 to combat the hyperuricemia occurring in the treatment of leukemias. YÜ and GUTMAN were able to confirm its effectiveness in the treatment of primary and secondary gout (1964). These same authors published their encouraging experience in the treatment of 108 patients with primary gout, myeloproliferative disease and neoplasms of other tissue origin. 70% of their patients had a pretherapeutic serum uric acid greater than 10 mg%. In 90% of the group allopurinol therapy was able to lower this value to less than 7 mg%. 50% of the 108 patients had a 24 hr urinary uric acid excretion in excess of 800 mg%, the normal limit, and indeed one third of them were excreting over 1 g/day at the beginning of treatment. By taking allopurinol, 19 patients achieved a 24 hr excretion of less than 600 mg. All 108 patients had been suffering from recurrent stones or gravel and colic. In 98 the complaints ceased on treatment. Numerous authors have since confirmed these findings (BOSS and SEEGMILLER 1979; KAVALACH 1974; MIANO et al. 1979; SPERLING and DE VRIES 1964; WALLACE 1978; FELLSTRÖM 1984).

In 1969, SMITH and BOYCE published data on a group of 92 patients they had treated with allopurinol for a period of six months. 48.5% had suffered from calculi of various types. None suffered a recurrence during the trial period. In a further 18.2% the frequency of attacks was reduced. These effects should not, however, be attributed to allopurinol alone, since the urinary pH was simultaneously either neutralised or alkalinised and diet was purine restricted. Promotion of diuresis by increased fluid intake is also a prerequisite for successful treatment.

Side Effects: Skin rashes with pyrexia and rigors have been described in 6% of patients (GUTMAN and YÜ 1964). In patients with primary gout there is a 10% chance of precipitating an acute arthropathy, usually preceded by pruritus and skin eruptions. Should such an episode occur, allopurinol must naturally be stopped. If the warning reaction is ignored, a severe hemorrhagic exfoliative dermatitis may ensue.

Other Side Effects: Diarrhea in 5% (GUTMAN), abdominal pains and colic. Jaundice due to granulomatous hepatitis in 1%. *Rare problems:* vasculitis, hypersensitivity reactions, toxic agranulocytosis, epidermolysis (BOSS and SEEGMILLER 1979).

Discussion: Allopurinol is a highly effective agent with relatively few hazards and has gained a permanent place in our therapeutic arsenal. It is useful both for disorders of uric acid metabolism and in the treatment of uric acid-, urate- and calcium stones.

(ii) The Treatment of Hyperuricemia and Hyperuricosuria with Uricosurics (Probenecid etc.)

Probenecid blocks tubular reabsorption of uric acid. By increasing uric acid excretion it therefore diminishes the endogenous pool. During probenecid treatment uric acid excretion will exceed the rate of production and the serum uric acid will then fall. The chief disadvantage of this approach is the initial temporary flooding of the tubular apparatus with uric acid. Intratubular precipitation and crystallisation may result with consequent acute renal failure or nephrolithiasis (BRAUN et al. 1977). The risk of exceeding the saturation concentration of uric acid (6.4 mg% at pH 7) is real, certainly at the beginning of treatment. Unless additional measures are taken to increase diuresis and raise urinary pH into the range 6.8 to 7.2, probenecid will be a hazardous way to guard against recurrent uric acid-, urate- or calcium oxalate calculi. We personally reject this approach altogether. Similar considerations apply to combinations of probenecid and allopurinol.

Neutralising the Urine: Neutralising urinary pH will improve the solubility of uric acid and its salts. The pH of this weak acid is 5.5, so it will be 50% dissociated at the same pH. At lower pH the decreasing dissociation rapidly leads to a marked fall in solubility. On the other hand, the latter is considerably better at pH 6.2. Uric acid stone patients may frequently be found to have a rather persistently acid urine, an effect caused by an abnormality of ammonia excretion, perhaps coupled to abnormal uric acid secretion (SIMMONDS 1976). Urinary pHs of 5.4 or less are frequently measured.

Dietary and pharmacologic measures aim to neutralize urine pH, achieving the optimal range of 6.2–6.8. Dietary control alone, such as increased intake of citrus fruit or its juice may suffice, but as a rule this does not provide enough base so that adjuvant medical treatment should be instituted.

Alkali treatment was proposed by HOWSHIP as early as 1861 (in SCULTETY and BALOGH 1967). Nowadays it is usual to use a combination of sodium bicarbonate and potassium citrate ("Uralyt-U®" in Europe) or acetazolamide. Citrates are salts of a weak acid and strong bases and therefore cause excretion of base and a dose dependent rise in urine pH. One should properly aim at urine *neutralisation*, since the concept of alkali excretion leads one to think in terms of an alkaline urine with its own risks of infective or ammonium urate stone precipitation.

BIBUS (1962) was the first author to describe citrates as oral dissolution therapy for uric acid lithiasis. His results were confirmed by ATSMON et al. (1963), both authors using Eisenberg solution. In the meantime there have been several reports of successful oral dissolution therapy for uric acid lithiasis (BAUMANN and RUTISHAUSER 1968; DE VRIES and SPERLING 1976). Treatment is controlled by continuous urinary pH profiles drawn up by the patient using indicator paper. The dose is then adjusted according to urine pH.

(iii) Side Effects of Urine Neutralization by Bicarbonates and Citrate Mixtures

Many authors (GUTMAN and YÜ 1968; SCHNEIDER et al. 1969; SCULTETY and BALOGH 1967) recommend adjusting the urine pH to 6.7–6.8. If values in excess of 7 are achieved and urinary tract infection should supervene, there is a risk of calcium phosphate stone formation. Neutralization treatment also tends to exacerbate infection. What is more, the original urate calculus may become encased in a phosphate mantle and resist subsequent chemolysis. It is essential to confirm the diagnosis of uric acid lithiasis before embarking on urine neutralization, since such treatment would be contraindicated for other types of stone and, of course, where the sometimes difficult differential diagnosis of urinary tract neoplasia was missed.

Patients with cardiac or renal failure are at risk from hyperkalemia. A dose of 10 g of commercial citrate mixture (Uralyt-U®) presents an absorbed potassium load of 0.8 g. Serum potassium must therefore be estimated at regular intervals.

Urinary tract infection may luxuriate in neutral urine and proven bacteruria therefore demands energetic antibiotic chemotherapy.

As long as these basic rules are adhered to, drug prophylaxis and chemical dissolution therapy for uric acid lithiasis are without serious side effects.

(iv) Chemolysis by Urine Neutralization and Blockade of Uric Acid Synthesis

This strategy combines a depression of uric acid excretion by allopurinol medication with maintenance of a urine pH between 6.8 and 7.2.

The dose of allopurinol will depend on the quantity of uric acid excreted. A daily diuresis of at least 2 liters must be maintained during treatment and bacterial urinary tract infection is to be eradicated. Oral chemolytic treatment presupposes a stone lying free in the lumen of the urinary tract where it can be bathed in urine. A radiologically or scintigraphically non-functioning kidney contraindicates dissolution therapy. The duration of treatment will depend on the size of the stone and the quality of urine neutralisation achieved – night-time included.

As a general rule it takes 4–8 weeks to dissolve the average stone, but size of stone and rate of diuresis will have an enormous influence.

4. Urate Calculi

Uric acid salts may give rise to one of two types of calculus, sodium hydrogenurate monohydrate or ammonium hydrogen urate.

a) Sodium Hydrogenurate Monohydrate

Drug treatment and recurrence prevention for this type of calculus are as for pure uric acid stones. Two principles already discussed are fundamental:

1. The urine should be neutralized with bicarbonate or citrate to a pH in the range 6.2–6.8. This improves the solubility of urates, since like all salts of weak acids, they are more soluble in a neutral or alkaline environment than at acidic pH.
2. Uric acid excretion is reduced by allopurinol blockade of the xanthine oxidase step in uric acid synthesis. A low purine diet and a high fluid intake to promote diuresis are self explanatory requirements.

It is, in principle, possible to dissolve these stones by such oral therapy. The basics are as for uric acid calculi, but dissolution may be slower, because the urates form tougher crystal aggregates. Success will depend on the duration of treatment, on the diuresis achieved and on the size and site of the calculus.

b) Ammonium Hydrogenurate

This type of calculus differs from the other uric acid- and urate stones, in that it occurs not in an acidic but rather in a mildly alkaline urine. Urease positive urinary pathogens generate ammonia from urea and the urine pH rises. If excessive uric acid excretion of any causation coincides with these events, the ammonium salt may crystallise out. Proper treatment depends on an understanding of this pathogenetic mechanism. The following points are to be born in mind:

1. Rigorous specific antibacterial chemotherapy. This should continue at a full dose for an adequate period. The presence of a stone predisposes to interstitial nephritis and pyelonephritis. In consequence urinary infection may be chronically relapsing or ineridicable.
2. Reduction of uric acid excretion by means of a low purine diet. Allopurinol blockade of uric acid synthesis if there is a metabolic disorder.
3. Neutralization or slight acidification of the urine. The optimal pH is between 6.2 and 6.6. Because of the risk of uric acid lithiasis, formal urine acidification is to be avoided.

The medication needed to control urine pH will depend on the initial alkalinity, and patients must be encouraged to keep a close watch themselves. Misconceived self-medication and poor monitoring potentiate the dangers of this type of calculus. Suitable acidifying agents include all those mentioned above under "Drug Treatment of Urinary Tract Infection: Urine Acidification – Dosage". Because their solubility is relatively independent of hydrogen ion concentration, *these calculi cannot be dissolved by oral treatment.*

5. The Treatment of Cystine Calculi

Cystinuria was one of the first inborn errors of metabolism to be described in relation to urolithiasis. WOLLASTON characterised the syndrome of cystinuria in 1810 without, however, appreciating its pathophysiology. It was left to GARROD (1908) to recognise a metabolic cause of the illness. First communications on the drug treatment of cystinuria are from MARGET (1817), TOEL (1855) and from V. UDRANSKY and BOUMANN (1889).

Cystinuria may present in a homozygous or a heterozygous form and consists of genetically determined excess excretion of cystine along with other dibasic amino acids such as arginine, ornithine and lysine. The three latter are, however, easily soluble in a slightly acid urine and do not therefore form calculi. Expression of the disorder will depend on hetero- or homozygosity, but in all events the abnormality concerns the *reabsorption mechanism* for the 4 dibasic amino acids in the distal renal tubule (Fig. 9).

Cystine normally has its own separate reabsorption mechanism in addition to the one shared with the other three acids. In cystinurics this dedicated mechanism is incompetent, with the result that all four acids compete for a single receptor. The capacity of the active transport mechanism is exceeded and only a concentration dependent fraction of each amino acid can be recovered, the majority spilling over into the urine.

According to HARRIS et al. (1955) the heterozygous and homozygous forms may be distinguished by the absorptive activity of a small intestinal biopsy specimen. Such differential diagnosis is, however, without therapeutic significance, since the choice and dose of agents will be determined by the level of cystine excretion.

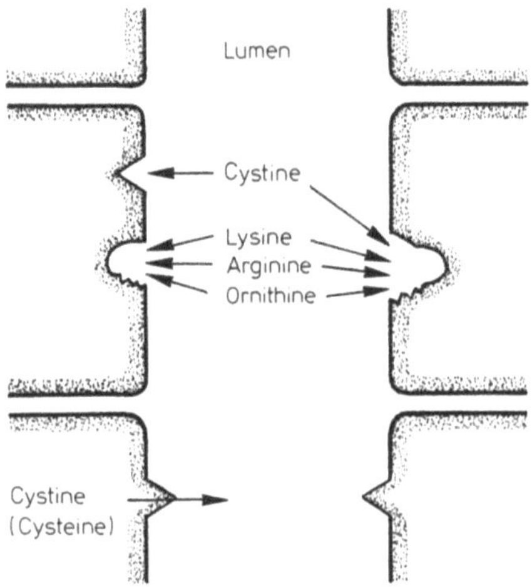

Fig. 9. The reabsorption mechanism in the distal renal tubule for the dibasic amino acids, ornithine, arginine, lysine and cystine (after HAUTMANN and TERHORST, HAUTMANN et al. 1977)

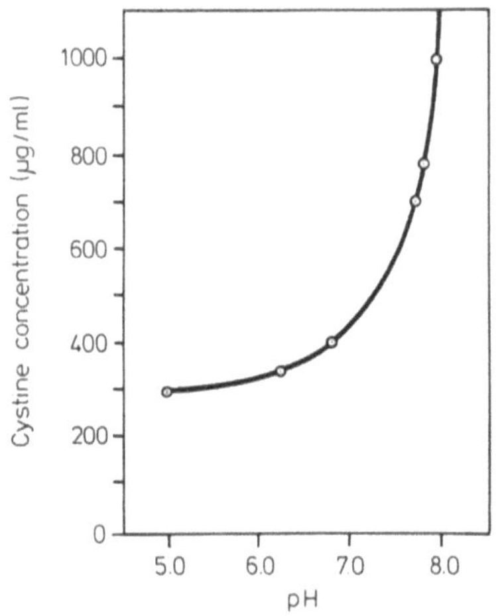

Fig. 10. The pH dependence of cystine solubility

DENT and SENIOR (1955) have pointed out that at 37 °C and pH 7 cystine remains in solution up to a concentration of 400 mg/l, its solubility being strongly pH dependent (Fig. 10), decreasing in acidic and improving in alkaline surroundings. Thus at pH 7.8 and 37 °C 800 mg/l may be held in solution. Homozygous patients, however, may excrete in the region of 1000 mg/l, so that they have a permanently supersaturated urine. A decrease in fluid intake, particularly at night, or a fall in urine pH will lead to crystallisation and stone formation.

Treatment is fundamentally symptomatic, since no remedy is available for the genetic transport defect. The following measures may be adopted:
1. Reduction in oral cystine intake.
2. Increase in daily diuresis by increased fluid intake – day and night.

3. Improvement of cystine solubility by urine alkalinisation.
4. Improvement of cystine solubility by binding poorly soluble cystine to more soluble molecules.

a) Cystinuria Diets and Associated Problems

Dietary restriction of cystine is only possible within certain limitations. On the one hand cystine is an essential amino acid, the restriction of which leads to cerebral- and growth impairment, at least in children. Thus growing children cannot be cystine restricted. In adults cystine excretion can be reduced by restricting methionine intake (SMITH et al. 1959).

DENT and SENIOR (1955) have pointed out that daily protein intake would have to be restricted to 20 g, if the urinary cystine output is to be lowered by one third. This view has been supported by LOTZ et al. (1965) and by KOLB et al. (1967), although ZINNEMANN and JONES (1966) think so harsh a restriction unnecessary. An intake as low as this barely escapes the risk of malnutrition, even in adults. In principle, an ultra low methionine diet ought to reduce urinary cystine output, but this approach has been rendered obsolete by modern drug therapy.

b) Fluid Intake, Volume, and Composition

Reducing urinary cystine concentrations by a massive increase in diuresis presents an alternative avenue of treatment. Yet to lower the cystine level below the critical value of 400 mg/l (at pH 7 and 37 °C) would require a fluid volume of 10–20 l/day! Depending on the rate of cystine excretion this quantity might even have to be increased. A number of factors make the oral intake of such large volumes undesirable.

The daily intake should, however, be increased to 4–7 l/24 hrs, particular attention being paid to nocturnal fluids, since cystinurics must maintain an adequate diuresis through the night. In choosing fluids the patient has to bear in mind the significance of maintaining a neutral or mildly alkaline urine, and for this reason citrus fruit and citrus juices are to be encouraged.

It should thus be plain that the intake volume is paramount. Adjustements in hydrogen ion concentration can be made pharmacologically.

c) Drug Treatment of Cystine Stones

The basic principles are to control the rate of cystine excretion and improve urinary cystine solubility by pH adjustment (alkali ingestion). Like that of uric acid, the solubility of cystine is markedly dependent on the pH, being worst in acid or weakly acid solution. One should therefore endeavour to raise urinary pH into the range 7.5–8.

Prior eradication of urinary tract infection will be mandatory, and simultaneous antibiotic maintenance therapy may be needed.

Urine alkalinisation can be achieved with sodium bicarbonate or a commercially available citrate concoction, such as Uralyt-U. The dose will be dictated by the starting pH of the urine. Side effects, guidelines for dosage and contraindications are all discussed in the section on uric acid lithiasis.

d) Chemical Conversion of Cystine to Cysteine

A number of groups of drugs are available which bind poorly soluble cystine and promote its conversion to the far more soluble substance cysteine. Chief among these are D-penicillamine, N-acetyl-D-L-penicillamine, acetylcysteine and alpha mercaptopropionylglycine (MPG). All these drugs undergo the following thio-exchange reactions with disulphide groups:

$$R_1{-}SH \rightarrow R_1{-}S^- + H^+$$

$$R_1{-}S{-}S{-}R_3 + R_1{-}S^- \rightarrow R_2{-}S{-}S{-}R_1 + R_3{-}S^-$$

These reactions result in poorly soluble cystine binding by its SH groups to D-penicillamine or to mercaptopropionylglycine. The resulting mercaptopropionylgylcine-cysteine-, D-penicillamine-cysteine-, mercaptopropionylglycine disulphide- or D-penicillamine-disulphide-D-penicillamine species are infinitely better soluble and no precipitation or crystallisation occurs at the concentrations involved. In 1963, CRAWHALL et al. reported effective depression of cystine excretion following oral D-penicillamine. The effect is largely maintained on long term treatment.

(i) D-Penicillamine

Dosage: The dose of D-penicillamine will mainly depend on the rate at which cystine is being excreted. Not more than 200 mg/g urinary creatinine should be given in 24 hrs and the usual daily dose is 1 g, occasionally 2 g, in divided doses.

CRAWHALL et al. recommend an initial dose of 150 mg eight hourly, increasing after three days to 450 mg three times a day. The final dose is adjusted according to the cystine output achieved on treatment, and may need revision at intervals.

Clinical Experience: Apart from the reduction in cystine excretion to normal levels described by CRAWHALL et al. (1963), by KING and BOYCE (1965) and by LOTZ et al. (1966), both McDONALD and FELLERS (1966), and the above authors achieved dissolution of cystine calculi with oral D-penicillamine. The latter effect, however, tended to take 6 months to a year to occur. CRAWHALL and WATTS succeeded in dissolving stones in only 3 of 19 patients with a litholytic dose of 450 mg eight hourly. Whether or not they employed additional measures such as alkalinisation of the urine or forced diuresis is unclear.

Side Effects: The clinical side effects seen at the beginning of treatment usually consist of allergic manifestations, noted by CRAWHALL et al. (1963) to set in around the tenth day. They usually comprise macular rash on the trunk and thighs accompanied by fever, arthralgia and generalized lymphadenopathy.

Laboratory findings may include thrombocytopenia and granulocytopenia. More severe forms of reaction usually appear to be related to racemic D and L isomeres and only rarely to pure D-penicillamines (CRAWHALL).

CORCOS et al. (1964) describe two cases of agranulocytosis, of which one ended fatally. This complication is rare. Both patients had been treated with penicillamine for rheumatoid arthritis.

The so-called hypersensitivity syndrome regresses when D-penicillamine is withdrawn. If fever or skin rash occur at the start of treatment, an antihistamine or prednisolone should be added.

Furthermore patients on penicillamine may develop proteinuria progressing to a frank nephrotic syndrome (ROSEMBERG and HAYSLETT 1967; FELTS et al. 1968). ADAMS et al. (1964) described focal glomerulonephritis presenting as a nephrotic syndrome and brought about by D-penicillamine treatment. STERNLIEB (1966) also reported the occurrence of nephrotic syndrome, but his report related to the use of racemic penicillamine.

As D-penicillamine binds the heavy metals iron, copper, zinc and mercury (for which reason it is also used in the treatment of Wilson's disease), one should be on the lookout for deficiency syndromes, although no cases have so far been described.

Note that pyridoxine deficiency may occur during penicillamine therapy. With this in mind, JAFFE et al. (1964) recommend pyridoxine replacement. However, neither iron- nor pyridoxine deficiency anemia has ever been observed during prolonged courses of treatment (CRAWHALL, WATTS).

Serious hematologic abnormalities such as agranulocytosis (CORCOS and colleagues), thrombocytosis (FAWCETT et al. 1966) or eosinophilia (McDONALD and HENNEMANN 1965) occur in the literature only as isolated case reports. These phenomena are reversible on withdrawing the drug. Severe skin changes including bullous epidermolysis have been described by BEER and COOKE (1967) and by KATZ (1967). Finally, EISER et al. (1968) came across impairment and occasionally total loss of taste sensation in patients on D-penicillamine.

As D-penicillamine has to be given on a life-long basis and in view of the wide variety of possible moderate or serious side effects, patients should be kept under close supervision and may need to switch to some other medication.

Contraindications to D-Penicillamine Treatment: D-penicillamine should not be given to patients with preexisting glomerular disease or nephrotic syndrome. Medication should also be avoided in pregnancy, unless absolutely necessary.

SHERWIN et al. (1960), CRAWHALL et al. (1967), and BOULDING (1961) continued D-penicillamine therapy for Wilson's disease throughout pregnancy. Teratogenicity was observed neither in the first nor in subsequent pregnancies. The only unusual finding was high D-penicillamine-cysteine excretion by the neonates on the first day after delivery, strong evidence that the drug crosses the placenta.

(ii) Alpha Mercaptopropionylglycin (MPG)

MPG has a similar effect to that of D-penicillamine in binding poorly soluble cystine in the urinary tract and converting it to MPG-cysteine, which is far more soluble. First reports of effective reduction in cystine excretion by MPG medication came from KING (1969). Numerous other reports followed, initially in the japanese literature (SONODA et al. 1970; KINOSHITA et al. 1972; NISHIMURA et al. 1972) and subsequently in America and Europe (THOMAS et al. 1970; TACCINOLI et al. 1973; REMIEEN et al. 1975; TERHORST and STUHLSATZ 1975; ZECHNER et al. 1976; HAUTMANN et al. 1977; MIANO et al. 1979), all testifying to the excellent clinical efficacy of this agent.

Dosage: The required daily dose will depend on the rate of cystine excretion, but generally lies in the range 0.5–2 g/day (HAUTMANN et al. 1977). The dose should be steadily increased until cystine excretion falls below the critical value of 100 mg/day.

Clinical Experience: Cystine excretion has been reduced in every case treated, the degree of reduction being correspondingly greater where previous cystine excretion was highest. Prophylactic MPG treatment achieved a recurrence rate of 3–5% or 9% (MIANO 1979). Stones dissolved in 9 out of 19 patients (47%) and regressed in a further 6 (32%) (MIANO). These results were achieved with simultaneous alkalinisation and increased diuresis.

Side Effects: In contrast to D-penicillamine there appears to be a virtual absence of serious side effects, even on long term treatment. In no case did side effects lead to treatment being interrupted.

Loose stools occurred sporadically. Spontaneously reversible skin rashes and pyrexia appeared in the initial phase. No serious complications are known to date.

Contraindications: None known.

Discussion: Unlike D-penicillamine, alpha mercaptopropionylglycine therapy is without serious side effects. The effectiveness appears to decrease, however, during prolonged administration, although this effect can be corrected by increasing the dose. Increases are needed at shorter and shorter intervals, and eventually an adequate depression of cystine excretion can no longer be attained. No such loss of effect is seen with D-penicillamine.

(iii) Ascorbic Acid in the Treatment of Cystinuria

High dose ascorbic acid therapy was launched as a new treatment of cystinuria in 1979 (ASPER et al. 1979). Oral intake of ascorbic acid shifts the redox potential of the urine to cause dose dependent conversion of poorly soluble cystine to soluble cysteine.

Dosage: 5 g per day.

Discussion: Ascorbic acid appears a promising agent for the treatment of cystinuria wherever D-penicillamine is contraindicated and the effect of MPG has been lost.

One potential side effect could be the conversion of ascorbic acid to oxalic acid and the subsequent development of hyperoxaluria. The above authors have seen no such event, albeit there is so far a lack of any large scale clinical trials that could confirm the long term effectiveness and absence of side effects from this treatment.

6. The Treatment of Rare Stones

a) Xanthine Lithiasis

Xanthine calculi are extremely rare, the frequency usually being quoted as 0.04% (HERRING 1962). PRIEN (1963) found not a single xanthine stone among 24,000 calculi analysed in the years 1948 to 1964. SEEGMILLER (1968) suspects an increasing incidence in the wake of the introduction of allopurinol as a treatment for uric acid lithiasis and primary gout. The blockade of uric acid synthesis at the hypoxanthine/xanthine stage might cause the formation of xanthine calculi, although both substances normally have good solubility at a slightly acid urinary pH. Two patients who did develop xanthine stones on allopurinol treatment were subsequently shown to have an enzyme defect that resulted in a six-fold increase in uric acid precursor production.

Endogenous xanthinuria arises from an inborn error of metabolism inherited as an autosomal recessive (DENT and PHILPOT 1954). Of a group of eight patients with this disorder three were stone formers. The biochemical lesion is a deficiency of xanthine oxidase, as a result of which neither xanthine nor hypoxanthine can be broken down to uric acid. With purine degradation thus effectively blocked, 50–80% of the purine load is excreted as xanthine, the remainder as hypoxanthine.

Patients with this syndrome classically have very low serum uric acid levels (less than 0.5 mg%) and a urinary uric acid loss less than 10 mg/day (normally up to 800 mg/day). Yet this excessive xanthine excretion alone cannot explain the formation of xanthine stones. As in calcium oxalate lithiasis, further unknown factors are generally considered to be involved in triggering xanthine crystal precipitation and the subsequent growth of calculi.

Treatment of Xanthine Lithiasis: The most important step is to secure a high fluid load, in the region of 3–4 liters a day and continuing through the night hours. In addition the urine must be meticulously held at an alkaline pH, even at nighttime, since xanthine is appreciably more soluble in an alkaline environment. The principles underlying urine alkalinisation are the same as those applying to cystine lithiasis. It is just as important in xanthinuria that the patient check his or her own urine pH several times daily and learn to correct the alkali dose as required. A low purine diet must be strictly adhered to, the permitted purine intake once again being matched to the degree of xanthinuria.

Medication: One might at first think allopurinol treatment illogical. Nevertheless, ENGELMANN et al. (1964) observed a fall in xanthine excretion and a compensatory rise in hypoxanthine loss after allopurinol administration. It should, however, be noted that their patient was not a stone former. In other cases soluble concretions of alloxanthine (an allopurinol-xanthine compound) may be formed, a step not possible in homozygous disease, since some xanthine oxidase is required to form the compound. In the heterozygous form of the disease, the formation of soluble alloxanthine suffices to reduce the xanthine concentration to a soluble level, thus preventing stone formation.

Recurrent xanthine calculi can be effectively prevented by maintaining an adequately high diuresis, by alkalinising the urine and by adhering to a low purine diet, as CIFUENTES-DELATTE and CASTRO-MENDOZA (1967) and DENT and PHILPOT (1954) have been able to demonstrate.

IV. Childhood Urolithiasis

Whilst in past centuries urolithiasis occurred quite commonly in children, improvements in nutrition have led to a steady decline in frequency – a marked contrast to the situation in adults (BARTONE and JOHNSTON 1977; BASS and EMANUEL 1966; BENNET and COLODNY 1973; CAMPBELL 1951; DAESCHNER et al. 1960; LATTIMER and HUBBARD 1951; MALEK and KELALIS 1975; MYERS 1957; TROUP et al. 1972; WILLNOW 1968)! In Norfolk, England, 2.9% of the overall population incidence of stones was contributed by children during the period 1772 to 1909, yet throughout the twentieth century the figure for the same region has only been 0.5% (GREEN and SHAW 1981). In contrast to the eighteenth century, when bladder stones were relatively common, the majority of cases are nowadays of renal or ureteric stones. The bladder stones of the old days were usually urate or uric acid. Most adult stones are nowadays calcific, being either infective in origin or else composed of pure calcium oxalate (HERING et al. 1981; MARQUARDT and NAGEL 1977; CAMPBELL 1951; VAHLENSIECK 1980; PASSMORE 1953; JOHNSTON 1973; MITCHEL 1981).

The frequency of urolithiasis among children is now less than 1% (CAMPBELL). There may be an additional unquantified population, since not all children with stones get admitted to hospital. For inpatient admissions CAMPBELL (1951) and WILLNOW (1968) give a figure of 0.5–1% of children, with a sex ratio similar to that for adult patients at 2:1 in favour of males.

Whilst in adults urinary tract infection is only involved in the formation of so-called infective stones, documented in 60% of suspected cases, infection is the dominant factor in childhood urolithiasis. 60–80% of these children have an active Proteus (38.0–51.2%), E. coli (15.0–28.2%) or Enterobacter (3.0–9.9%) urinary tract infection. Infection is frequently associated with an anatomical abnormality of obstructive type. The strong prevalence of infection among juvenile stone patients also determines the composition distribution of their calculi, which is fundamentally different to that found in adult groups (MINKOV et al. 1981):

Table 6. The composition of juvenile uroliths

Calcium oxalate calculi	54.7%
Uric acid and urate stones	19.3%
Phosphates (infective)	22.1%
Cystine stones	3.9%

Whilst infection is extremely common, true metabolic disease is rare as a cause of stones in children:

Table 7. Metabolic disorders causing urolithiasis in children

1. Primary oxalosis and hyperoxaluria (< 1%)
2. Cystinuria (approx. 3%)
3. Disorders of purine metabolism (Lesch-Nyhan-Syndrome) (2.5%)
4. Renal tubular acidosis (< 1%)
5. Hyperparathyroidism (< 0.5%)
6. Hypercalciuria, e.g. vitamin D intoxication (< 0.5%)
7. Adenosine phosphoribosyltransferase deficiency (SIMMONDS et al. 1976 and 1979) (5 cases)

1. Dietary and Medical Treatment of Oxalosis and Hyperoxaluria

Primary oxalosis is a genetically determined disorder of glyoxalate metabolism (WILLIAMS 1976). The hallmark of the disease is recurrent malignant urolithiasis with early oxalosis of all the internal organs. Nephrocalcinosis and uremia or cardiomyopathy and congestive cardiac failure are the usual causes of death, since massive oxalate deposition inhibits basic organ functions. Two distinct types are recognised:

Type I (glycoluria): This condition is characterised by excessive oxalate excretion, combined with excess output of glycolate and glyoxalate. The cause is glyoxalate dehydrogenase deficiency.

Type II (gylcinuria): There is increased urinary oxalate-, glyoxalate and glycine excretion.

Both types are inherited as autosomal recessives and the cause is untreatable by drug or diet. Early dialysis is the only therapeutic avenue, renal transplantation being of little avail in a condition where the implant rapidly undergoes nephrocalcinosis.

2. Dietary and Medical Treatment of Cystinuria

The etiology and pathogenesis are as already described for adults. Cystinuria is the commonest metabolic disorder to cause stones in children. Treatment and recurrence prevention are once again based on the following principles, each of which will receive varying emphasis, depending on age and weight of the child (PAVANELLO et al. 1981).

1. Fluid intake is increased to 2–3 liters/day, depending on the age of the child.
2. The urine is alkalinised up to pH 7.5–8. Existing urinary tract infection requires energetic antibiotic therapy.
3. Poorly soluble cystine is converted into more soluble cysteine by SH-binding. Alpha mercaptopropionylglycine is a less toxic agent more appropriate for children at a dose of 20–40 mg/kg.

Although nephrotic syndrome has also been documented for mercaptopropionylglycine therapy, D-penicillamine causes a far wider spectrum of serious side effects and should be avoided in children. The aim of medical treatment is to depress urinary cystine excretion to under 150–100 mg/day.

Dietary methionine restriction, as sometimes advocated for adults, is quite unacceptable in children, since it results in retarded brain development.

a) Disorders of Purine Metabolism

Primary gout rarely occurs in combination with childhood stones. Uric acid stones occur more commonly as part of a secondary hyperuricemia and hyperuricosuria. The chief cause is chemotherapy of malignancy (e.g. of the various leukemias or of Wilm's tumor). Tumor necrosis results in an increased purine nucleotide load for conversion into uric acid. Primary hyperuricemia occurs in children virtually only in the Lesch-Nyhan syndrome.

In 1964, LESCH and NYHAN described two young brothers with a severe syndrome of choreoathetosis, spasticity, mental retardation and self mutilation. In collaboration with ROSENBLOOM and KELLY, SEEGMILLER was able to demonstrate (SEEGMILLER et al. 1967) a deficiency in the enzyme hypoxanthine guanine phosphoribonuclease. This enzyme is required for the utilization of guanine and hypoxanthine in purine nucleotide synthesis, and in its absence guanine and hypoxanthine are irreversibly converted to uric acid by xanthine oxidase. Excessive uric acid production causes both the neurologic picture and a hyperuricosuria associated with recurrent stones. The condition is X-linked.

Hyperuricosuria should be treated along the same lines as have been established for adults:
1. Fluid intake is increased to 1–2 liters/day, according to age.
2. Urine neutralisation.
3. Blockade of xanthine oxidase with allopurinol, the dose being adjusted to age and weight of the child. The dose is usually in the range 50–100 mg mane.

b) Renal Tubular Acidosis

The etiology and pathogenesis are those described for the adult form, but the syndrome is invariably more severe in children. Medical treatment is directed at correcting the metabolic acidosis by giving bicarbonate. The dose of bicarbonate must be determined according to the degree of base deficit, as calculated from blood gas analysis. Potassium replacement should be given for hypokalemia; calcium and vitamin D supplements are necessary in longstanding disease, or where there is proven renal osteodystrophy and skeletal demineralization.

Untreated cases die of nephrocalcinosis and uremia, although for the homozygous form treatment does not radically improve this gloomy outlook.

Hyperparathyroidism: Primary hyperparathyroidism is excessively rare in children. Suspicion should be aroused by the combination of recurrent stones, reduced renal function, polydipsia and polyuria with isosthenuria and a (frequently chance) finding of hypercalcemia. Further investigation should be carried out along adult lines.

The treatment of proven hyperparathyroidism is surgical exploration of the parathyroid glands.

(i) *Hypercalciuria*

In children such a condition is quite uncommon, the quoted frequencies varying from 2% to 10% (APLAS et al. 1981; BORGMANN and NAGEL 1981; HERING et al. 1981). These figures are significantly lower than among the adult population, for whom 20–40% is often given (YENDT et al. 1960; COE and KAVALACH 1974; PAK 1976). Causes of hypercalciuria include hyperparathyroidism, vitamin D toxicity, bone pathology and, presumably, overresponsiveness to vitamin D.

Vitamin D toxicity is a manifestation either of extreme sensitivity of the intestine to vitamin D metabolites or of true intoxication resulting from overdosage with multivitamin preparations. The latter arises if the daily dose exceeds 50,000 i.u. for any lentgh of time. Vitamin D overdose or increased intestinal responsiveness to vitamin D and its metabolites result in increased uptake of dietary calcium with temporary hypercalcemia and hypercalciuria. The clinical picture is one of anorexia, vomitting, thirst and polyuria. The hypercalcemia results in calcification of blood vessels, kidney and skin.

Treatment comprises stopping the culprit medication, phosphate and sulphate infusions and, in severe cases, intravenous EDTA in 5% dextrose combined with corticosteroids. Cases of extreme hypercalcemia may require hemodialysis.

Other hypercalciurias of either unclassifiable or of so-called idiopathic etiology, including syndromes caused by bone pathology, respond well to thiazide treatment. The daily dose will depend on age and weight of the patient, up to a maximum of 25–50 mg/day by mouth. The side effects of longterm thiazide therapy must be looked for and corrected as they arise.

(ii) *APRT Deficiency*

CARTIER and HAMET first described the homozygous form of this autosomal dominant genetic disorder in 1974 in a four year old girl with nephrolithiasis. A total of 450 g of calculous material was removed transurethrally and was found to consist of 10% uric acid and 90% 2,8-dihydroxyadenine. Urinary adenine levels were found to be raised by a factor of 40 (normally up to 1.5 mg/24 hrs). Further children with the same metabolic disorder have since been described (SIMMONDS et al. 1976; SIMMONDS 1979; ASPER and SCHMUCKI 1982).

Adenine is poorly soluble in urine and therefore tends to crystallise out to form stones. As xanthine oxidase is involved in the synthesis of adenine, allopurinol treatment is both indicated and effective, as demonstrated by the children SIMMONDS has treated.

(iii) Infective Calculi

Since the majority of childhood stones are of infective etiology (SCHNEIDER 1979), their successful removal and the correction of predisposing anatomical abnormalities must be followed by vigorous antibiotic therapy if infection is to be eradicated. Treatment should continue for at least half a year, the dose being lowered from an initial high level to a maintenance regime after 14 days. The purpose of this procedure is to deal with soft tissue infection, the presence of which can invariably be demonstrated in patients with infective stones.

Care should be exercised in any attempt at drug induction of urine acidification, since metabolic acidosis is easily precipitated. Regular blood chemistry is mandatory.

The choice of agent and the principles underlying its use are those described in relation to adults. The dose will need adjustment to keep the pH around 6.

3. General Comments on the Drug Treatment of Juvenile Urolithiasis

Children with urolithiasis require closer supervision than adults, especially during medical treatment. The clinical effectiveness, the severity of side effects and the general acceptability of any drug need continual reassessment. Investigations such as full blood count, ESR, serum electrolytes, urea and creatinine, perhaps liver function, urinary lithogen excretion, urine microscopy and culture should all be performed at regular intervals. A full reassessment is required at least every six months, three-monthly if at all possible, so that side effects come to be noticed at an early juncture. Children must be treated flexibly, not just following a rigid plan. The choice of medication and its dosage will have to be carefully considered, and adjustments made as they suggest themselves, taking the date of the next consultation into account. Special diets should be strictly avoided, since they present a real risk of inducing growth disorders. On the other hand an adequate fluid intake properly distributed over day and night remains the mainstay of prophylaxis.

V. Conclusion

The primary cause of urinary calculi can only be treated where the pathogenetic mechanism of stone formation is adequately understood. Only then can recurrence be prevented in such a fundamental way. At the time of writing only cystine- and uric acid lithiasis and perhaps, with certain exceptions, infective calculi fall within that category. The formation of intrarenal calcium oxalate and calcium phosphate is, by way of contrast and despite intensive research effort, still beyond our intellectual grasp. Computer aided analysis has not helped to understand the significance behind excretion patterns of urinary lithogens and stone inhibitors, since the differences between normal subjects and stone sufferers are often subtle. Improved mathematical models for calculating urinary saturation that take account of both lithogenic and inhibitory factors have failed to show a way forward. By measuring the tissue concentration of lithogenic substances and on the basis of scanning electron microscopy one is led to suspect that primary stone forming events take place not only within the lumen but equally in the peritubular domain. In this light it seems that to base ones therapeutic strategy on measurements of urine composition is not to aim at the pathogenetic mechanism but at mere circumstance. As long as the fundamental risk factors and the primary site of urolithogenesis remain equally obscure, all our standard treatment, set out in the above chapter for specific pictures such as hypercalciuria or hyperoxaluria, must be regarded with deep suspicion. It must be pointed out that factors like calcium, oxalate or uric acid, to name but a few, will all bind in a wide variety of different combinations, depending on urinary pH, ionic charge, temperature and molar concentration. Any attempt to influence the excretion of individual substances is therefore likely to remain problematic in the very least, as long as we fail to consider overall urine composition. This picture is further complicated by the fact that treatment aimed at preventing recurrence is only initiated once a stone has already occurred. By this time the excretion pattern of urinary lithogens and stone inhibitory may in no way any longer reflect the conditions under which the stone was generated. Preventive drug therapy is, what is more, only ever based on point observations of sequential events which may be substantially affected by eating and drinking habits.

The conclusion from these considerations must be that any treatment should be preceded by several days devoted to mapping out the excretion pattern, both in time and in chemical diversity. Whilst financial and laboratory constraints might seem to limit this ambition, there is no other obvious way to eliminate the spurious effects of external factors. After all, it has become standard practice only to give hypotensive agents when hypertension has been repeatedly detected on a number of occasions under varying circumstances. If the urinary supersaturation concept is to prevail, it will also be necessary to demonstrate to what extent, for example, increased calcium excretion so increases urinary saturation as to present a risk of stone formation. Only where a single factor can be shown to make a substantial contribution within the context of overall urine composition to raising this risk above a critical threshold should medical treatment be aimed at that factor. Computer programs are nowadays available that facilitate this calculation. Recent studies have shown further that such computations of relative saturation provide a means of distinguishing normal subjects from stone sufferers and patients with a first attack from those with a recurrence. The presence of any substance in abnormal quantities but without substantial effect on overall relative saturation could then not be considered a risk factor worthy of pharmacologic intervention. In that case diet alone would suffice.

Yet as long as we are unable to measure intrarenal or intratubular concentrations of the principle lithogens and until mathematical models for calculating relative saturation and supersaturation are unable to give unequivocal risk probabilities, the excretion pattern of 24 hour- or fractional urines will remain the basis of medical and dietary treatment, however, unsatisfactory that may be.

References

Acker KJ van (1977) Complete deficiency of adenine phosphoribosyltransferase: Report of a family. N Engl J Med 297:127–132
Adams DA, Goldman R, Maxwell M, Latta H (1964) Nephrotic syndrome associated with penicillamine therapy of Wilson's disease. Am J Med 36:330–336
Adams TH, Norman AW (1970) Studies on the mechanism of action of calciferol I. Basic parameters of Vit D-mediated calcium transport. J Biol Chem 245:4421–4431
Albrecht KF, Moncada F (1981) Radiographic search for renal calculi during nephrolithotomy by the Renodor-technique. In: Schulman CC (ed) Advances in diagnostic urology. Springer, Berlin Heidelberg New York, p 80
Alken CE (1967) Die konservative Behandlung des Nierensteinleidens. Wien Klin Wochenschr 79:657–658
Alken P, Hutschenreiter G, Günther R, Marberger M (1981) Percutaneous stone manipulation. J Urol 125:463–466
Altmann RD, Johnston CC, Khairi MRA, Wellman H, Seratini AN, Saukey RR (1973) Influence of disodium etiolsonate on clinical and laboratory manifestations of Paget's disease of bone (osteitis deformans). N Engl J Med 289:1379–1384
Anderson E, Rundles RW, Silbermann HR, Metz EN (1967) Allopurinol control of hyperuricosuria. J Urol 97:344–347
Aplas G, Schrott KM, Böwing B (1982) Ursachen, Therapie und Verlauf der Urolithiasis im Kindesalter (eine Analyse von über 170 Fällen). In: Kaufmann J (Redg von) Verhandlungsberichte der Deutschen Gesellschaft für Urologie, 33. Tagung, Köln 1981. Springer, Berlin Heidelberg New York, S 256–261
Archer HE, Dormer AE, Slowen EF, Watts RWE (1957) Studies on the urinary excretion of oxalate by normal subjects. Clin Sci 16:405–411
Asper R, Schmucki O (1982) Diagnostik und Therapie der 2,8-Dihydroxyadenia-Lithiasis. In: Gasser G, Vahlensieck W (Hrsg) Fortschritte der Urologie und Nephrologie, Bd 20, Pathogenese und Klinik der Harnsteine IX. Steinkopff, Darmstadt, S 274–282
Asper R, Schmucki O, Eggli R, Rosenmund H (1979) Die medikamentöse Beeinflussung des Cystein/Cystin-Verhältnisses im Urin: Eine neue Cystinurietherapie. In: Gasser G, Vahlensieck W (Hrsg) Fortschritte der Urologie und Nephrologie, Bd 14, Pathogenese und Klinik der Harnsteine VII. Steinkopff, Darmstadt, S 417–421
Atsmon A, Vries A de, Frank M (1963) Uric acid lithiasis. Elsevier, Amsterdam
Backmann U, Danielson BG, Fellström B, Johansson G, Ljunghall S, Wikström B (1981) The clinical importance of renal tubular acidosis in recurrent renal stone formers. In: Smith LH, Robertson WG, Finlayson B (eds) Urolithiasis. Plenum Press, New York London, p 67–69
Band RP, Silverberg DS, Henderson IF, Ulan RA, Wensel RH, Bauerjee TK, Little AS (1970) Xanthine nephropathie in a patient treated with allopurinol lymphosarcoma. N Engl J Med 283:354–357
Bartone FF, Johnston JH (1977) Staghorn calculi in children. J Urol 118:76–79
Bass HN, Emanuel B (1966) Nephrolithiasis in childhood: Clinical and etiologic considerations. Clin Pediatr (Phila) 5:79–85
Bass HN, Emanuel B (1966) Nephrolithiasis in childhood. J Urol 95:749–753
Baumann JM, Rutishauser G (1968) Die Behandlung der Harnsäuresteine. Ther Umsch 25:249–254
Baumann JM, Ganz U, Bisaz S, Fleisch H, Rutishauser G (1975) Ergebnisse der Ethan-Hydroxy-Diphosphonat-Studie nach einjähriger Steinprophylaxe. In: Vahlensieck W, Gasser G (Hrsg) Fortschritte der Urologie und Nephrologie, Bd 7. Pathogenese und Klinik der Harnsteine IV. Steinkopff, Darmstadt, S 171–173
Becker BA, Swift JG (1959) Effective reduction of the acute toxicity of certain pharmacological agents by use of synthetic ion exchange resins. Toxicol Appl Pharmacol 1:42–54
Beer WE, Cooke KB (1967) Epidermolysis bullosa induced by penicillamine. Br J Dermatol 79:123–125
Benedict JD, Forsham PH, Stetten D jr (1949) The metabolism of uric acid in the normal and gouty human, studied with the aid of isotopic uric acid. J Biol Chem 181:183–193
Bennet AH, Colodny AH (1973) Urinary tract calculi in children. J Urol 109:318–320

Berger L, Yü TF (1975) Renal function in gout IV. An analysis of 524 gouty subjects including long term follow up studies. Am J Med 59:605–613
Bibus B (1962) Beitrag zur Zitronentherapie der Uratsteine. Urol Int 14:28–41
Binder HJ (1974) Intestinal oxalate absorption. Gastroenterology 67:441–446
Blacklock N, Macleod MA (1974) The effect of cellulose phosphate on intestinal absorption und urinary excretion of calcium. Br J Urol 46:385–392
Blaschke R, Maar K (1977) Kugelförmige Calciumphosphat-Konkremente im Harn und in der Kernzone von Oxalatsteinen. In: Vahlensieck W, Gasser G (Hrsg) Fortschritte der Urologie und Nephrologie, Bd 11: Pathogenese und Klinik der Harnsteine VI. Steinkopff, Darmstadt, S 84–89
Borgmann V, Nagel R (1982) Urolithiasis im Kindesalter. In: Kaufmann J (Redg. von) Verhandlungsberichte der Deutschen Gesellschaft für Urologie, 33. Tagung, Köln 1981. Springer, Berlin Heidelberg New York, S 251–255
Boss GR, Seegmiller JE (1979) Hyperuricemia and gout. N Engl J Med 26:1459–1468
Boulding JE (1961) Treatment of Wilson's disease with D-penicillamine. In: Walsh JM, Cummings JN (eds) Wilson's disease. Some current aspects. Blackwell Scientific Publications, Oxford, p 224
Boyce WH, Elkins IB (1974) Reconstructive renal surgery following anatrophic nephrolithotomy: Followup of 100 consecutive cases. J Urol 111:307–312
Braun J, May P, Samberger N (1977) Vergleichende Untersuchungen über Harnsäure- und Elektrolytkonzentrationen im Serum und Urin unter Benzbromaron und Allpurinol. In: Vahlensieck W, Gasser G (Hrsg) Fortschritte der Urologie und Nephrologie, Bd 11, Pathogenese und Klinik der Harnsteine VI. Steinkopff, Darmstadt, S 345–350
Brock WA, Nachtsheim DA, Parsons CC (1980) Hemiacridin imigation of renal pelvic calculi in patients with ideal conduit urinary diversion. J Urol 123:345–347
Bruce RR, Griffith DP (1981) Retrospective follow-up of patients with struvite calculi. In: Smith LH, Robertson WG, Finlayson B (eds) Urolithiasis. Plenum Press, New York London, p 191–193
Budevski G (1975) Die Harnsteinbildung bei Harnwegsinfektionen in unserem Krankengut. IV. Jenaer Harnsteinsymposion, Symposiumsbericht Jena 1975, S 65–68
Buelow H, Frohmüller H (1976) Der Rezidiv-Harnstein. Med Klin 71:449–457
Burghele T, Rugendorff EW, Covaliu T (1967) Zur Harnsteinprophylaxe mit Ionenaustauschern. Urologe 6:234–238
Butt AJ (1960) History of the treatment of urinary lithiasis. In: Butt AJ (ed) Treatment of urinary lithiasis. Charles C. Thomas Publisher, Springsfield Ill, p 3
Campbell MF (1951) Clinical pediatric urology. Saunders, Philadelphia
Carrod AB (1853) Gout, 2. Aufl. London
Cartier R, Hamet M (1974) Une nouvelle maladie metabolique: Le deficit complet en adenine phosphoribosyl-transferase avec lithease de 2,8-dihydroxyadenine. CR Acad Sci 297:883–887
Caspary WF (1979) Oxalaturolithiasis bei gastroenterologischen Erkrankungen. Pathogenese, Klinik und Therapie. Therapiewoche 29:2158–2165
Cattel WR, Spencer AG, Taylor GW, Watts RWE (1962) The mechanism of the renal excretion of oxalate in the dog. Clin Sci 22:43–52
Chaussy CH, Schmiedt E, Jocham D, Brendel W, Forssmann B, Walther W (1982) First clinical experience with extra-corporeally induced destruction of kidney stones by shock waves. J Urol 127:417–420
Cifuentes-Delatte L, Castro-Mendoza H (1967) Xanthinuria familiar. Rev Clin Esp 107:244–248
Cochran M, Hodgkinson A, Zarembski PM, Anderson CU (1968) Hyperoxaluria in adults. Br J Surg 55:121–128
Coe FL, Kavalach AG (1974) Hypercalcuria and hyperuricosuria in patients with calcium nephrolithiasis. N Engl J Med 19:1344–1350
Coe FL, Raisen L (1973) Allopurinol treatment of uric acid disorders in calcium stone formers. Lancet I:129–131
Cohanim M, Yendt ER (1981) Reduction of urinary oxalate excretion during chronic thiazide therapy. In: Smith LH, Robertson WG, Finlayson B (eds) Urolithiasis. Plenum Press, New York London, p 235–239

Cook DA (1975) Letter: Treament of renal stones: cellulose phosphate or magnesium. N Engl J Med 291:1034–1035
Corcos JM, Soler-Beghara J, Mayer K, Freyberg RH, Goldstein R, Jaffe F (1964) Neutrophilic agranulocytosis during administration of penicillamine. JAMA 189:265–268
Cram RL, Geho WR, Ray RD (1971) Diphosphonate treatment of calcinosis universalis. N Engl J Med 285:1012–1013
Crawhall JC, Watts RWE (1968) Cystinuria. Am J Med 45:736–755
Crawhall JC, Scowen EF, Watts RWE (1963) Effect of penicillamine on cystinuria. Br Med J (Clin Res) 1:588–590
Crawhall JC, Scowen EF, Thompson CJ, Watts RWE (1967) Dissolution of cystine stones during D-penicillamine treatment of a pregnant patient with cystinuria. Br Med J (Clin Res) 1:216–221
Daeschner CW, Singleton EB, Curtis JC (1960) Urinary tract calculi and nephrocalcinosis in instants and children. J Pediatr 57:721–724
Danielson BG (1985) Drugs against kidney stones: effects of magnesium and alkali. In: Schwille PO, Smith LH, Robertson WG, Vahlensieck W (eds) Urolithiasis and related clinical research. Plenum Press, New York and London, pp 525–532
Deetjen P, Boylan JW, Kramer K (1975) Physiology of the kidney and water balance. Springer, New York Heidelberg Berlin
Dempsey E, Caroll EL, Albright F, Hennemann PH (1958) A study of factors determining fecal electrolyt excretion. Metabolism 7:108–114
Dent CE, Philpot GR (1954) Xanthinuria, an inborn error (or deviation) of metabolism. Lancet I:182–185
Dent CE, Senior B (1955) Studies on the treatment of cystinuria. Br J Urol 27:317–332
Dent CE, Harper CM, Parfitt AG (1964) The effect of cellulose phosphate on calcium metabolism in patients with hypercalciuria. Clin Sci 27:417–425
Dirks IH, Onamme GA, Sutton RAL (1976) Filtration and Reabsorption von Kalzium in der Niere. Internationales Harnsteinsymposion, Davos 1976. In: Feldmann U, Mewes D (Hrsg) Urolithiasis. Straube, Erlangen, S 26–28
Dirks J (1984) Renal handling of calcium. Vth International Symposion on urolithiasis and related clinical research, Garmisch-Partenkirchen
Dock W, Frank NR (1950) Cation exchangers: Their use and hazards as aids in managing edema. Am Heart J 40:638–645
Dosch W (1976) Ionenaustauscher. Symposion Nierensteinleiden, München 1976
Dosch W (1978) Mineralogische Grundlagen der Harnsteinbildung. Med Welt 29:39–43
Duarte CG, Bland JH (1965) Changes in metabolism of calcium, phosphorus and uric acid after oral administration of chlorothiazide. Metabolism 14:899–903
Dulce HJ (1965) Die Phosphattherapie des Harnsteinleidens. Urologe 4:163–164
Dulce HJ, Dulce MC, Butz M (in Druck) Einfluß von Säure- und Basenbelastung auf Harnzusammensetzung und Löslichkeitsverhältnisse. In: Gasser G, Vahlensieck W (Hrsg) Klinik und Pathogenese der Harnsteine, Harnsteinsymposion Bonn–Wien, XI. Symposion, Wien, 21.–23. 3. 85, Steinkopff, Darmstadt
Earnest DL, Johnson G, Williams HE, Admirand WH (1974) Hyperoxaluria in patients with ileal resection. An abnormality in dietary oxalate absorption. Gastroenterology 66:1114–1122
Edwards NA, Russel RGG, Hodgkinson A (1965) The effect of oral phosphate in patients with recurrent renal calculus. Br J Urol 37:390–398
Eisenberger F, Schmiedt E, Peifer KJ, Chaussy Ch, Rothe R, Klein V, Reidl P (1973) In-situ-Perfusion und Kühlung der Niere bei Ausgußsteinen. Münch Med Wochenschr 115:404–409
Elder TD, Wyngaarden JB (1960) The biosynthesis and turnover of oxalic acid in normal and hyperoxaluria subjects. J Clin Invest 39:1337–1344
Elefant E, Brodsky M, Jelinek J (1966) Urolithiasis in infants. Ann Pediatr (Basel) 199:581–587
Elliot JS, Ribeiro ME (1970) Magnesium and calcium oxalate solubility. Invest Urol 8:396–390
Elomaa I, Karonen SL, Kairento AL, Pelkonen R (1981) Seasonal variation of urinary calcium and oxalate excretion, serum 25(OH)D_3 and albumin level in relation to renal stone for-

mation. In: Gasser G, Vahlensieck W (Hrsg) Fortschritte der Urologie und Nephrologie, Bd 17, Pathogenese und Klinik der Harnsteine VIII. Steinkopff, Darmstadt, S 121–126
Engelmann K, Watts RWE, Klinenberg JP, Sjoerdsma A, Seegmiller JE (1964) Clinical, physiological and biochemical studies of a patient with xanthinuria and pheochromocytoma. Am J Med 37:839–861
Ettinger B (1976) Recurrent nephrolithiasis: Natural history and effect of phosphat therapy. Am J Med 61:200–206
Ettinger B (1976) Recurrent nephrolithiasis: Natural history and effect of phosphate therapy. JAMA 61:200–206
Fam B, Rossier AB, Yalla S, Berg S (1976) The role of hemiacridin in the management of renal stones in spinal cord injury patients. J Urol 48:531–537
Fawcett NP, Nyhan WL, Anderson WW (1966) Thrombocytosis during treatment of cystinuria with penicillamine. J Pediatr 69:976–979
Fellström B (1985) Allopurinol treatment in urolithiasis. In: Schwille PO, Smith LH, Robertson WG, Vahlensieck W (eds) Urolithiasis and related clinical research act, Plenum Press, New York and London, pp 505–512
Felts JH, King JS, Boyce WH (1968) Nephrotic syndrome after treatment with penicillamine. Lancet I:53–54
Finlayson B (1974) Renal lithiasis in review. Symposion on renal lithiasis. Urol Clin North Am 1:181–211
Fishbeim WN (1981) Urease inhibitors in the treatment of infection induced stones: Some chemical, pharmacologic and clinical considerations. In: Smith CH, Robertson WG, Finlayson B (eds) Urolithiasis. Plenum Press, New York London, p 209–214
Fitzpatrick JM, Marberger M, Wickham JEA (1981) A study of the effectiveness of inosine in renal transplantation. Eur Urol 7:16–18
Flanagan TL, Sax MF, Heming AE (1951) Toxicity studies on amberlite XE-96, a carboxylic type cation exchanger resin. J Pharmacol Exp Ther 103:215–222
Fleisch H, Bisaz S (1961) Isolation from urine of pyrophosphate, a calcification inhibitor. Am J Physiol 203:671–678
Fleisch H, Bisaz S (1966) Pathophysiologie der Urolithiasis. Z Urol 59:785–791
Fleisch H, Russel RGG, Bisaz S, Mühlbauer RC, Williams DA (1970) The inhibitory effect of phosphonates on the formation of calcium phosphate crystal in vitro and on aortic and kidney calcification in vivo. Eur J Clin Invest 1:12–18
Garrod AB (1853) Nature and treatment of gout and rheumatic gout, 2nd edn. London
Garrod AE (1908) Inborn errors of metabolism. Lancet II:73–79, 142–148, 214–220
Gebhardt M, Bastian HP (1976) Harnsteingruppierung und Analysengenauigkeit. Urol Int 31:217–229
Genot R (1956) Nor moyen d'action sur hypercalcurie des lithiase urinaires. Semin Hop (Paris) 32:2978
Gershoff SN (1964) Vitamin B_6 and oxalate metabolism. Vitam Horm 22:581–589
Gil-Vernet J (1965) New surgical concepts in removing renal calculi. Urol Int 20:255–259
Gil-Vernet JM (1981) Three-dimensional radiography of the kidney. In: Schulman CC (ed) Advances in diagnostic urology. Springer, Berlin Heidelberg New York, p 87–100
Glazenburg J (1972) The effect of hydrochlorothiazide on the renal excretion of oxalic acid and on the formation of oxalate stone in the urinary tract. Archivum Chirurgicum Nederlandicum 23:217–223
Godfrey RG, Rankin TJ (1969) Uric acid renal lithiasis: Management by allopurinol. J Urol 101:643–647
Goldberg A, Smith JA, Lockhead A (1963) Treatment of lead poisoning with oral penicillamine. Br Med J 1:1270–1275
Green NA, Shaw AB (1981) Bladder stones in children. The Norwich School of Lithotomy. Eur Urol 3:126–131
Griffith DP (1978) Struvite stones. Kidney Int 13:372–382
Griffith DP, Musher DM, Campbell JW (1973) Inhibition of bacterial urease. Invest Urol 11:234–238
Griffith DP, Musher DM, Itin Ch (1976) Urease. The primary cause of infection induced urinary stones. Invest Urol 13:346–350

Griffith DP, Gibson JR, Clinton CW, Musher DM (1978) Acetohydroxamine acid: Clinical studies of a urease inhibitor in patients with staghorn renal calculi. J Urol 119:9–15

Griffith DP, Moskowitz P, Feldman S (1981) Infection, induced stones: Status of clinical trials with Urostat™ (Acetohydroxamic acid). In: Smith LH, Robertson WG, Finlayson B (eds) Urolithiasis. Plenum Press, New York London, p 199–208

Gutman AB, Yü TF (1957) Renal function in gout with a commentary on the renal regulation of urate excretion, and the role of the kidney in the pathogenesis of gout. Am J Med 23:600–608

Gutman AB, Yü TF (1968) Uric acid nephrolithiasis. Am J Med 45:756–759

Hagmaier V, Flückiger B, Pauvic N, Vortisch H, Lauffenburger T, Rutishauser G, Remagen W (1978) Auswirkungen eines oral verabreichten calciumbindenden Kationenaustauschers auf den Calcium- und Knochenstoffwechsel der Ratte. In: Gasser G, Vahlensieck W (Hrsg) Fortschritte der Urologie und Nephrologie, Bd 11, Pathogenese und Klinik der Harnsteine VI. Steinkopff, Darmstadt, S 257–260

Hagmaier V, Werness P, Smith LH (1984) Enteric hyperoxaluria: Risk factors for urolithiasis in addition to hyperoxaluria. In: Ryall R, Brockis JG, Marshall V, Finlayson B (eds) Urinary Stone, Churchill Livingstone, Melbourne–New York, pp 241–247

Hallson PC, Rose GA, Samuell CT (1981) Inhibitors of calcium oxalate and calcium phosphate crystal formation in urine – a critique and reappraisal. In: Smith LH, Robertson WG, Finlayson B (eds) Urolithiasis. Plenum Press, New York London, p 589–600

Hammarsten G (1928) On calcium oxalate and its solubility in the presence of inorganic salts with special reference to the occurrence of oxaluria. CR Lab Carlsberg 17:1–36

Hammarsten G (1929) On calcium oxalate and its solubility in the presence of inorganic salts with special reference to the occurence of oxaluria. CR Trav Lab Carlsberg 17:1–85

Harris H, Mittwoch U, Robson EB, Warren FL (1955) Phenotypes and genotypes in cystinuria. Ann Hum Genet 20:57–61

Harrison HE, Harrison HC (1963) Sodium, potassium and intestinal transport of glucose, l-tyrosine phosphate and calcium. Am J Physiol 205:107–111

Hartung R (1975) Die Bedeutung der Harnsäure bei der Kalziumoxalatnephrolithiasis. Münch Med Wochenschr 117:387–390

Hartung R, Leskovar P, Allgayer R, Schneider H, Bender O, Wellnhofer E, Simmel M (1981) Inhibited precipitation and growth of calcium oxalate crystals in the presence of alkaline salts of some polyhydroxycarboxylic acids. In: Smith LH, Robertson WG, Finlayson B (eds) Urolithiasis. Plenum Press, New York London, p 663–667

Hatch M, Bourke E, Costello J (1977) New enzymic method for serum oxalate determination. Clin Chem 23:76

Hauser W, Frick J (in Druck) Erste Ergebnisse einer Metaphylaxe mit Natrium-Kalium-Zitrat an rezidivierenden Kalziumoxalatsteinträgern. In: Gasser G, Vahlensieck W (Hrsg) Klinik und Pathogenese der Harnsteine. Harnsteinsymposion Bonn–Wien, XI. Symposion, Wien, 21.–23. 3. 85. Steinkopff, Darmstadt

Haussler M, Hughes M, Baylink D, Littledike ET, Cork D, Pitt M (1977) Influence of phosphate depletion on the biosynthesis and circulating level of 1-alpha, 2,5 dihydroxyvitamin D. In: Massry SG, Ritz E (eds) Phosphate metabolism. Plenum Press, New York, p 233–250

Hautmann R (1980) Oxalatstoffwechsel, Hyperoxalurie, Oxalose. In: Hautmann R, Lutzeyer W (Hrsg) Harnsteinfibel. Deutscher Ärzteverlag, Köln, S 62–71

Hautmann R, Terhorst B, Stuhlsatz HW, Lutzeyer W (1977) Mercaptopropionylglycine: A progress in cystine stone therapy. J Urol 117:628–630

Hautmann R, Hering F, Lutzeyer W (1978) Effects and side effects of cellulose phosphate and succinate in long term treatment of hypercalcuria or hyperoxaluria. J Urol 120:712–715

Hayashi Y, Kaplan RA, Pak CYC (1975) Effect of sodium cellulose phosphate therapy on crystallization of calcium oxalate in urine. Metabolism 24:1273–1278

Heidbreder E, Hennemann H, Krempien B, Heidland A (1972) Solidiaretische Behandlung der renal-tubulären Azidose und ihrer Komplikationen. Dtsch Med Wochenschr 97:1504–1507

Helbig W, Findeisen B (1971) Serum- und Harngehalt bei Haemoblastosen und Gicht sowie seine Beeinflussung durch Allopurinol. Z Inn Med 26:233–237

Hering F (1980) Spezielle Maßnahmen beim Harnsäurestein. In: Hautmann R, Lutzeyer W (Hrsg) Harnsteinfibel. Deutscher Ärzteverlag, Köln, S 156–159
Hering F, Lutzeyer W (1979) Resorptive and absorptive hypercalcuria. Therapy with sodium cellulose phosphate or thiazides. Eur Urol 5:29–31
Hering F, Hautmann R, Lutzeyer W (1979) Wirksamkeit und Nebenwirkungen einer differenzierten Hypercalciurie-Therapie. Ein Vergleich zwischen Thiaziden, Natrium-Cellulosephosphat, Campanyl und deren Kombination. In: Gasser G, Vahlensieck W (Hrsg) Fortschritte der Urologie und Nephrologie, Bd 14, Pathogenese und Klinik der Harnsteine VII. Steinkopff, Darmstadt
Hering F, Nowak H, Lutzeyer W (1980) Neues Konzept der Harnsteinprophylaxe – Computerprogramm zur Kalkulation des Löslichkeitsproduktes im Harn. In: Frohmüller H (Redg von) Verhandlungsberichte der Deutschen Gesellschaft für Urologie, 31. Tagung, München 1979. Springer, Berlin Heidelberg New York, S 474–475
Hering F, Burschard G, Pyhel N (1981) The relation between relative supersaturation and crystal aggregation in urine – a SEM study and a computerized calculation of the ion equilibrium. In: Smith LH, Robertson WG, Finlayson B (eds) Urolithiasis. Plenum Press, New York London, p 441–445
Hering F, Frank M, Lutzeyer W (1981) Urolithiasis im Kindesalter. In: Frohmüller H (Redg von) Verhandlungsberichte der Deutschen Gesellschaft für Urologie, 32. Tagung, Berlin 1980. Springer, Berlin Heidelberg New York, S 274–277
Herring LC (1962) Observations on the analysis of 10,000 urinary calculi. J Urol 88:545–562
Hesse A, Böhmer I, Classen A, Vahlensieck W (in Druck) Steigerung der inhibitorischen Wirkung des Harns durch Verabreichung eines Natrium-Kalium-Zitrat-Gemisches (Oxalyt C) In: Gasser G, Vahlensieck W (Hrsg) Klinik und Pathogenese der Harnsteine. Harnsteinsymposion Bonn–Wien, XI. Symposion, Wien, 21.–23. 3. 85. Steinkopff, Darmstadt
Hodgkinson A (1977) Oxalic acid in biology and medicine. Academic Press, London New York San Francisco
Hodgkinson A, Zarembski PM (1968) Oxalic acid metabolism: A review. Calcif Tissue Res 2:115–132
Hodgkinson A, Wilkinson R, Nordin BEC (1973) The concentration of oxalic acid in human blood. In: Delatte LC, Rapado A, Hodgkinson A (eds) Urinary calculi. Karger, Basel, p 18–23
Hodgkinson A, Bisset P, Tye J (1975) Effect of succinimide and other drugs on oxalate excretion by rats. Urol Int 30:465–471
Holländer E, Schwarczmann P (1969) Hemmung der endogenen Harnsäuresynthese mit Allopurinol. Münch Med Wochenschr 111:1623–1626
Horn HD (1971) Basis-Diagnostik und konservative Therapie bei Kranken mit Kalziumstein-Diathese. Dtsch Med J 21:506–512
Howard JE, Thomas WC (1968) Control of crystallization in urine. Am J Med 45:693–699
Hutschenreiter G, Riedmiller H, Thüroff J, Alken P (1982) Intraoperative, sonographische Sternlokalisation und dopplergesteuerte Nephrotomie – das Ende von Ischaemie und Kühlung. In: Kaufmann J (Redg von) Verhandlungsberichte der Deutschen Gesellschaft für Urologie, 33. Tagung, Köln 1981. Springer, Berlin Heidelberg New York, S 357
Jacobs STC, Gittes RF (1976) Dissolution of residual renal calculi with hemiacridin. J Urol 115:2–4
Jacobson AL, Singhal PC, Mandin H, Hyne JB (1979) Urinary ionic calcium and binding sites in normocalciuric idiopathic calcium urolithiasis. Invest Urol 17:218–222
Jaffe IA, Altmann K, Merryman P (1964) The antipyridoxin effect of penicillamine in man. J Clin Invest 43:1869–1873
Johansson G, Backman U, Danielson BG, Fellström B, Ljunghall S, Wikström B (1981) Prophylactic treatment with magnesium hydroxide in renal stone disease. In: Smith LH, Robertson WG, Finlayson B (eds) Urolithiasis. Plenum Press, New York London, p 267–273
Johnston JH (1973) Etiologic puzzle: Calculous disease in children. Med World News (Urology) 15
Kallistratos G (1972) Physicochemical principles and clinical results concerning the conservative treatment of kidney stones in urinary calculi. International Symposion renal stone research, Madrid 1972, p 198–205

Katz R (1967) Penicillamine-induced skin lesion, a possible example of human lathyrism. Arch Dermatol 95:196–198

Keiser HR, Henkin RI, Bartter FC, Sjoerdsma A (1968) Loss of taste during therapy with penicillamine. JAMA 203:381–383

Kelley WN, Rosenbloom FM, Miller J, Seegmiller JE (1968) An enzymatic basis for variation in response to allopurinol. Hypoxanthine-guanine-phosphoriboxyltransferase deficiency. N Engl J Med 278:287–293

King JS jr (1969) Treatment of cystinuria with alpha-mercaptopropionylglycine. A preliminary report with some notes on calcium chromatography of mercaptants. Proc Soc Exp Biol Med 129:927–932

King JS (1971) Currents in renal stone research. Clin Chem 17:971–982

King JS, Boyce WH (1965) Effect of penicillamine on cystinuria. Invest Urol 2:595–597

Kinoschita K, Yachiku S, Takenhi N, Kotake T, Sonoda T (1972) Treatment of cystinuria with alpha-mercaptopropionylglycine. Proceedings 2nd International Symposion on Thiola, Sauten, Osaka 1972, p 50–54

Klauwers J, Wolf PL, Cohn R (1969) Failure of renal transplantation in primary oxalosis. JAMA 205:551

Knappworst A, Broschk P, Weinkopf F, Weinkopf J (1978) Zur Herkunft des Harnoxalats, insbesondere über den Anteil des exogenen Oxalats. In: Gasser G, Vahlensieck W (Hrsg) Fortschritte der Urologie und Nephrologie, Bd 11, Pathogenese und Klinik der Harnsteine VI. Steinkopff, Darmstadt, S 53–56

Kohler FP (1962) Renacidin and tissue reaction. J Urol 87:102–108

Kolb FO, Earll JM, Harper HA (1967) Disappearance of cystinuria in a patient treated with prolonged low methionine diet. Metabolism 16:378–381

Kollwitz AA, Brauer R (1968) Die Harnsäuresteinbildung aus der Sicht des Urologen. Urol Int 23:411–427

Krakoff IH, Meyer RL (1965) Prevention of hyperuricemia in leukemia and lymphoma. Use of allopurinol, a xanthine oxidase inhibitor. JAMA 193:1–6

Lattimer JU, Hubbard M (1951) Pediatric urological admissions. J Urol 66:89–93

Lesch M, Nyhan WL (1964) A familial disorder of uric acid metabolism and central nervous system function. Am J Med 39:561–570

Lichtwitz A, Parlier R, Seze S de, Hioco D, Miravet L (1961) L'effet hypocalcin reque des sulfonamides duretiques. Sem Hop Paris 37:2350–2362

Ljunghall S, Backmann U, Danielson RG, Fellström B, Johansson G, Willström B (1981) Long-term treatment with bendroflumethiazide for prevent of stones. Metabolic effects. In: Smith LH, Robertson WG, Finlayson B (eds) Urolithiasis. Plenum Press, New York London, p 245–248

Lotz M, Potts JT (1964) Quantitation of the effects of penicillamin therapy in cystinuria. J Clin Invest 43:1293–1296

Lotz M, Potts JT, Bartter FC (1965) Recent advances in the therapy of cystinuria. Milit Med 130:768–774

Lotz M, Potts JT, Holland JM, Kieser WS, Bartter FC (1966) D-penicillamine therapy in cystinuria. J Urol 95:257–261

Luca HF de (1979) Vitamin D metabolism and function. Springer, Berlin Heidelberg New York

Lytton B (1979) Surgery of the kidney. In: Harrison JH, Gittes RF, Perlmutter AD, Stamey TA, Walsh PC (eds) Campbell's urology. Saunders, Philadelphia London Toronto, p 1993–2046

Lytton B, Glazier WB, Chudry IH, Bane AE (1979) The use of ATP-Mg Cl_2 in the treatment of post-ischemic renal injury. Trans Am Assoc Gen Surg 70:145–148

Mac Donald WB, Fellers FX (1966) Penicillamine in the treatment of patients with cystinuria. JAMA 197:396–402

Malek RS, Kelalis PP (1975) Pediatric nephrolithiasis. J Urol 113:545–551

Malluche HH, Tschöpe W, Ritz E, Meyer W, Massry S (1981) Disturbed terminal mineralisation of bone in idiopathic hypercalcuria. In: Smith LH, Robertson WG, Finlayson B (eds) Urolithiasis. Plenum Press, New York London, p 841–845

Mandel NS, Mandel GS (1981) Epitaxis between stone-forming crystals at the atomic level. In: Smith LH, Robertson WG, Finlayson B (eds) Urolithiasis. Plenum Press, New York, p 469–480
Marberger M, Eisenberger F (1980) Regional hypothermia of the kidney: Surface or transarterial cooling? A functional study. J Urol 124:179–183
Marberger M, Stackl W (1981) Renal hypothermia in situ. In: Resnick MI (ed) Current trend in urology, vol 1. William and Wilkins, Baltimore London, p 70–76
Marberger M, Günter R, Mayer EJ, Wiestler MA (1976) A simple method for in situ preservation of the ischemic kidney during renal surgery. Invest Urol 14:191–193
Marberger M, Stackl W, Hruby W (1982) Percutaneous litholapaxy of renal calculi with ultrasound. Eur Urol 8:236–242
Marget A (1817) An essay on chemical history and medical treatment of calculus disorders. London
Marquardt H, Nagel R (1977) Das Harnsteinleiden im Kindesalter. 19. Nordd. Urologentag, Braunlage 1977
Martin DL, Luca HF de (1969) Calcium transport and the role of vitamin D. Arch Biochem Biophys 134:139–148
May P, Braun J (in Druck) Zitratausscheidung rezidivierender Kalziumoxalatsteinbildner vor und während einer alkalisierenden Behandlung. In: Gasser G, Vahlensieck W (Hrsg) Klinik und Pathogenese der Harnsteine. Harnsteinsymposion Bonn–Wien, XI. Symposion, Wien, 21.–23. 3. 85. Steinkopff, Darmstadt
McChesney EW, McAuliff JP (1950) Effects of some ion exchange resins on the mineral metabolism of rats. Am J Physiol 160:164–276
McDonald JE, Henneman PH (1965) Stone dissolution in vivo and control of cystinuria with D-penicillamine. N Engl J Med 273:578–584
Melchior H, Lang G (1981) Three-dimensional intraoperative stone localisation. In: Schulman CC (ed) Advances in diagnostic urology. Springer, Berlin Heidelberg New York, p 101–105
Melnick I, Landes RR, Hoffman AA, Burch JF (1971) Magnesium therapy for recurring calcium oxalate urinary calculi. J Urol 105:119–122
Miano L, Galluci M, Petta S (1976) Dissoluzione di litiasi renale cistiniar mediante terapia medica. Prog Med 32:207–212
Miano L, Galluci M, Petta S (1979a) Results of medical treatment of cystine lithiasis. Eur Urol 5:265–272
Miano L, Petta S, Galluci M (1979b) Allopurinol in the prevention of calcium oxalate renal stones. Eur Urol 5:229–232
Millis RM (1971) Severe hypersensitivity reactions associated with allopurinol. JAMA 3:799–802
Minkov N, Konstantinov D, Gatser G (1981) Urolithiasis in children. Eur Urol 3:132–133
Mitchel JP (1981) Lithiasis in children. Eur Urol 3:121–124
Mulvaney WP (1960) Clinical use of renacidin in urinary calcifications. J Urol 84:206–212
Myers NA (1957) Urolithiasis in childhood. Arch Dis Child 32:48–54
Nemoy NJ, Stamey ThA (1976) Use of hemiacridin in management of infection stones. J Urol 116:693–695
Nicolayson R (1937) Studies upon the mode of action of vitamin D. II. The influence of vitamin D on the faecal output of endogenous calcium and phosphorus in the rat. Biochem J 31:106–113
Nishimura R, Ishido T, Takai S (1970) Effect of alpha-mercaptopropionylglycine. Proceedings 1st International Symposion on Thiola, Sauten, Osaka 1970, p 235–237
Nishimura R, Ishido T, Takai S (1972) Studies on cystinuria. Proceedings 2nd International Symposion on Thiola, Sauten, Osaka 1972, p 47–49
Nordin BEC (1976) Calcium phosphate and magnesium metabolism. Churchill-Livingstone, Edinburgh
Osler W (1912) Section XI nephrolithiasis. The principles and practice of medicine. Appleton, Oxford, p 717
Pak CYC (1972) Effects of cellulose phosphate and sodium phosphate on formation product and activity product of brushite in urine. Metabolism 21:447–455

Pak CYC (1973) Sodium cellulose phosphate. Mechanism of action and effect on mineral metabolism. J Clin Pharmacol 13:15–27
Pak CYC (1973) Hydrochlorothiazide therapy in nephrolithiasis: Effect on urinary activity product and formation product of brushite. Clin Pharmacol Ther 14:209–217
Pak CYC (1975) A simple test for the diagnosis of absorptive, resorptive and renal hypercalcuries. N Engl J Med 292:497–500
Pak CYC, Arnold LH (1975) Heterogenous nucleation of calcium oxalate by seeds of monosodium urate. Proc Soc Exp Biol Med 149:930–952
Pak CYC, Peacock M (1984) Need for classification of calciurias in stone patients – pros. and cons. Vth International Symposion on urolithiasis and related clinical research, Garmisch-Partenkirchen
Pak CYC, Cox JW, Powel E, Barter FC (1971) Effect of oral administration of ammonium chloride, sodium phosphate, cellulose phosphate and parathyroid extract on the activity product of brushite in urine. Am J Med 50:67–76
Pak CYC, Delen CS, Bartter FC (1974) Successful treatment of recurrent nephrolithiasis (calcium stones) with cellulose phosphate. N Engl J Med 290:175–180
Pak CYC, Tolentino R, Stewart A, Galosy RA (1978) Enhancement of renal excretion of uric acid during long term thiazide therapy. Invest Urol 16:191–193
Parfitt AM, Higgins BA, Nassim JR, Collins JA, Hilf A (1964) Metabolic studies in patients with hypercalcuria. Clin Sci 27:463–482
Passmore R (1953) Observation on epidemiology of stone in the bladder in Thailand. Lancet I:638–640
Pavanello L, Rizzoni G, Dussini N, Zaccello G, Passerini G, Tasca A, Pagano F (1981) Cystinuria in children. Eur Urol 3:139–143
Pietrek J, Kokot F (1973) Treatment of patients with calcium containing renal stones with cellulose phosphate. Br J Urol 45:136–143
Pinto B, Bernshtam J (1978) Diethylaminoethanol-cellulose in the treatment of absorptive hyperoxaluria. J Urol 119:630–632
Pinto B, Pujol J (1981) Identification of a small molecular weight inhibitor of the oxalate precipitation. In: Smith LH, Robertson WG, Finlayson B (eds) Urolithiasis. Plenum Press, New York London, p 637–639
Potter CF, Cadenhead A, Simmonds HA, Cameron JS (1979) Differential absorption of purine nucleosides and bases. In: Rapado A, Watts RWE, Bruyn CHMM de (eds) Purine metabolism. Plenum Press, New York London
Prien EL (1955) Studies in urolithiasis. J Urol 73:627–652
Prien EL (1963) Crystallographic analysis of urinary calculi: A 23-year survey study. J Urol 89:917–924
Prien ES, Gershoff SF (1974) Magnesium oxide-pyridoxine therapy for recurrent calcium oxalate calculi. J Urol 112:509–512
Rapado A (1970) Treatment of idiopathic hypercalcuria with sodium cellulose phosphate. Rev Clin Esp 119:61–68
Rapado A, Calle H de la, Castrillo JM, Mancha A, Traba ML, Cifuentes-Delatte L (1976) Nephrolithiasis bei Hypercalcurie und Hyperparathyreoidismus. Münch Med Wochenschr 118:799–804
Remieen A, Kallistratos G, Burchardt P (1975) Treatment of cystinuria with thiola (alpha-mercaptopropionylgylcine). Eur Urol 1:227–230
Riedmiller H, Thüroff J, Alken P, Hutschenreiter G, Hohenfellner R (1981) Gefäß- und Steinlokalisation durch Ultraschall – das Ende von Ischämie und Kühlung in der Nierensteinchirurgie? Akt Urol 12:210–215
Ries SW, Malament M (1962) Renacidin: A urinary calculus solvent. J Urol 87:657–661
Riet B van't, O'Rear CE (1981) Interaction of dyes with inorganic constituents of kidney stones. In: Smith LH, Robertson WE, Finlayson B (eds) Urolithiasis. Plenum Press, New York London, p 669–672
Ritz E, Schmidt-Gayk H, Möhring K (1975) Zur Pathophysiologie und Therapie der Hypercalcurie bei rezidivierenden Oxalatsteinen. In: Vahlensieck W, Gasser G (Hrsg) Fortschritte der Urologie und Nephrologie, Bd 7, Pathogenese und Klinik der Harnsteine IV. Steinkopff, Darmstadt, S 138–143

Robertson WG (1976) Urinary excretion. In: Nordin BEC (ed) Calcium, phosphate and magnesium metabolism. Churchill-Livingstone, Edinburgh, p 113–161

Robertson WG, Knowles F, Peacock M (1976) Urinary acid mucopolysaccarides inhibitors of calcium oxalate crystallisation. In: Fleisch H (ed) Urolithiasis research. Plenum Press, New York London, p 331

Robertson WG, Peacock M, Heyburn PJ, Speed R, Hanes F (1978) The role of affluence and diet in the genesis of calcium containing stones. In: Gasser G, Vahlensieck W (Hrsg) Fortschritte der Urologie und Nephrologie, Bd 11, Pathogenese und Klinik der Harnsteine VI. Steinkopff, Darmstadt, S 5–14

Robertson WG, Peacock M, Heyburn PJ (1979) Epidemiological risk factors in calcium stone formation. In: Gasser G, Vahlensieck W (Hrsg) Fortschritte der Urologie und Nephrologie, Bd 14, Pathogenese und Klinik der Harnsteine VII. Steinkopff, Darmstadt, S 105–116

Robertson WG, Peacock M, Heyburn PJ, Rutherford A, Sergeant VJ, Bambach CP (1981 a) A risk factor model of stone-formation: Application to the study of epidemiological factors in the genesis of calcium stones. In: Smith LH, Robertson WG, Finlayson B (eds) Urolithiasis. Plenum Press, New York London, p 303–307

Robertson WG, Peacock M, Ouiment D, Heyburn PJ, Rutherford A (1981 b) The main risk factor for calcium oxalate stone disease in man: Hypercalcuria or mild hyperoxaluria. In: Smith LH, Robertson WG, Finlayson B (eds) Urolithiasis. Plenum Press, New York London, p 3–12

Robertson WG, Peacock M (1985) Pathogenesis of Urolithiasis. In: Schneider H-J (Ed) Urolithiasis: Etiology, Diagnosis. Springer, Berlin Heidelberg New York Tokyo (Handbook of Urology, Vol. 17/I, p 185–334)

Rodgers A, Garside J (1981) The effect of some urinary constituents on the in vitro nucleation and growth kinetics of calcium oxalate. In: Smith LH, Robertson WG, Finlayson B (eds) Urolithiasis. Plenum Press, New York London, p 641–650

Rodman J (1984) Secondary urolithiasis. Vth International Symposion on urolithiasis and related research, Garmisch-Partenkirchen

Rohde M, Bach D, Dewes W, Schneeberger W, Vahlensieck W, Zilleken F (1978) Zur Gesetzmäßigkeit, Abhängigkeit und Beeinflußbarkeit des Oxalatgehaltes in Harnen von Patienten mit rezidivierender Calciumoxalat-Nephrolithiasis. In: Gasser G, Vahlensieck W (Hrsg) Fortschritte der Urologie und Nephrologie, Bd 11, Pathogenese und Klinik der Harnsteine VI. Steinkopff, Darmstadt, S 280–287

Rose GA (1982) Hyperoxaluria and recurring stone formation apparently cured by short courses of pyridoxin. In: Gasser G, Vahlensieck W (Hrsg) Fortschritte der Urologie und Nephrologie, Bd 17, Pathogenese und Klinik der Harnsteine VIII. Steinkopff, Darmstadt, S 376–380

Rose GA, Harrison AR (1974) The incidence, investigation and treatment of idopathic hypercalcuria. Br J Urol 46:261–274

Rose GA, Harrison AR, Kasidas GP (1981) Hyperoxaluria and recurrent stone formation apparently cured by short courses of pyridoxine. In: Gasser G, Vahlensieck W (Hrsg) Fortschritte der Urologie und Nephrologie, Bd 17, Pathogenese und Klinik der Harnsteine VIII. Steinkopff, Darmstadt, S 376–380

Rose GE, Arthur LJH, Kasidas GP, Scott IV (1982) Primary hyperoxaluria in a neonate. In: Gasser G, Vahlensieck W (Hrsg) Fortschritte der Urologie und Nephrologie, Bd 20, Pathogenese und Klinik der Harnsteine IX. Steinkopff, Darmstadt, S 35–39

Rosemberg LE, Hayslett JP (1967) Nephrotoxic effects of penicillamine in cystinuria. JAMA 201:698–700

Rugendorff EW, Schneider HJ, Hallwachs O (1981) Long term effects of campanyl in the treatment of patients with calcium urinary stone. In: Smith LH, Robertson WG, Finlayson B (eds) Urolithiasis. Plenum Press, New York London, p 283–286

Rundles RW, Wyngaarden JB, Hitchings GH, Ellion GB, Silberman HR (1963) Effect of a xanthine oxidase inhibitor on thiopurine metabolism, hyperuricemia and gout. Tr A Am Physicians 76:126–130

Russel RGG, Edwards BA, Hodgkinson A (1964) Urinary pyrophosphate and urolithiasis. Lancet I:1446

Ryall RL, Marshall VR (1981) The effect of normal and stone forming urine on the growth and aggregation of calcium oxalate crystals in relation to urinary glycosaminoglycans and urate concentrations. In: Smith LH, Robertson WG, Finlayson B (eds) Urolithiasis. Plenum Press, New York London, p 611–618

Sallis JD, Bichler KH, Korn S, Haussmann A (1981) Urinary glycosaminoglycan excretion in patients with urolithiasis. In: Smith LH, Robertson WG, Finlayson B (eds) Urolithiasis. Plenum Press, New York London, p 619–622

Samberger N, Braun J, Lux B, May P (1979) Harnsäuresteinbildung und Uratverstopfung der ableitenden Harnwege durch Urikosurika. Akt Urol 10:21–26

Schachter D, Rosen SM (1959) Active transport of Ca^{45} by the small intestine and its dependence an vitamin D. Am J Physiol 196:357–359

Schmucki O, Asper R, Weibe WH (1979) Streßinduzierte Veränderung der Elektrolytkonzentrationen im Urin bei der Ratte. In: Gasser G, Vahlensieck W (Hrsg) Fortschritte der Urologie und Nephrologie, Bd 14, Pathogenese und Klinik der Harnsteine VII. Steinkopff, Darmstadt, S 126–134

Schneider HJ (1979) Epidemiologische Aspekte der Urolithiasis. Urologe [Ausg B] 19:54–61

Schneider HJ (1980) Spezielle Maßnahmen der Therapie und Prophylaxe bei Infektsteinen. In: Hautmann R, Lutzeyer W (Hrsg) Harnsteinfibel. Deutscher Ärzteverlag, Köln, S 181–190

Schneider HJ, Klotz L, Horn G (1969) Die Herstellung eines Zitratgranulats und seine Verwendung in der Therapie der Harnsäurelithiasis. Z Urol Nephrol 62:351–355

Scholz D, Schwille PO, Sigel A (1981) Experience with thiazides in a double blind study. In: Smith LH, Robertson WG, Finlayson B (eds) Urolithiasis. Plenum Press, New York London, p 249–252

Schrier EE, Rubin JL, Lee KE, Werness PG, Smith LH (1981) Characterization of the calcium oxalate crystal growth inhibitors in human urine. In: Smith LH, Robertson WG, Finlayson B (eds) Urolithiasis. Plenum Press, New York London, p 579–588

Schulte KE, Rendic S, Henke G, Mrongovius RJ (1979) Pharmacokinetics and disposition of orally administered 3,4-C^{14} succinimide in the rat. Vortrag Arbeitstagung Succinimid, Iserlohn 1979

Schwille PO (in Druck) Orales Alkali-Zitrat bei Gesunden – Ergebnisse einer Dosis-Wirkungsstudie. In: Gasser G, Vahlensieck W (Hrsg) Klinik und Pathogenese der Harnsteine. Harnsteinsymposion Bonn–Wien, XI. Symposion, Wien, 21.–23. 3. 85. Steinkopff, Darmstadt

Schwille PO, Semberger NM (1975) Cyclisches Adenosinmonophosphat (3′-s′-c AMP) in Urin und Plasma von Harnsteinkranken unter besonderer Berücksichtigung des primären HPT. In: Vahlensieck W, Gasser G (Hrsg) Fortschritte der Urologie und Nephrologie, Bd 7, Pathogenese und Klinik der Harnsteine IV. Steinkopff, Darmstadt, S 184

Scott JT (1966) Allopurinol. Am Rheum Dis [Suppl] 25(6)

Scott JT, Holloway VP, Glass HI (1966) Studies of uric acid pool and turn over rate. Am Rheum Dis 38:366–373

Scott R, Patterson PJ, Smith M, Mathiesen A (1979) Reduction in urinary oxalate values by allopurinol. Urology 12:212–214

Scultety S, Balogh ES (1967) Zur Auflösung und Prophylaxe der Uratsteine. Z Urol Nephrol 60:843–852

Scurr DS, Bridge CM, Robertson WG (1981) Studies on inhibitors and promoters of the crystallization of calcium oxalate in urine and in matrix from calcium oxalate stones. In: Smith LH, Robertson WG, Finlayson B (eds) Urolithiasis. Plenum Press, New York London, p 601–605

Seegmiller JE (1968) Xanthine stone formation. Am J Med 45:780–783

Seegmiller JR, Rosenbloom FM, Kelley WN (1967) Enzym defect associated with a sex-linked human neurological disorder and excessive purine synthesis. Science 155:1682–1684

Segura JW, Erickson SB, Wilson DM, Berg CJ van den, Smith LH (1981) Infected renal lithiasis: Results of long-term surgical and medical management. In: Smith LH, Robertson WG, Finlayson B (eds) Urolithiasis. Plenum Press, New York London, p 195–198

Shah BG, Draper HH (1966) Depression of calcium absorption in parathyroid-ectomized rats. Am J Physiol 211:963–966

Sherwin AL, Beck IT, McKenna RD (1960) The course of Wilson's disease (hepatolenticular degeneration) during pregnancy and after delivery. Canad Med Assoc 83:160–166

Silbermann HR (1967) A new approach to the treatment of uric acid stones with comments on xanthinuria and calculi. Mod Treatment 4:531–538

Simmonds HA (1956) Harnsteine bei Kindern. Münch Med Wochenschr 121:1654–1656

Simmonds HA (1979) Diskussionsbeitrag in: Proceedings 3rd International Symposion on Pursia: Metabolism in man, Madrid/Spain 1979

Simmonds HA, Barrat TM, Webster DR, Sahota A, Acker KJ van, Cameron JS, Dillon M (1976) Spectrum of dihydroxyadenine urolithiasis in complete APRT deficiency. Purine metabolism in man. In: Rapado A, Watts RWE, Bruyn CHMM de (eds) Advances in experimental medicine and biology. Plenum Press, New York London, p 337–341

Smith AD, Lange PH, Miller RP, Reinke DB (1979) Dissolution of cystine calculi by imigation with acetylcysteine through percutaneous nephrostomy. J Urol 13:422–423

Smith DR, Kolb FO, Harper HA (1959) Management of cystinuria and cystine-stone disease. J Urol 81:61–64

Smith L (1985) Effects of orthophosphates and ion binders. In: Schwille PO, Smith LH, Vahlensieck W (eds) Urolithiasis and related clinical research. Plenum Press, New York and London, pp 483–489

Smith MJ (1977) Placebo versus allopurinol for renal calculi. J Urol 117:690–692

Smith MJ, Boyce WH (1969) Allopurinol and urolithiasis. J Urol 102:750–753

Sommerkamp H (1977) Diagnostik der renal tubulären Azidose. In: Gasser G, Vahlensieck W (Hrsg) Fortschritte der Urologie und Nephrologie, Bd 9, Pathogenese und Klinik der Harnsteine V. Steinkopff, Darmstadt, S 165–167

Sommerkamp H (1981) Therapie der renal tubulären Azidose mit Ethacrynsäure. In: Gasser G, Vahlensieck W (Hrsg) Fortschritte der Urologie und Nephrologie, Bd 17, Pathogenese und Klinik der Harnsteine VIII. Steinkopff, Darmstadt, S 419–421

Sonoda T, Kinoschita K, Kotake T, Sunao Y, Takenki N (1970) Effect of thiola on cystinuria. Proceedings 1st International Symposion Thiola, Sauten, Osaka 1970, p 231–234

Sorenson L (1968) Seminars on the Lesh-Nyhan-Syndrom. Management and treatment, discussion. Fed Proc 27:1099

Sperling O, Vries A de (1964) Studies on the etiology of uric acid lithiasis. Part 2: Solubility of uric acid in urine specimens from normal subjects and patients with idiopathic uric acid lithiasis. J Urol 92:331–334

Stark H, Savir A (1980) Dissolution of cystine calculi by pelvic caliceal irrigation with D-penicillamin. J Urol 124:895–898

Sternlieb I (1966) Penicillamine and the nephrotic syndrome. Results in patients with hepatolenticular degeneration. JAMA 198:1311–1312

Suby HJ, Albright F (1943) Dissolution of phosphatic urinary calculi by the retrograde introduction of citrate solution containing magnesium. N Engl J Med 228:81–91

Sur BK, Pandey HN (1981) Effect of different urinary constituents on inhibiting or acceleration calcium oxalate crystallisation. In: Smith LH, Robertson WG, Finlayson B (eds) Urolithiasis. Plenum Press, New York London, p 607–610

Sutor DJ (1969) Growth studies of calcium oxalate in the presence of various ions and compounds. Br J Urol 41:171–178

Sy WA de, Osterlinck W (1981) Bidimensional radioscopy: A rapid method for peroperative localisation of residual calculi. In: Schulman CC (ed) Advances in diagnostic urology. Springer, Berlin Heidelberg New York, p 83–86

Taccinoli M, Lotti T, Miano L, Laurenti C (1973) La calcolosi urinaria nell'infanzia. Relaz Uff 46 ° Congres Soc Ital Urol

Terhorst B, Lutzeyer W (1973) Möglichkeiten der medikamentösen Oxalatsteinprophylaxe. Z Urol Nephrol 65:815

Terhorst B, Melchior HJ (1972) Die medikamentöse Behandlung des Harnsteinleidens. Urol Int 27:230–244

Terhorst B, Stuhlsatz HW (1975) Cystinsteintherapie mit Mercaptopropionylglycine MPG. Urologe [Ausg A] 14:190–193

Tew WP, Malis CD, Lehninger AL, Walker GW, Howard JE (1981) Inhibition of PTH-induced nephrocalcinosis by phosphocitrate. In: Smith LH, Robertson WG, Finlayson B (eds) Urolithiasis. Plenum Press, New York London, p 559–568

Thannhausers Lehrbuch des Stoffwechsels und der Stoffwechselkrankheiten, 2. Aufl. Herausgegeben von Zöllner N. Thieme, Stuttgart (1952)
Thannhauser SJ (1956) Über die Pathogenese der Gicht. DMW 81:492–496
Thomas J, Lemonnier A, Charpentier C, Lelne R, Melon J, Steg A, Aboulker P (1970) Lithiase cystinique – première résultats cliniques avec l'alpha-mercaptopropionylgylcine. Première résultats biologiques avec le dithiosalicylate de sodium. J Urol Nephrol 76:823–828
Thomas J, Melon JM, Steg A, Aboulker P (1972) Traitement hyperoxalurique par le succinimide dans la lithiase oxalique rénale de l'homme. Therapie 26:999–1005
Thomas J, Charpentier C, Thomas E (1976) Traitement de la lithiase cystinique par l'alphamercaptopropionylglycine. Therapie 31:623–629
Thomas J, Melon JM, Duburque MT, Thomas E, Desgrez P, Aboulker P (1977) Elimination urinaire de l'acide oxalique et de l'acide glycolique chez le sujet sain et le sujet atteint de lithiase renale oxalique. Rein Foil Nutr 173
Thomas WC (1978) Use of phosphates in patients with calcareous renal calculi. Kidney Int 13:390–396
Timmermann A, Kallistratos G (1966) Modern aspects of chemical dissolution of human renal calculi by irrigation. J Urol 95:469–475
Timmermann A, Kallistratos G (1968) Gefahren und Kontraindikationen der instrumentellen Nierensteinchemolyse. Urol Int 23:236–243
Timmermann A, Kallistratos G (1973) Instrumentelle Nierensteinchemolyse. In: Hienzsch E, Schneider HJ (Hrsg) Der Harnstein. VEB Gustav Fischer, Jena
Tiselius HG, Larson L (1981) Inhibition of calcium oxalate crystal growth in patients with urolithiasis. In: Smith LH, Robertson WG, Finlayson B (eds) Urolithiasis. Plenum Press, New York London, p 623–629
Toel F (1855) Beobachtungen über Cystinbildung. Ann Chem Pharmacol 96:247–251
Troup CW, Lawnicki CC, Bourne RB, Hodgson NB (1972) Renal calculus in children. J Urol 107:306–307
Tschöpe W, Beck C, Christ D, Schmidt-Gayk H, Ritz E (1979) Phosphatstoffwechsel unter Basalbedingungen und nach Phosphatbeladung. In: Gasser G, Vahlensieck W (Hrsg) Fortschritte der Urologie und Nephrologie, Bd 14, Pathogenese und Klinik der Harnsteine VII. Steinkopff, Darmstadt, S 147–153
Udransky L von, Boumann E (1889) Über das Vorkommen von Diaminen, sogenannten Ptomainen bei Cystinurie. Z Physiol Chemie 13:562
Vabusek M (1976) Zur Prophylaxe von Harnsteinen bei Hyperurikaemie und Gicht. In: Feldmann U, Mewes D (Hrsg) Urolithiasis. Straube, Erlangen, S 162–165
Vahlensieck W (1976) Diät beim Harnsteinleiden. Infusionstherapie 3:243–248
Vahlensieck W (1980) Kindliche Harnsteine. In: Hautmann R, Lutzeyer W (Hrsg) Harnsteinfibel. Deutscher Ärzteverlag, Köln, S 211–218
Vries A de, Sperling O (1976) Uric acid stone formation: Basic concepts of etiology and treatment. In: Williams DI, Chisholm GD (eds) Scientific foundation of urology. Heinemann Medical Books, London, p 297–302
Vries A de, Frank M, Atsmon A (1962) Inherited uric acid lithiasis. Am J Med 33:880–886
Wallace SL (1978) The treatment of gout, arthritis. Rheum 15:317–332
Watts RWE (1973) Oxalate biosynthesis in primary hyperoxaluria. Internationales Harnstein-Symposion, Madrid 1972. In: Cifuentes-Delatte L, Rapado A, Hodgkinson A (eds) Urinary calculi. Karger, Basel, p 13–17
Watts RWE, Watkins PJ, Matthias JQ, Gibbs DA (1966) Allopurinol and acute uric acid nephropathy. Br Med J 1:205–208
Wellhöner HH (1976) Allgemeine und systematische Pharmakologie und Toxikologie. Springer, Berlin Heidelberg New York
Westenfelder M, Galanos C, Madsen PO (1975) Experimental lipid. A induced nephritis in the dog. Invest Urol 5:337–345
Wilkinson R (1976) Absorption of calcium, phosphorus and magnesium. In: Nordin BEC (ed) Calcium phosphate and magnesium metabolism. Churchill-Livingstone, Edinburgh, p 36–112

Williams G, Sallis JD (1981) The sources of phosphocitrate and its role as an inhibitor of calcium phosphate and calcium oxalate crystallisation. In: Smith LH, Robertson WG, Finlayson B (eds) Urolithiasis. Plenum Press, New York London, p 569–577

Williams HE (1974) Calcium nephrolithiasis and cellulose phosphate. N Engl J Med 290:224

Williams HE (1976) Oxalsäure: Absorption, Exkretion and Mebabolismus. Internationales Symposion, Davos 1976. In: Feldmann U, Newes D (Hrsg) Urolithiasis. Straube Erlangen, S 87–91

Williams HE (1977) The causes of kidney stones – their diagnosis and treatment. Med Times 105:55–59

Williams HE, Smith LH jr (1968) Primary hyperoxaluria. Am J Med 45:196–219

Williams HE, Johnson GA, Smith LH (1971) The renal clearance of oxalate in normal subjects and patients with primary hyperoxaluria. Clin Sci 41:213–218

Willnow U (1968) Nephrolithiasis im Säuglings- und Kindesalter. DMW 92:1668–1674

Wolf M (1969) Kationenaustauscher als Diuretica. In: Herken H (Hrsg) Diuretica. Springer, Berlin Heidelberg New York (Handbuch der experimentellen Pharmakologie, Bd XXIV, S 574–593)

Wolff HP (1954) Die Therapie mit Kationenaustauschern im Lichte fünfjähriger Erfahrung. Klin Wochenschr 32:761–770

Wollaston WH (1810) On cystic oxide, a new species of urinary calculus. Philos Trans R Soc Lond [Biol] 100:223–230

Worthmann RL, Kelly WN (1977) Gout and hyperuricemia: A rational approach to management. Clin Ther 1:159–184

Wrong O, Davies HEF (1959) The excretion of acid in renal disease. Q J Med 28:259–363

Yendt ER (1985) Effects of thiazides. Vth International Symposion on urolithiasis and related clinical research, 1984. Plenum Press, New York (in press)

Yendt ER, Cohanim M (1973) Ten years experience with the use of thiazides in the prevention of kidney stones. Am Clin Climat Assoc 85:65–75

Yendt ER, Gagné RJA, Cohanim M (1966) The effect of thiazides on idopathic hypercalcuria. Am J Med Sci 251:449–460

Yü TF (1965) Secondary gout associated with myeloproliferative diseases. Arthritis Rheum 8:765–771

Yü TF (1974) Milestones in the treatment of gout. Am J Med 56:673–677

Yü TF, Gutman AB (1964) Effect of allopurinol (4-hydroxypyrazol[3,4-d]pyrimidine) on serum and urinary uric acid in primary and secondary gout. Am J Med 37:885–898

Zarembski PM, Hodgkinson A (1969) Some factors influencing the urinary excretion of oxalic in man. Clin Chir Act 25:1–10

Zechner O, Latal D, Grundig E, Muller M (1976) Klinische Aspekte der Cystinurie und ihre Behandlung mit Thiola. Wien Klin Wochenschr 88:101–105

Zilleken F (1975) Wirkungsweise des Succinimids im Intermediärstoffwechsel. Symposium zur Succinimidtherapie, veranstaltet von der Firma Medice, Iserlohn 1975

Zinnemann HH, Jones JE (1960) Dietary methionine and its influence on cystine excretion in cystinuric patients. Metabolism 15:915–921

Zöllner N (1960) Moderne Gichtprobleme. Ergeb Inn Med Kinderheilk 14:321–389

Zöllner N, Griebsch A (1973) Influence of various dietary purines on uric acid production. International Symposion on renal stone research, Madrid 1973, p 84–88

Zöllner N, Schattenkirchner M (1967) Allopurinol in der Behandlung der Gicht und der Harnsäurenephrolithiasis. DMW 92:654–660

Zöllner N, Griebsch A, Gröbner W (1972) Einfluß verschiedener Purine auf den Harnsäurestoffwechsel. Ernährungsumschau 3:79–82

The Treatment of Ureteric Colic and Promotion of Spontaneous Passage

D. BACH

I. Introduction

When a calculus travels from the renal pelvis into the ureter, complete or partial obstruction results, with characteristic accompanying symptoms. The predominant feature is colic, usually an acute event leading to early medical intervention. As the colic subsides the aim of further treatment becomes the reduction of obstruction, be it by conservative drug therapy, by instrumentation or by surgery. Where shape, level and size of the stone are favorable, specific conservative therapy will result in spontaneous passage in about 60–90% of cases (BACH et al. 1983; BANDHAUER 1970; MADERSBACHER et al. 1975; SCHNEIDER 1985; VAHLENSIECK 1970, 1973; VAHLENSIECK and BASTIAN 1973). Any conservative treatment of ureteric colic or to promote spontaneous passage should be founded on pathophysiological understanding of the obstructed ureter.

II. Pathophysiology

1. Innervation of the Ureter

Recent publications (HANNAPPEL 1984; HANNAPPEL et al. 1982) have demonstrated the smooth muscle of the renal pelvis and ureter to be a functional syncytium. Primary pacemaker cells in the most intrarenal domains of the renal pelvis generate an intrinsic myogenic rhythm of ureteric peristalsis. Variations in diuresis affect this pacemaker rate only marginally. The primary myogenic excitation and conduction in the pyeloureter is, however, subject to modification by central nervous activity mediated via the autonomic nerves. Apart from factors within the ureter such as diuresis, obstruction and inflammation, ureteric motility will depend on sympathetic activity in the renal plexus, hypogastric nerves, spermatic and iliac plexuses. The parasympathetic, on the other hand, has little direct effect on the ureter, except for changes in detrusor activity, which spread from the bladder into the lower ureter (Fig. 1).

Sympathomimetics stimulate and sympathetic blocking agents inhibit ureteric peristalsis (MELCHIOR and TERHORST 1969). Sympathetic activity affects the ureteric smooth muscle by the action of adrenotropic transmitter substances

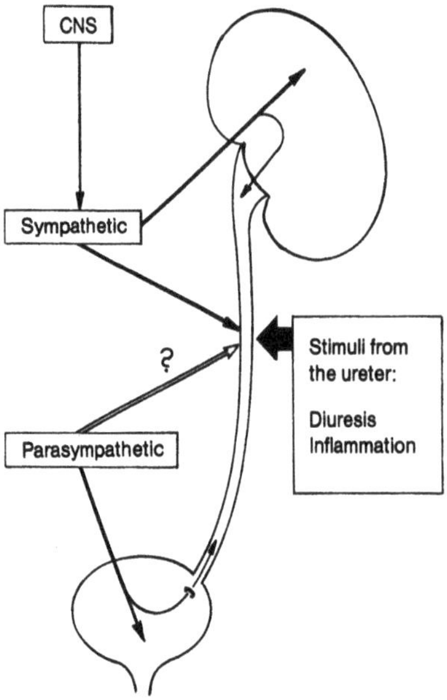

Fig. 1. Pathways controlling ureteric activity (after MELCHIOR and TERHORST 1969)

on alpha- and betaadrenergic receptors. Stimulation of alpha receptors increases muscle tone and beta stimulation relaxes it. Blockade of the appropriate receptor has the opposite effect.

The sharing of segmental innervation by ureter and intestine (excluding duodenum and jejunum) suggests that the disordered intestinal motility often seen during ureteric colic may be due to viscero-visceral reflexes. Viscerocutaneous reflexes may occur in selected areas (Zones of Head) of the corresponding dermatomes. The genitofemoral nerve, which sends twigs to the ureter, is said to be responsible for the testicular pain frequently experienced by men with low-lying ureteric calculi.

2. Urodynamics of Obstruction

Modern rheomanometric, electromanometric and electromyographic studies have largely disproved classical concepts of ureteric colic: The idea can no longer be upheld that uncoordinated spasms result from hyperperistalsis of the obstructed segment of the pelviureteric system and are directed at expelling the stone.

Following complete occlusion of the ureter by a calculus intraluminal pressure starts to rise immediately until the so-called effective filtration pressure or maximum ureteric pressure (20 – 80 mm Hg) is reached. The frequency of peristaltic waves increases and the amplitude of contraction decreases. Finally, only frequent waves of ineffectively low amplitude remain and urinary flow is either markedly reduced or comes to a complete standstill (BOYARSKI and LABAY 1972; MELCHIOR and RATHERT 1969; RUTISHAUSER 1970). Although the effective filtration pressure initially rises, the rise in pressure is not necessarily associated with colic (SÖKELAND and MAY 1970). The cause of colic has therefore to be thought not only in the increase in intraluminal pressure but also in local distension of the ureteric wall, in spasm due to local irritation and in localized ischemia of the ureter. Afferent impulses are conducted by sympathetic pain fibers to give rise to the characteristic pain. Distension of the renal capsule by urinary obstruction and alterations in renal perfusion may also contribute.

III. The Treatment of Colic (Initial Analgesia)

The pathophysiology of acute urinary tract obstruction and clinical experience in urologic practice both point to early parenteral administration of effective centrally acting analgesic. The indications are twofold: to control pain symptoms and to correct the autonomic disturbances of acute ureteric colic. An analgesic agent with a central action and sympathomimetic properties is thus the mainstay of treatment in the acute colic phase (BRÜHL and BACH 1978; BRÜHL 1975).

Inadequate pain relief during colic is often due to the route of administration. "Initial analgesia" should be intravenous. Reduced absorption often delays and attenuates the effect of intramuscular injection, oral or rectal administration. These routes should therefore be eschewed for pain control in urology (BRÜHL and BACH 1978). If a single intravenous bolus proves inadequate one may be forced to continue analgesic therapy by continuous infusion, which should always be carried out under inpatient supervision.

1. Metamizole (Novaminsulfone)

Metamizole (e.g. as Novalgin) has stood the test of decades of use in urologic practice and remains a first line analgesic of choice for ureteric colic. The dose is one ampoule (2.5 g) intravenously. Apart from an excellent analgesic effect this agent also has a weak spasmolytic activity on smooth muscle. Metamizole occasionally gives rise to hypersensitivity reactions with bronchospasm, dose-dependent hypotension and occasionally profound shock (in rare cases with a fatal outcome). Agranulocytosis occurs sporadically, especially after repeated and oral administration. For these reasons pyrazolone hypersensitivity should always be enquired after and the agent should be injected slowly with emergency equipment at the ready. In the presence of proven pyrazolone hypersensitivity oral treatment should be discontinued because of the risk of allergy.

Although metamizole has been in use as an analgesic since 1972 and is available in 182 commercial preparations and 343 presentations, a final verdict by the Federal Health Ministry is not yet to hand. No further guidance is likely to emerge until the availability of results from the "Boston Study" on agranulocytosis and aplastic anemia commenced in 1977 (Bekanntmachung der Bundesärztekammer 1981, 1982).

2. Pentazocine

If metamizole proves inadequate to abolish pain a more powerful analgesic should be employed. The drug pentazocine (Fortral) has proved reliable in this role (BRÜHL 1975), once again in a dose of one ampoule (30 mg) intravenously. The risk of hypotensive circulatory disturbances following administration must be born in mind. Patients should remain lying for some time following injection and not be allowed to drive themselves after outpatient treatment.

3. Morphine

Sadly, opiates continue in frequent use on the grounds that symptoms are uncontrollable by any other means. Although it is true that morphine or its derivatives usually control colic or tenesmus, the effect rests first and foremost on the central action of these drugs. The alkaloid morphine – and to a less degree its derivatives hydromorphone (Dilaudid) or oxycodone (Eukodal) – cause respiratory depression and markedly increase gastrointestinal tone. Despite this increased tone the excitability of the intestine by stretch stimuli is substantially reduced, peristalsis is decreased and transit time increased. Repeated administration not infrequently leads to ileus and marked meteorism, the latter, rather than urological symptoms often precipitating hospital admission. Opiates also increase sphincter tone and may precipitate retention of urine, which, in the presence of effective analgesia, may lead to diagnostic errors. As well inhibiting already disordered peristalsis opiates may cause vomitting. These factors, the risk of dependence and the probability that the colic and bladder spasms arising during attempted onward passage of the stone will require repeated medication all militate against the opiates and their use in the treatment of acute ureteric colic should be deprecated.

IV. Passage of the Stone

The period following abolition of colic symptoms should be devoted to promoting spontaneous passage of the stone. In the presence of a favorable stone the aim of this treatment is to decompress the ureter, restore normal urinary tract tone and reinitiate the peristaltic activity that will be needed for the successfull expulsion of the stone (Table 1).

1. Spasmoanalgesia

Spasmoanalgesia should be reserved for the *post-colic* phase. The term "spasmoanalgesia" as applied to the treatment of ureteric colic is the subject of urodynamic debate. As already pointed out, colic is not due to increased peri-

Table 1. The treatment of ureteric colic and promotion of spontaneous passage

I. Initial analgesia (Treatment of colic)	
Parenteral analgesics:	
Metamizole and/or pentazocine (1 ampoule slowly i.v.)	
consider infusion therapy	
II. Extented spasmoanalgesia (Promotion of spontaneous passage)	
1. Metamizole	3×20–30 drops/day
and/or	
2. Spasmo-Cibalgin comp.	3×1 suppos./day
and/or	
3. Urol	3×2–3 caps./day
III. Adjuvant therapy	
1. Anti-edema therapy	
Reparil	3×2 tabs./day
and/or	
Urol	3×2 caps./day
2. Increased diuresis	
Increased oral intake to give a urine volume of at least 2 liters/24 hrs	
(recommended medicinal teas: Nieron, Solubitrate, Teecura)	
and/or	
Diuretics:	
Furosemide	20–40 mg/day (1–2 tabs)
or Hydrochlorothiazide	50 mg/day (2 tabs)
(beware of electrolyte disturbances)	
3. Physical exercise	

stalsis or tone of the proximal ureter but to overdistension of the renal pelvis and ureteric wall, with consequent stimulation of sympathetic pain fibers running in the splanchnic nerves (RUTISHAUSER 1970). Local irritation of the ureteric mucosa, with resulting spasm at the level of the stone has also been postulated as a cause of colic. The combination of an analgesic with an atropine-like spasmolytic is aimed at abolishing viscero-visceral reflexes related to the colic, such as the bladder spasms which may occur during transit of the stone. Spasmolytics also have an important role in restoring normal pressure and flow relationships. These factors taken together represent the rationale of "spasmonanalgesia".

Spasmolytics: A fundamental distinction should be made between spasmolytic agents acting directly on muscle and those acting on nerve fibers. Either group is suitable for combination with analgesics.

Papaverine and its derivatives are the prototype of the former group (e.g. Spasmo-Cibalgin), whereas N-butyl-scopolamine (Buscopan) is the most frequently employed exponent of the latter.

Agents of either group are commercially available in combination with analgesics and denoted by the suffix "comp." (compositum) (e.g. Spasmo-Cibalgin comp., Baralgin-comp., ect.).

Agents acting on the Sympathetic: The rationale for using this type of agent in combination with an analgesic lies in the sympathetic control of ureteric activity. There is certainly an experimental foundation for the use of some members of this group, such as beta-sympathomimetics (e.g. Alupent) or alpha-receptor blockers (e.g. Dibenzyran) (MELCHIOR and TERHORST 1969). However, little clinical experience has yet been gained and side-effects are not infrequent, so the routine use of such substances cannot be regarded as established practice.

2. Extended Spasmoanalgesia

For cases where initial analgesia has rid the patient of his pain and if the stone is potentially capable of pass spontaneous passage, VAHLENSIECK recommends continuous spasmoanalgesic medication to prevent the recurrence of colic and to hasten the stone on its way (Table 1). The same author has coined the term "extended spasmoanalgesia", meaning continuous administration of a drug combination at regular intervals, so as to avoid or reduce the need for strong analgesics, even if a long period of outpatient treatment ensues (VAHLENSIECK and BASTIAN 1973).

3. Herbal Remedies

Herbal remedies have been used in the treatment of urolithiasis for centuries and have proved of particular value in preventing recurrence and in promoting spontaneous passage of ureteric calculi. One such product, Urol, has been in use for many years and its effectiveness in promoting spontaneous passage has been tested in randomized multicenter studies. The preparation contains anthraquinone derivatives of madder root, which are said to dissolve and "corrode" the surface of stones (GEBHARDT 1979). It also contains khellin, which has a spasmoanalgesic effect (WESTENDORF and VAHLENSIECK 1981). Most of the other components have been shown to have a diuretic effect, promoting in toto an eightfold increase in diuresis in animal experiments (DEETJEN 1979). Another component, aescine, also has powerful antiedematous properties. The

Table 2. The effect of Urol compared to that of classical "extended spasmoanalgesia" in promoting spontaneous passage of ureteric calculi

	BACH et al. (1983)		SCHNEIDER (1982)	
	Urol	Spasmo-analgesia	Urol	Spasmo-analgesia
Patients treated	55	56	105	77
Proportion recurrent cases %	36	31	45	37
Mean stone transit time (days)	18	17	22	21
Spontaneous passage rate (%)	89	86	89	88
Cost to time of passing stone (DM)	45	84		

preparation may be used as a single agent or in combination with other traditional spasmoanalgesics.

Two comparative studies on the conservative treatment of ureteric stones were unable to demonstrate a difference in spontaneous passage rate between the Urol treated group and the group receiving "classical" spasmoanalgesic therapy (Table 2) (BACH et al. 1983; SCHNEIDER 1982). Since the success rate is the same and both the side effects and the price give Urol an advantage, the latter should be the first line of treatment to promote spontaneous passage. If pain recurs on this regime, a parenterally administered spasmoanalgesic should be added.

4. Adjuvant Therapy

a) Anti-Edematous Drugs

The aim of anti-edema therapy is to abolish local edema in the ureteric wall at the site of an impacted calculus, thus promoting onward transit of the stone. The active principle aescine, isolated from the horse chestnut, has been shown in clinical studies to have a marked anti-edema action. Aescine can be administered as a single agent (e.g. Reparil 3 × 1 ampoule/day intravenously in the acute phase, then 3 × 1 tablet/day) or in combination with a herbal extract (e.g. Urol).

b) Increased Diuresis

Adequate diuresis is of fundamental importance for the onward transit of calculi, the stone being carried forward in a bolus of urine. Certain basic principles should be born in mind when seeking to promote diuresis:

Because of the risk of forniceal rupture so-called "forced diuresis" should only be instituted (e.g. by infusion therapy) during colic-free spells. Under no circumstances should "drinking bouts" be prescribed, because patients with a previous cardiac history are all too easily overloaded in this way.

A steady intake of 2–3 litres should be spread evenly over the day. Special teas with diruretic properties are of value here (e.g. Nieron tea, Solubitrat tea, Teecura tea).

If there is no other way of achieving adequate diuresis, the gentle administration of diuretics may be indicated. Proven agents include furosemide (Lasix) and hydrochlorothiazide (Esidrix). During diuretic therapy a balanced fluid intake and careful monitoring of plasma electrolytes are essential (beware of hypokalemia!).

c) Physical Activity

Adequate physical activity stimulates renal perfusion and therefore diuresis. Clinical experience shows that exercise promotes passage of stones.

V. Complications of Conservative Treatment

How long conservative treatment is persisted with will depend on the rate at which the stone progresses and on the possible occurrence of complications during treatment.

1. Urinary Obstruction

If the outflow from the renal pelvis is completely obstructed by a stone increasing distension and cessation of urine flow will require conservative treatment to be abandoned and replaced by instrumentation or surgery.

Shortterm decompression of the collecting system may be achieved by percutaneous nephrostomy.

The anatomy of the renal pelvis and the site of the stone will together affect the degree of distension. An extrarenal pelvis is better able to compensate for rises in pressure than an intrarenal pelvis. Thus a case with a high located stone and an intrarenal pelvis will require earlier intervention than one with a low located stone and an extrarenal pelvis.

2. Infection

Any patient with an ureteric calculus is at risk of sepsis, both because of the obstruction and accumulation of stagnant urine above it and because of inflammatory change in the ureter. Stagnant urine is an ideal culture medium for bacteria. Thus the clinical pictures that may develop from a urinary tract infection include pyelonephritis, renal carbuncle, perinephric abscess, pyonephrosis and, most serious and life-treatening of all, urinary septicemia. If therefore, the diagnosis of urinary infection is made in the presence of an obstructing ureteric calculus, the greatest caution should be exercised and early intervention seriously considered.

References

Bach D, Hesse A, Feuereisen B, Vahlensieck W, Joost J, Lehmann H-D, Wegner G (1983) Optimierung der konservativen Harnsteinaustreibung. Fortschr Med 101:337–342
Bandhauer K (1970) Therapie des Uretersteins. Akt Urol 1:42
Bekanntmachungen der Bundesärztekammer (1981) Dtsch Ärzteblatt 78:918
Bekanntmachungen der Bundesärztekammer (1982) Dtsch Ärzteblatt 79:39
Boyarski S, Labay P (1972) Ureteral Dynamics. Williams and Wilkins, Baltimore
Brühl P (1975) Zur Pharmakotherapie urologischer Schmerzen. In: Neuhaus GA, Kubicki StK (Hrsg) Pentazocin. Thieme, Stuttgart, S 36
Brühl P, Bach D (1978) Kreuzschmerzen aus der Sicht des Urologen: Klinik, Diagnostik, Therapie. Therapiewoche 28:3829

Deetjen P (1979) Die besondere Art der Diurese unter dem Einfluß von Urol. Fortschr Urol Nephrol [Suppl] 14:1

Gebhardt M (1979) Erste, vorläufige Ergebnisse einer Studie über die litholytische Wirksamkeit von Urol auf Calcium-Oxalatsteine. Fortschr Urol Nephrol [Suppl] 14:34

Hahn E, Sökeland J, Wolters A (1979) Kolikbehandlung und pharmazeutische Harnsteinaustreibung. In: Vahlensieck W (Hrsg) Urolithiasis 2. Springer, Berlin Heidelberg New York, S 1–18

Hannappel J (1984) Physiologie der oberen Harnwege. Therapiewoche 34:6488

Hannappel J, Golenhofen K, Hohnsbein J, Lutzeyer W (1982) Pacemaker process of ureteral peristalsis in multicalyceal kidneys. Urol Int 37:240

Madersbacher H, Frick J, Bartsch G (1975) Ergebnisse der konservativen Behandlung von Uretersteinen. Fortschr Urol Nephrol 5:199

Melchior H, Rathert P (1969) Die Steuerung der Ureterperistaltik. In: Lutzeyer W, Melchior H (Hrsg) Ureterdynamik. Thieme, Stuttgart, S 32

Melchior H, Terhorst B (1969) Die Wirkung sympathicotroper Substanzen auf die Ureterdynamik. Urologie [Ausg A] 8:348

Rutishauser G (1970) Druck und Dynamik in den oberen Harnwegen. Steinkopff, Darmstadt

Schneider H-J (1982) Phytopräparate in der Behandlung des Harnsteinleidens. MMW 125:365

Schneider H-J (1985) Phytopharmaka in der Harnsteintherapie – Ergebnisse einer multizentrischen Studie mit Urol. Bonn-Wiener Harnsteinsymposium, Wien 21.–23.03.1985

Sökeland J, May P (1969) Physiologische und pathophysiologische Gesichtspunkte der Elektromanometrie und Elektromyographie. In: Lutzeyer W, Melchior H (Hrsg) Ureterdynamik. Thieme, Stuttgart, S 114

Vahlensieck W (1970) Behandlung des „akuten Harnsteins“. Dtsch Med Wochenschr 95:529

Vahlensieck W (1973) Das Harnsteinleiden. Wien Med Wochenschr 123:561

Vahlensieck W, Bastian H-P (1973) Der „akute“ Harnstein. Fortschr Med 91:905

Westendorf J, Vahlensieck W (1981) Spasmolytische und kontraktile Einflüsse eines Kombinationspräparates auf die glatte Muskulatur des isolierten Meerschweinchendarms. Arzneimittelforsch 31:40

Surgical Treatment of Renal Calculi

M. MARBERGER and W. STACKL

I. Introduction

"If you would rise aloft, first shed ballast" ... (Ernst Trier)

Nowhere in urology are these words more applicable than to the surgery of kidney stones. For the period 1970 to 1980 the Index Medicus lists 393 scientific papers on the subject, a figure which reflects not only the magnitude of the whole problem but also the immense efforts that continue to be made to improve the results of treatment. There is a corresponding state of flux in clinical practice. The last five years in particular have witnessed the ever more rapid application of new technologies to clinical problems. It is therefore no longer really possible to treat the subject in an encyclopedic fashion and still retain any claim to completeness or absolute authority. With this in mind we have limited ourselves to giving a contemporary overview of current practice, in an account somewhat modified by our own clinical experience. Even by this approach we will inevitably present a number of techniques which may rapidly loose importance in the near future.

II. The Classification of Kidney Stones

As in every other field of clinical practice, the results of surgery can only be assessed if individual cases are properly classified prior to treatment according to clearly defined criteria. Only such data will permit comparisons both between individual groups of cases within a series and between series reported by different authors. Although long accepted as fundamental in the field of oncology, this principle has hitherto found only scant observance in stone surgery. Wide variations, for example, in the entity meant by the term "staghorn calculus" go a long way to explaining how residual stone rates after operation by comparable techniques can be reported as anything from 8% to 41% (MARBERGER and STACKL 1981).

Despite its key significance for the recurrence rate, the mineral composition of a stone is of minor importance for its surgical removal, compared to its size, shape, topography, and to anatomical relationships (BLANDY and MARSHALL 1976; HINMAN and CATTOLICA 1983). Surgical management further depends to

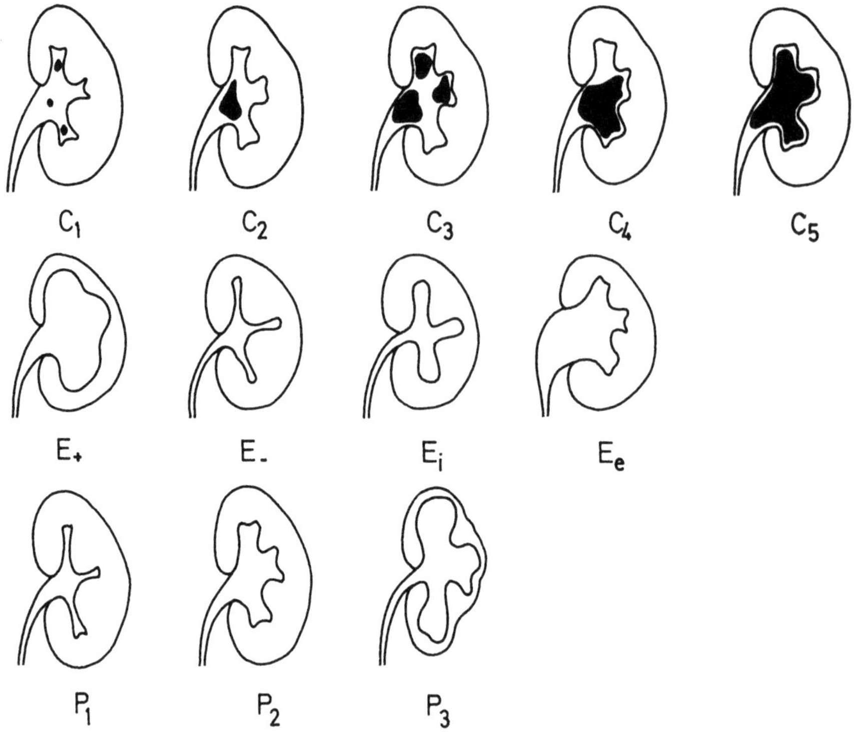

Fig. 1. Classification of kidney stones according to ROCCO: C = extent of calculus, E = lumen of collecting system (+: dilated, −: not dilated; *i:* intrarenal, *e:* extrarenal), P = parenchyma

a great extent on the functional state of the kidney. WICKHAM (1979) has attempted to cover these considerations in the following simple classification:

Grade I: Small immobile calculus in a calyx or a small stone mobile in the pelvis and capable of passing spontaneously.

Grade II: Intrapelvic stone that will not pass.

Grade III: Staghorn calculus filling the entire pelvocalyceal system or multiple calyceal and renal pelvis stones in an otherwise normal kidney.

Grade IV: Similar calculous disease as grade III, combined with atrophic or pyelonephritic destruction of wide areas of the renal parenchyma.

Despite its clinical usefulness this classification is too vague for comparing the results of different authors. More precise systems, both restricted to staghorn calculi have been proposed by MOORES and O'BOYLE (1976) and by FAURE and SARRAMON (1982). The classification of ROCCO (1983) is modelled on the UICC TNM system and seems adequate for all purposes. Depending on the history, on the IVU findings and on quantitative isotope renography the stone is assigned to a category "C", the collecting system to a category "E" and the parenchyma to a category "P" (Fig. 1). Recurrent stones receive the additional suffix "R (1, 2, 3...)" and solitary kidneys the suffix "Pu". The system has been officially accepted and recommended by the European Society for Intrarenal Surgery since 1983.

III. The Indication for Surgery

The spontaneous dissolution of renal calculi has only been observed in exceptional circumstances, e.g. immobilization stones in children (ELLIOT 1954; PYRAH 1979). Whilst uric acid stones are easily dissolved by oral alkalinisation, oral dissolution of cystine stones fails rather more frequently (see chapter on "Drug Therapy of Urinary Calculi and Prevention of Recurrence") and struvite calculi will only ever disappear if urinary tract infection and bacterial urease activity are eliminated (GRIFFITH 1978). Any other type of renal stone disease can only be cured by spontaneous passage, percutaneous dissolution or operative removal. Spontaneous passage depends on the relation of the stone size to the narrowest diameter of the urinary tract. According to UENO et al. (1977) stones with a length of over 12 mm or over 9 mm in diameter have little prospect of passing spontaneously; with a iatrogenic ureteric stricture or a congenital anomaly, such as an abnormal uretero-pelvic junction even smaller stones will be retained. Smooth rounded calculi pass more easily than sharp irregular ones, which cause promote reaction (BOYARSKI and LABAY 1979). In a series of 1948 clinical stone episodes in 538 patients WILLIAMS (1963) recorded a need for operative intervention in 28%, a figure similar to that of 32.9% given by SCHNEIDER and HIENSCH (1975) for their patients.

In principle therefore surgery is indicated for every symptomatic stone that will not pass. Naturally the age and fitness for surgery of the patient must be taken into account, but the low morbidity of percutaneous operative techniques, some of which can be carried out under local anesthesia, nowadays permits a liberal view to be taken even in high-risk patients.

Problems arise more easily over asymptomatic stones, particularly where their removal implies intricate surgery. Even staghorn calculi may remain clinically silent for long periods of time and only come to light in the course of investigations for loin pain or urinary tract infection. However stable the clinical picture may remain for years at a time such a stone nevertheless spells doom for the kidney (Fig. 2). BLANDY et al. (1976) have traced the fate over a period of up to twenty years of 40 patients in whom surgery was not chosen as the first line of treatment. Sixteen patients lost the kidney, usually as an emergency procedure for pyonephrosis, and 11 patients ultimately died as a result of their renal calculi. The experience of KUESS et al. (1979), BENNET and HARRISON (1972), WOJEWSKI and ZAJACZKOVSKI (1973), METZNER and BOYCE (1974), ROUS and TURNER (1977), CONSTANTINOPLE et al. (1979) and of VARGAS et al. (1982) has been uniformly the same. Despite a high recurrence rate the results of surgery are significantly better (BOYCE and ELKINS 1974; WICKHAM et al. 1975; BLANDY et al. 1976; GIL-VERNET and CARRALPS 1979; MARBERGER 1979), so that one should nowadays on principle remove "asymptomatic" staghorn calculi. Simpler pelviceal stones have a high tendency to obstruct and therefore rarely remain asymptomatic over a longer period indicating early surgery. Calyceal stones may, however, remain unchanged and asymptomatic for years (Fig. 3). Surgery is only indicated for such stones if they start to grow, cause urinary tract infection (CIBERT et al. 1972; REDMAN et al. 1975) or under special

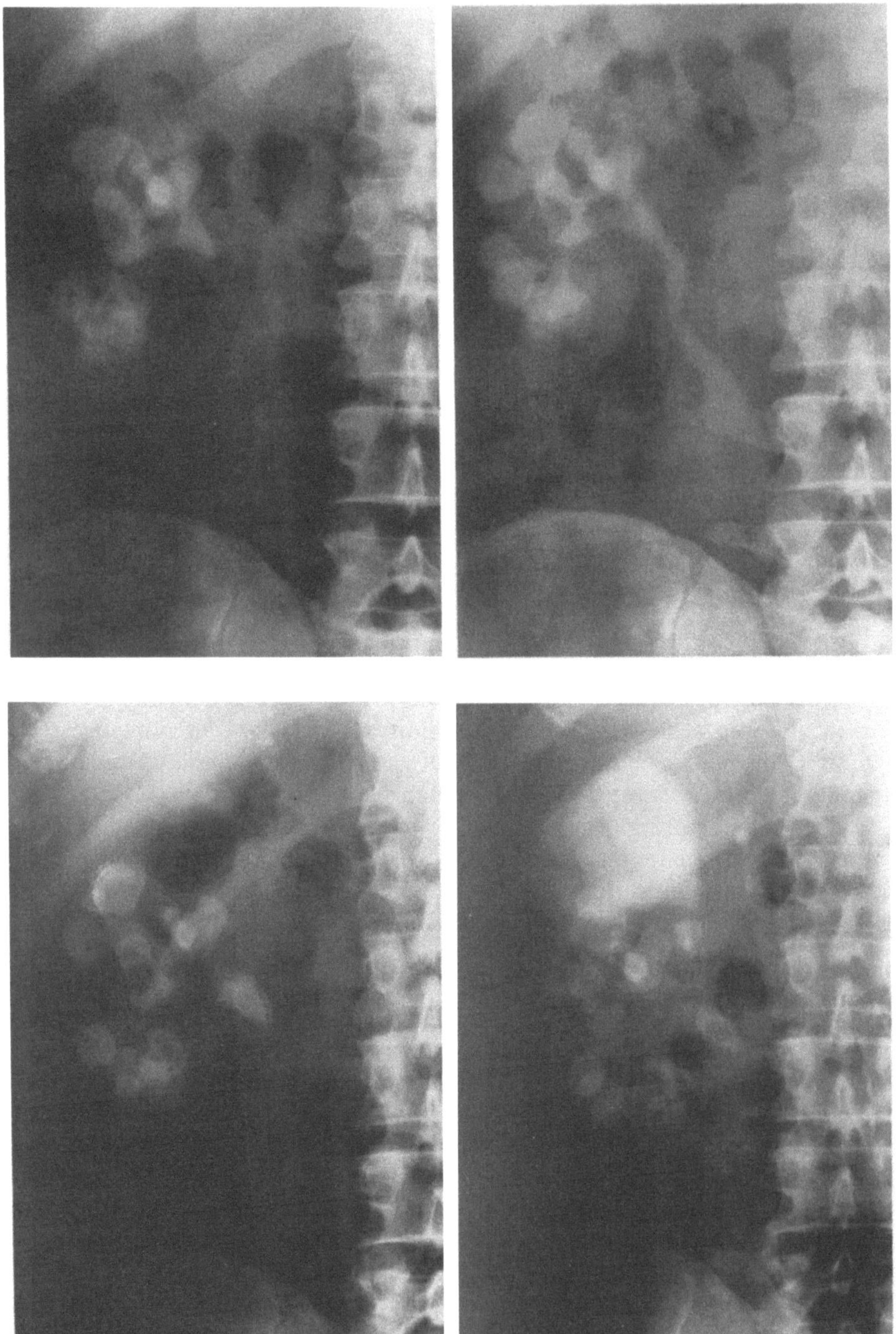

a

b

Fig. 2. **a** Right sided staghorn calculus with minor impairment of renal function. **b** Ten years later: the size of the stone has hardly altered and the patient has not experienced major symptoms, but the function of the kidney has deteriorated markedly

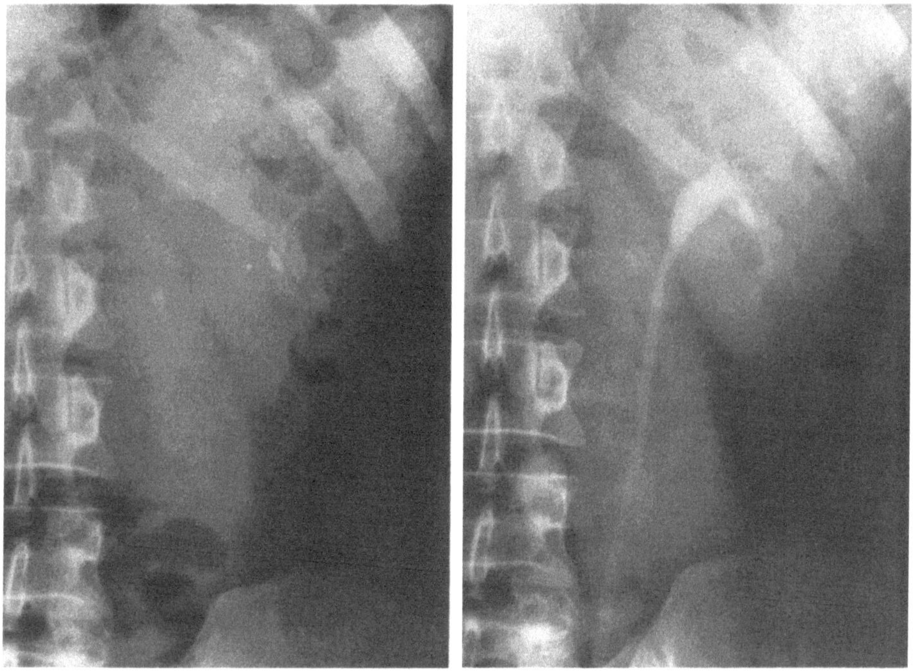

a

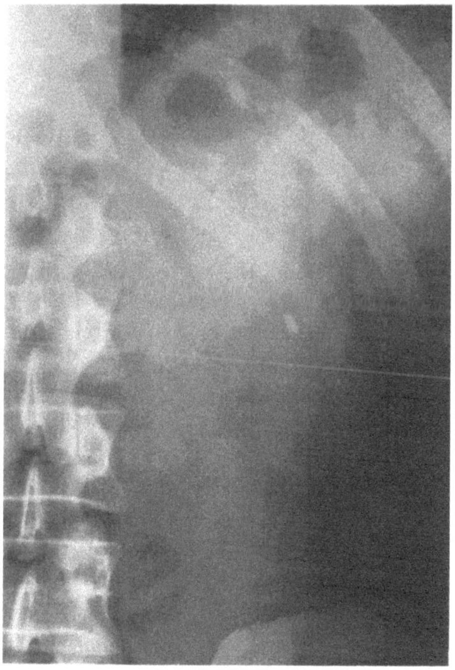

b

Fig. 3. **a** Asymptomatic non obstructing calyceal stone. **b** Unchanged plain film fifteen years later

circumstances, e.g. in airline pilots, whose fitness to fly depends on their freedom from stones.

The urgency to intervene surgically depends on the symptoms, on the size and position of the stone, on the degree of obstruction and on the presence or absence of urinary tract infection.

Anuria demands immediate restoration of urinary flow, since morbidity and mortality both rise in direct relation to the level of azotemia (HAMBURGER et al. 1966; DEES 1976; WILSON et al. 1979). Where, on the other hand, a normal contralateral kidney guarantees adequate excretion and where the symptomatology permits there is time enough to plan an elective procedure. Indeed in borderline cases of possible spontaneous passage a trial of conservative treatment may even be appropriate.

The chief factor determining obstructive damage to the kidney is the rise in intraluminal pressure in the system above the point of obstruction, which depends on the extent and duration of obstruction (MICHAELSON 1974), on the capacity and elasticity of the collecting system (WALKER et al. 1980) and on the flowrate within the system (SCHWEIZER 1973; DJURHUUS and STAGE 1976; JOHNSTON 1969). In the presence of complete obstruction renal pelvis pressure may rise from 6–25 mm Hg to 60 mm Hg, especially where the pelvis is small and intrarenal (MICHAELSON 1974; GILLENWATER 1979). The consequences for renal function have been thoroughly investigated in animal models: Depending on the pressure rise and the duration of obstruction, glomerular filtration rate, urine production, urinary concentrating capacity, T_m PAH, T_m glucose, potassium excretion and sodium reabsorption all fall within hours, with an initial transient rise in renal blood flow (WOODY et al. 1977; GILLENWATER 1979; WALKER et al. 1981). The pathophysiologic process appears similar to that of ischemic damage (ENGBERG et al. 1983). With the subsequent fall in renal blood flow, secondary tissue damage results from malperfusion, whilst pressure within the pelvis and proximal tubuli gradually normalizes. In the dog tubular function falls to 70% of baseline at 24 hours, 50% at 72 hours, 30% at 6 days and 20% at 14 days. The glomerular filtration rate falls in a similar fashion (VAUGHAN and GILLENWATER 1971; WALKER et al. 1980). The reversibility of parenchymal damage depends chiefly on the duration of complete obstruction: after up to seven days of total obstruction the dog kidney is capable of complete recovery. After longer periods some loss of function is inevitable, although even after 28 days of obstruction progressive partial functional recovery can be observed over a period of months (KERR 1954; VAUGHAN and GILLENWATER 1971; WILSON 1977).

These laboratory findings have only limited applicability to the clinical situation, where complete obstruction is the exception. The work of HOLM-NIELSEN et al. (1981), however, suggests a sensitivity of the human kidney broadly similar to that of the dog. 72 patients with obstructed kidneys and reduced renal function recovered completely if the obstruction was relieved within 2 weeks, whereas after 2–4 weeks 3 out of 17 kidneys were permanently damaged, a quota rising to 11 out of 33 after obstruction for over 4 weeks. As long as there is no infection therefore and if there appears any prospect of spontaneous passage, even cases of severe obstruction may safely be left 2–3 weeks without risk of permanent damage. The collecting system compensates pressure rises better if the pelvis is extrarenal or the obstruction lower down the tract, so that a conservative treatment attempt may be carried out even longer (STECKER 1978). Where there is little prospect of the stone passing on its own, delay is pointless.

The danger to the kidney from obstruction rises dramatically in the presence of infection (HOLM-NIELSEN et al. 1981). Bacteria proliferate explosively within the obstructed system, especially following iatrogenic infection by ureteric instrumentation, and may within hours produce multifocal suppurative pyelonephritis, Gram-negative septicemia (DAVIDSON and TALNER 1973; CARL and SCHMIEDT 1974; HASCHEK et al. 1974) and severe parenchymal destruction (DAVIDSON and TALNER 1978). Symptoms of an infected obstructed kidney, such as fever and rigors, therefore demand urgent action to relieve obstruction. Cardiovascular shock symptoms or a fall in platelet count are cardinal signs of Gram-negative endotoxic shock and indicate a condition with a mortality of up to 50–70%, despite appropriate therapy (BLANDY et al. 1976; SKOLUDA et al. 1977; KOFLER et al. 1977; YOUNG 1979). Antibiotics alone will not control the situation, even where the causative organism and its sensitivity are already known (SEIDENFELD and LUBY 1982), unless adequate urine drainage is provided (CORRIERE and SANDLER 1982). This must therefore be achieved within hours as an emergency procedure (FINGERHUT et al. 1982).

Where the stone promises no technical difficulties the treatment of choice is immediate operative removal of the stone. In more problematic cases, such as recurrent stones in a patient in poor general condition, a percutaneous nephrostomy may tide over a critical phase, allowing the patient to recover and the stone to be removed on another occasion under more favorable conditions (BARBARIC et al. 1976). Such a course of action is, however, conditional on early primary intervention before abscesses have formed within the parenchyma: focal infiltration and necrosis appear on ultrasound as sonographically poorly defined, relatively sonolucent areas and on CT as poorly defined wedge-shaped areas of reduced contrast enhancement (CORRIERE and SANDLER 1982; Fig. 4). Decompression of the upper tract by a ureteric catheter is usually inadequate, because the long thin catheter drains purulent urine poorly (CARL and SCHMIEDT 1974). Surgical intervention, however, is urgent, even if pyelonephritis runs a less dramatic course. An infected and obstructed kidney may still be extensively damaged in the absence of severe symptoms. Systemic toxic manifestations such as loss of appetite, weight loss, anemia and a deteriorating general condition eventually make the diagnosis of pyonephrosis inescapable (BLANDY et al. 1976; RATHERT et al. 1977). Finally, about 60% of all perinephric abscesses ensue from infected renal or ureteric calculi either by direct extension of parenchymal infection or from the extravasation of infected urine after spontaneous perforation of the collecting system (TRUESDALE et al. 1977). Since in this situation the extent of inflammatory changes rarely permits precise anatomical dissection, the stones are best left in situ for a second operation once the abscess has been drained and eradicated.

The overall therapeutic aim of renal stone surgery must be the complete removal of all calculi and the restoration of normal urinary drainage with a minimum loss of renal function. Multiple stones may require multiple operations.

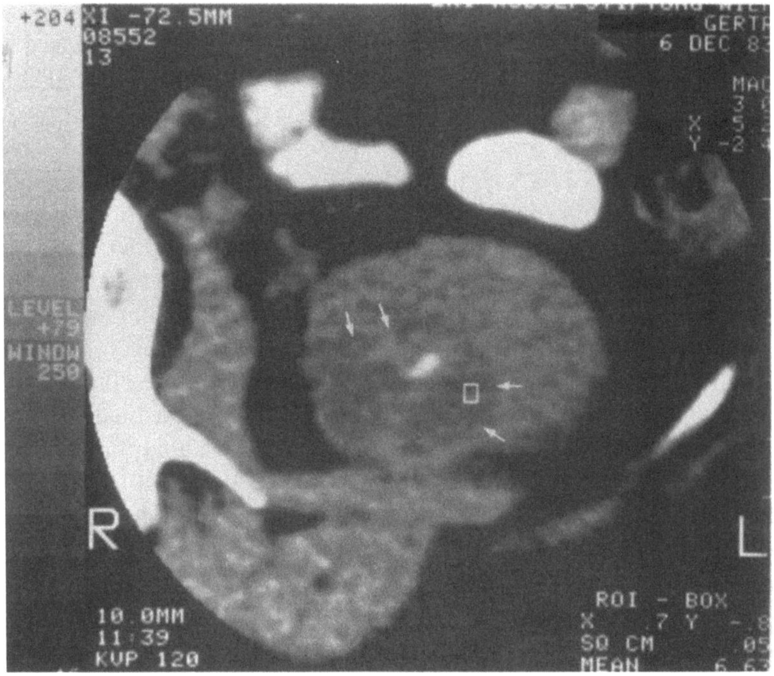

Fig. 4. Focal suppurative infiltration in stone bearing kidney: The CT scan shows a poorly delineated wedge shaped area of reduced enhancement (*arrows*)

Surgical management should therefore not center on a rigid set of rules but rather be adapted to suit the individual situation, taking into account the anatomical conditions, the size and distribution of the stones and the clinical circumstances.

Technically easy, bilateral pelviceal or high ureteric calculi in a fit patient may be removed in one session (STREENEVASAN 1974). Because it involves less muscle trauma a bilateral modified posterior lumbotomy is to be preferred in this situation, with the patient in a prone position (WARD 1976). A median upper transverse abdominal (chevron) incision permits the removal of more complicated bilateral calculi in a single operation without turning the patient. In the experience of DEMLER et al. (1973) the morbidity of this procedure is no greater than that of extensive unilateral operations. A bilateral flank incision is however less advisable because of the need to reposition the patient during the procedure and because of the effects on respiration of pain and postural factors (SCHRAMM 1980). In patients operated by this approach regional anesthesia of the 11th and 12th intercostal nerves is absolutely indispensible (CRAWFORD et al. 1978). Generally, however, a second procedure after 8–14 days is preferable (RESNICK and BOYCE 1980). Either the more symptomatic side or the kidney more severely threatened by partial or complete obstruction should then take precedence. Where there is a marked difference in technical difficulty, e.g. a difficult recurrent stone on one side and a simple pelviceal stone on the other, removing the simple stone first will allow the more demanding procedure to be undertaken in the safe knowledge of a well functioning contralateral kidney. Where preserving a kidney is of doubtful merit, the opposite side should, by the same token, be operated first, since nephrectomy may appear a less grave step if this first procedure has proceeded without mishap (MICHALOWSKI et al. 1970).

Multiple unilateral stones at various levels should whenever possible all be removed at once, since leaving a distal obstruction behind will promote extravasation from the more proximal incision in the collecting system. If a supravesical ureteric calculus inaccessible from above but amenable to a transurethral approach is only noticed during nephrolithotomy, a fine gauge nephrostomy (GIL-VERNET 1977) or pyelostomy tube should be left in situ until the distal stone has been removed. Where the diagnosis was made preoperatively the distal stone should be removed first, prior to open surgery. Conversely residual obstruction proximal to an incision into the urinary tract promotes postoperative stenosis due to the reduced urinary flow. Emergency nephrostomies should for the same reason be removed as early as possible after definitive removal of the distal obstruction.

For stones in solitary kidneys the indications for surgical interventions are only altered to the extent that any risk of damage by obstruction or infection renders surgical remedy even more urgent. STACKL et al. (1983) were unable to confirm experimentally the clinical impression of others (GOLDSTEIN and GOLDSTEIN 1968; JAMES et al. 1980) that solitary kidneys are more resistant to extraneous damage, but the low complication rate of modern surgical techniques does not justify a more conservative approach (BISCHOFF 1969; REDMAN and BISSADA 1976; BOYCE et al. 1978; PERRY et al. 1980). Even advanced renal failure should not preclude surgical intervention. Relieving obstruction and controlling infection frequently stabilizes renal function, so that chronic dialysis can be avoided (PROCA 1970; WITHEROW and WICKHAM 1980; MEBEL et al. 1982; Fig. 5). Removing obstructing stones may even be indicated in dialysis patients to preserve residual renal function and reduce the risk of pyonephrosis, thus significantly improving quality of life.

IV. Preoperative Investigations and Patient Preparation

The diagnosis of renal calculous disease is dealt with in detail in the chapter by VAHLENSIECK (1985). Once the decision has been taken to operate, the surgeon must obtain unequivocal preoperative information on position, number and shape of the calculi, on the anatomical configuration and function of the affected kidney and on complicating factors such as urinary tract infection. This data is essential for planning the operation and frequently exceeds the information required in merely developing the indications for surgery per se. The clinical situation of urolithiasis is prone to sudden dramatic change, e.g. a change in the position of an apparently immobile stone,

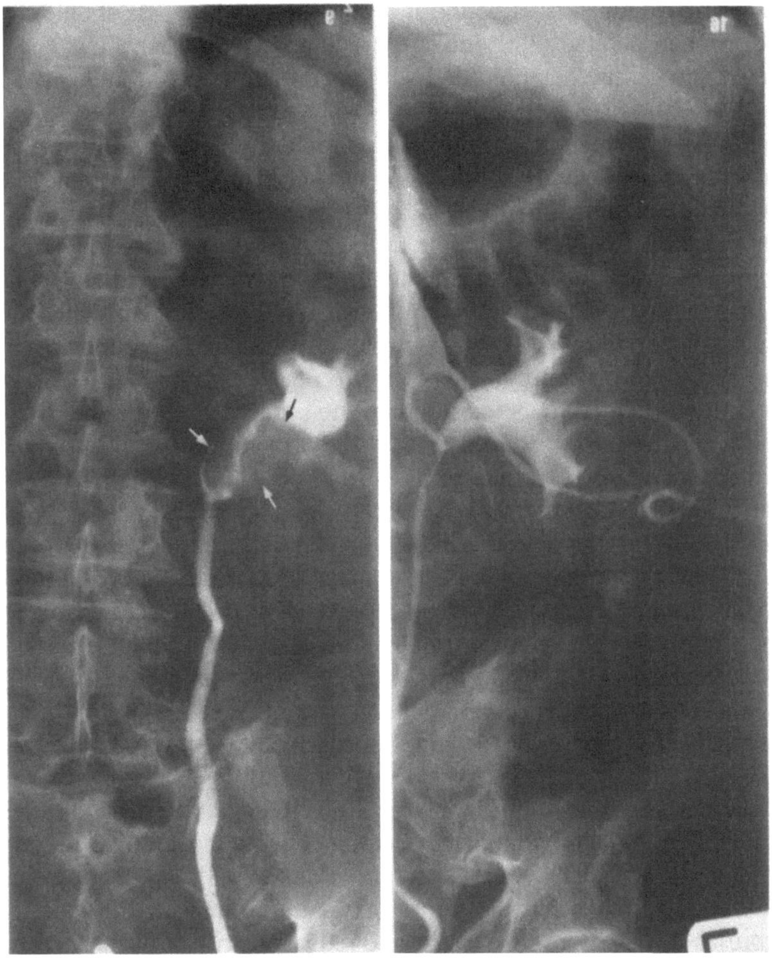

a b

Fig. 5. **a** Retrograde pyelogram: the solitary left kidney of a 61-years old male contains an obstructing, poorly opaque pelviceal stone (*arrows*); serum creatinine 18 mg%. **b** Antegrade examination: there is free drainage following surgical removal with perioperative hemodialysis; serum creatinine 6,5 mg%, no further dialysis required

and the appropriate preoperative investigations are therefore at the exclusive responsibility of the surgeon. In this context the unaffected contralateral kidney merits special attention.

A recent intravenous urogramme, and a plain control film performed immediately preoperatively represent the core investigations, capable, if correctly performed, of supplying all the necessary information including a rough estimate of renal function in the vast majority of cases (MARBERGER 1983). It is of the very greatest importance to confirm unequivocally that the shadow considered to be a calculus lies within the lumen of the urinary tract. This can frequently only be documented by multiple views in different radiologic planes, by a constant relationship of the shadow to the renal parenchyma and lumen or indirectly by defining the level of urinary obstruction. Obstruction distal to the calculus, e.g. by another ureteric calculi, must be excluded. Where an increased volume of contrast dye, delayed oblique, and post-micturition films fail to demonstrate this, retrograde pyelography is still required.

For complicated calculi full three-dimensional localization within the kidney is desirable, especially where parenchyma may have to be incised. Computerized tomography (CT) without and with contrast enhancement is ideal as it provides accurate simultaneous delineation of the stone, parenchyma and collecting system (WICKHAM et al. 1978; FEDERLE et al. 1981). In this way information becomes available preoperatively e.g. on whether the stone lies in an anterior or posterior group of calyces or whether the overlying parenchyma is thinned (Fig. 6). Attenuation measurements allow the clear identification of calculi as such even when their coefficients of linear X-ray absorption are only slightly above that of water, and they are therefore invisible on plain films (SEGAL et al. 1978; ALTER et al. 1979; GREENBERG et al. 1982; Fig. 7). Depending on the inherent contrast of the stone, the limit of resolution is reached at 1 – 3 mm diameter. By examining the pixel pattern and the absolute CT values measured at 77 and 125 kVp (E) even the chemical composition of calculi may be predicted radiologically with an accuracy of at least 70% (MITCHESON et al. 1983). The rather rare poorly opaque uric acid and cystine stones may thus be distinguished from struvite calculi and treated conservatively by dissolution therapy. Finally, dynamic sequential CT permits semiquantitative evaluation of renal function from the time-dye density curves registered over the renal parenchyma during contrast enhancement. This even provides values for specific regions of interest (WALZ et al. 1981; YOUNG et al. 1981; WALZ et al. 1982; YOKOYAMA et al. 1982).

Where CT is unavailable calyceal calculi up to a diameter of approx. 0.5 cm may nevertheless still be accurately located by ultrasound, especially where there is calyceal dilatation (EDEL 1978; WALZ, HUTSCHENREITER and HOHENFELLNER 1980). Alternatively, plain tomography may be employed with a slice thickness of 0.5 cm. As an aid to the surgeon's spatial orientation the planes at which the various parts of the calculi are best seen (i.e. the distances of the relevant planes from the plane of the film) may be marked on a plain film. The model becomes even more clear if anterior, median and posterior portions of the stone are drawn in different colors on transparent film (GREGOIR 1975). Stereoscopic imaging reduces the radiation dose but requires stereoscopic viewing equipment (GEORGI and MARBERGER 1976). The introduction of intraoperative Doppler sonography (RIEDMILLER et al. 1981, 1983; BOYCE 1982; THUEROFF et al. 1982) has definitively rendered renal angiography obsolete in assessing renal vascular anatomy for anatrophic nephrotomy (DRACH 1975). Although the deleterious effects of an intraarterial bolus contrast medium on borderline renal function can be largely overcome by using non-ionised contrast agents and by adequate hydration (EISENBERG et al. 1981) the procedure remains elaborate and invasive out of all proportion to the possible benefits for surgery.

The assessment of renal function mainly influences surgical management as to the question whether relieving obstruction is likely to improve function and

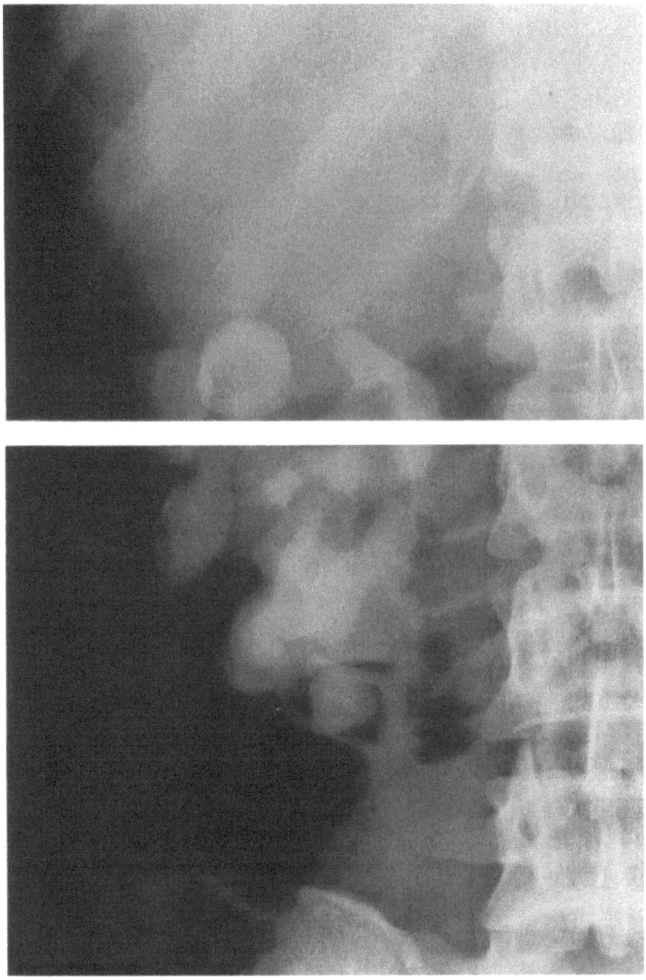

a

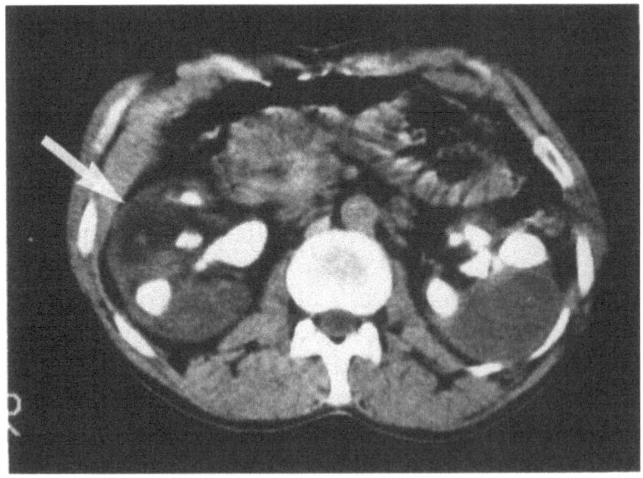

b

thus render a stone-bearing kidney of border-line function worth saving. Split clearance studies under steady state conditions with ureteric catheterization are accurate, but invasive and nowadays clinically obsolete. Where complete ureteric obstruction has been relieved by temporary percutaneous nephrostomy unilateral clearance of endogenous creatinine may conveniently be estimated using the nephrostomy urine. An accurate assessment of glomerular filtration of the stone-bearing kidney is then available. Otherwise, if dynamic CT is not available, resort must be taken to split radioisotope function studies.

^{131}I-Hippuran renography is the technique most commonly used. Using an array of collimators, or more accurately, the gamma camera a scintigram is recorded from each kidney. After subtraction of extrarenal activity as estimated from a whole body uptake curve (Oberhausen 1971) or by means of a second radionuclide that remains in the circulation (Britton and Braun 1968), the percentage contribution of each kidney to the total clearance may be calculated. In acute obstruction this technique tends to overestimate function (Doppelfeld and Weissbach 1979), but with chronic obstruction there is excellent correlation of the values obtained before and after decompressing the kidney by percutaneous nephrostomy (Alken et al. 1977). The technique is ideal for establishing a preoperative baseline and for subsequent followup after stone surgery (May 1974; Heidenreich et al. 1976; Schlegel 1977; Marberger and Eisenberger 1980), but only allows statements to be made about function at the time of examination and not the possible functional reserve (Ofstad et al. 1973; Mogensen et al. 1976; Heinze et al. 1977; Bueschen et al. 1978; Walker et al. 1982). The use of ^{123}I-iodohippuran reduces radiation and permits the investigation to be combined with sequential dynamic scintigraphy and – where the computing capacity is available – with compartmental analysis of the renogram (Buttermann et al. 1979).

The higher count yield emitted by the radionuclide ^{99m}Tc-DTPA (diethylene triamine pentaacetic acid) permits early phase pictures to be taken on a seconds time scale, giving improved morphological evaluation of the blood supply (Georgi 1982). Deconvolution analysis permits calculation of radionuclide renal transit time and separate imaging of renal parenchyma and renal pelvis differentiates between parenchymal lesions and obstruction (Diffay et al. 1976; Buck et al. 1980; Whitfield et al. 1981). 50% of an injected dose of ^{99m}Tc-DMSA (Technetium dimercaptosuccinic acid) becomes fixed to the tubules within one hour, its distribution being proportional to the differential renal blood flow (Daly et al. 1979). The substance is extensively bound to plasma proteins and shows minimal early excretion. Thus the renal pelvis urine is virtually devoid of activity, even with complete obstruction. The technique permits good assessment of the residual functional parenchyma in obstructed kidneys by simple static scintigraphy (Parker et al. 1981; Kawamura et al. 1983).

Fig. 6. **a** Right sided staghorn stone. **b** CT scan in the plane marked by white line on the plane film (a) showing stones in the renal pelvis and in an anterior, medial and posterior calix; note the thinned out parenchyma (*arrow*)

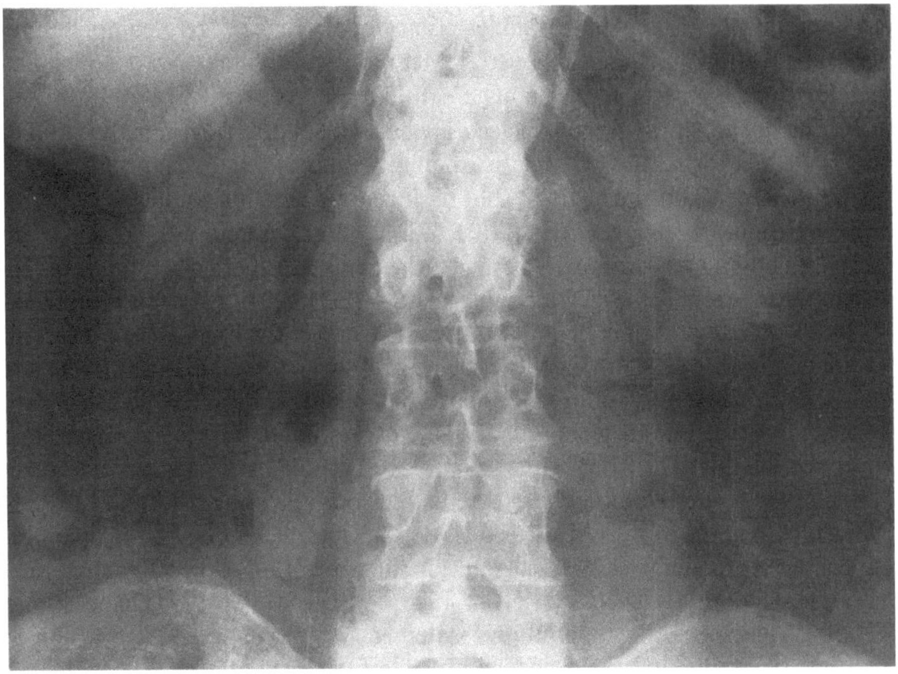

a

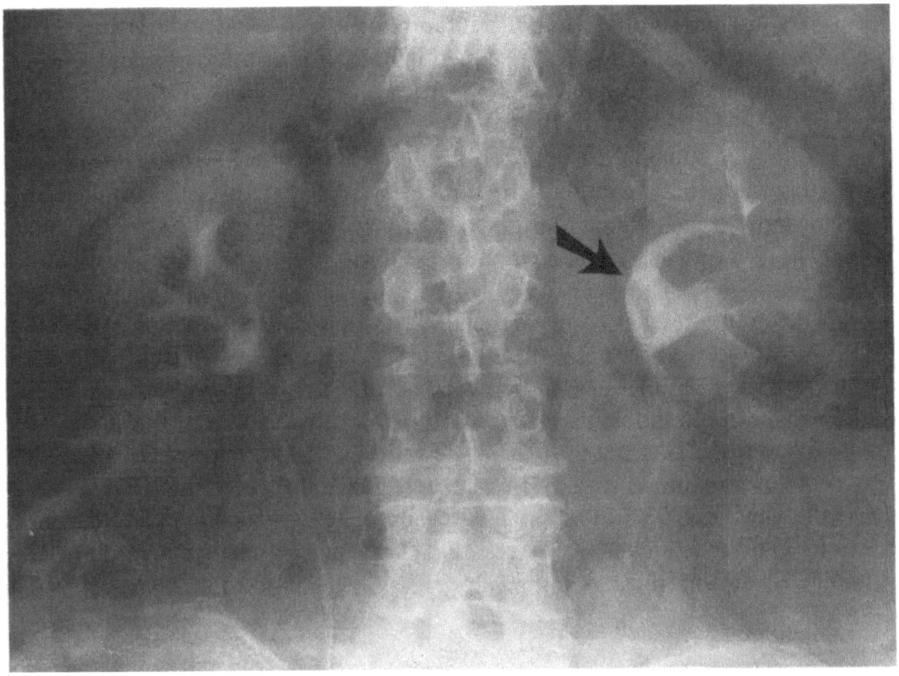

b

Fig. 7. Non-opaque renal pelvis stone in the left kidney. **a** Plain film, **b** IVP with filling defect in the renal pelvis (*arrow*). **c** Sonogram with for stone (+ . . . +) typical sound-shadow, **d** CT scan showing unmistakably the stone in the renal pelvis (*arrow*); the renal pelvis is surrounded by fatty tissue

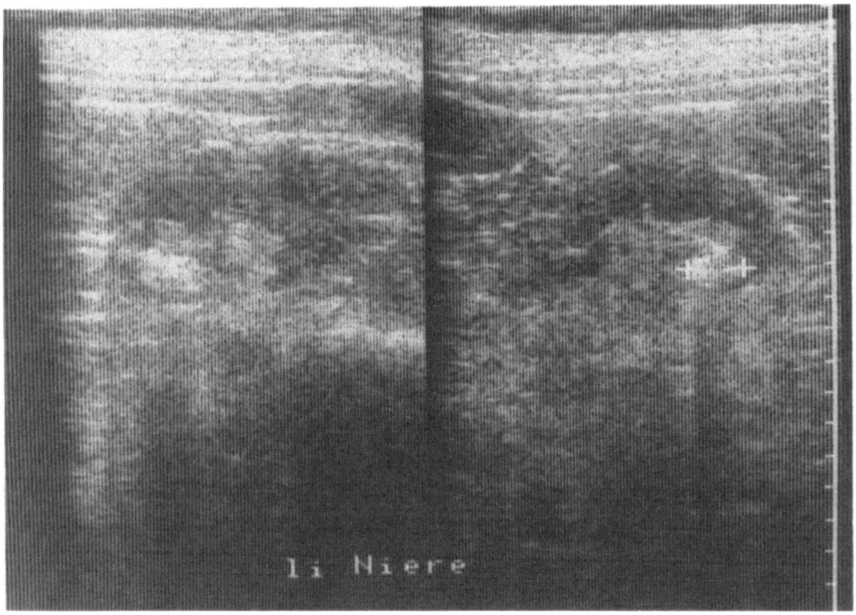
li Niere

c

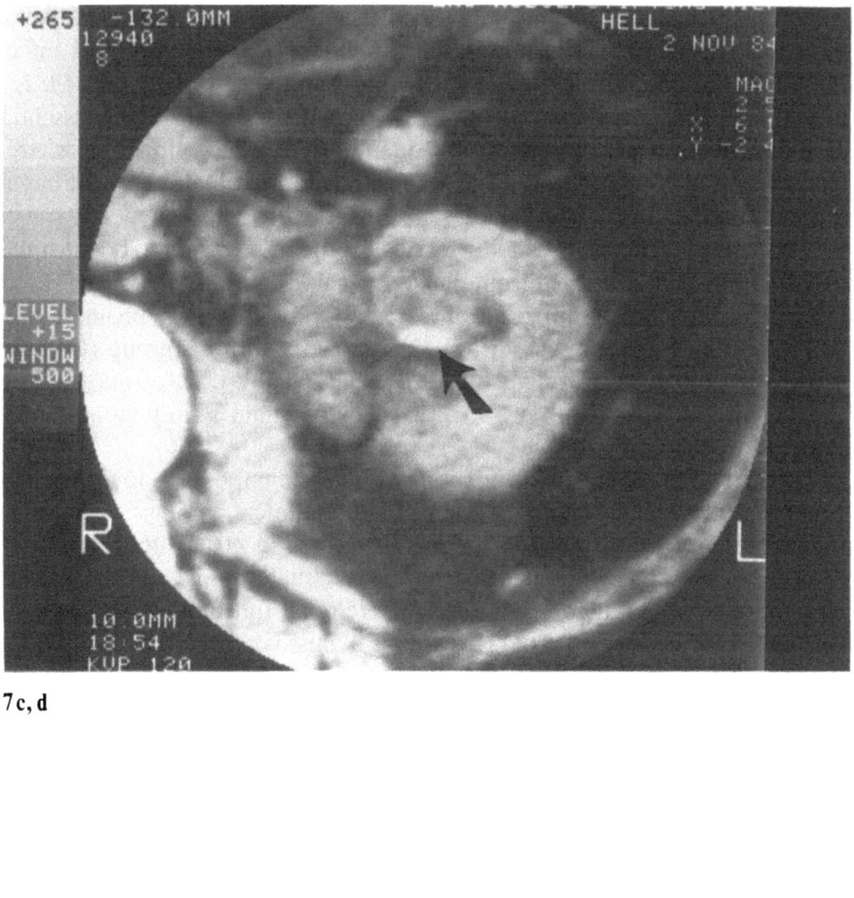
+265
-132.0MM
12940
8
HELL
2 NOV 84
LEVEL
+15
WINDW
500
R
L
10.0MM
18:54
KVP 120

d

Fig. 7 c, d

Whether or not a kidney is worth preserving cannot be decided on a strict percentage figure of the residual function (MERIDIES 1973; EISEN et al. 1974; MAY 1974; PARKER et al. 1981; KAWAMURA et al. 1983), since a variety of other factors such as the state of the opposite kidney, age and general condition of the patient, technical difficulty and probable outcome of an organ-saving procedure also have to be considered (WALKER et al. 1981; JEFFS 1981). As 28% of all patients with unilateral stone disease will experience a stone episode on the opposite side at some time during their remaining lifetime (WILLIAMS 1963), and since a residue of only 15–20% of the normal parenchymal still provides renal function essentially still superior to dialysis (SIGEL 1965; SEMB 1968; BISCHOFF 1969), the decision must favor organ preservation whereever possible. Under no circumstances should nephrectomy be justified solely by the presence of a technically difficult recurrent stone. The younger the patient the more frugally nephrectomy should be resorted to, even where organ preservation carries a high risk of recurrence. For patients over 70 years of age with a staghorn and a normal opposite kidney, on the other hand, nephrectomy may be more reasonable, as it solves the problem for years at a low complication rate. The principle indication for nephrectomy in the management of urolithiasis remains pyonephrosis, i.e. an organ completely destroyed by suppurating infection (BLANDY et al. 1976; RATHERT et al. 1977).

Urinary tract infection remains among the gravest complications of nephrolithiasis (see page 91) and carries a significantly increased postoperative complication rate in terms of suppurating pyelonephritis and perirenal infection (CORRIERE and SANDLER 1982), septicemia (SEIDENFELD and LUBY 1982) and wound infection (ALLO and SIMONS 1983). It is therefore absolutely essential to exclude infection preoperatively by quantitative urine culture or where infection is already present, to institute specific antimicrobial treatment based on the sensitivity pattern of the causative organism.

As in other urological pathology, E. coli is the most common organism identified in cases of rather uncomplicated renal calculi. Proteus and Pseudomonas predominate with recurrent stones and after instrumentation, and E. coli accounts for only one third of the infections in this group (COX 1974). Four fifths of all staghorn calculi are infected at the time of diagnosis: COX (1974) cultured E. coli in only 13%, whereas 23% had Pseudomonas and 43% Proteus.

With an urgent indication for surgery it may be impossible to await the outcome of culture and sensitivity testing. If the clinical findings and urinalysis suggest urinary tract infection, parenteral broad spectrum antibiotic therapy should be instituted without delay and at adequate dosage, as soon as specimens have been obtained for culture. Where renal function is impaired or surgery involving temporary renal ischemia is planned, nephrotoxic substances are to be avoided (BOYCE 1975; MARBERGER 1978). The cephalosporins, carbenicillin, aminopenicillins or acylaminopenicillins are therefore the agents of choice, whereas the aminoglycosides, polymixins and tetracylines are less suitable. An emergency operation is scarcely ever required for a complicated staghorn, the most common infected calculus. 2–3 days are therefore usually available for specific treatment of the infection with antibiotics according to the sensitivity pattern of the individual organism, parenterally and in high dose. Where renal function is impaired the dose has to be modified according to the GFR; serum antibiotic levels may need to be determined regularly. Rarely is it possible to sterilise the urinary tract in this way, but the bacteria count may be significantly reduced. In obstructed kidneys the effectiveness of the antimicrobial therapy is increased by temporary diversion via a percutaneous nephrostomy (MARBERGER 1979) or by a ureteric catheter (BOYCE 1975). Unlike colonic surgery, however, there is no justification for giving prophylactic preoperative antibiotics routinely in the absence of infection (ALLO and SIMONS 1983).

The kidney is more resistant to exogenous injury, e.g. temporary ischemia or incision of the parenchyma under conditions of forced diuresis and salt loading (SCHILLING et al. 1980; HULAND 1983; OOSTERLINCK and DESY 1983). In patients with a normal renal function therefore the preoperative period of no oral fluid intake should be covered by intravenous infusion of 1000 ml saline. With impaired renal function and a salt loosing diathesis it may occasionally also be necessary to ensure adequate hydration with saline (TASKER et al. 1974), but because of these patients' latent tendency to pulmonary edema this should not be a routine measure.

Reduced renal function is not a contraindication to surgical intervention (WITHEROW et al. 1980; MEBEL et al. 1982), but the patient requires careful pretreatment with the aim of achieving the best possible preoperative homeostasis. An exact estimate of the residual function, best evaluated by endogenous creatinine clearance is the first step (WILSON et al. 1979). Hypertension must be treated and water and electrolyte unbalances carefully corrected. Patients whose creatinine clearance lies below 15 ml/min may require measurement of central venous or pulmonary artery pressure before this can safely be achieved (KASIKE and KJELLSTRAND 1983). Because of the risk of cardiac arrest during induction of anesthesia, hyperkalemia must be regarded as the most dangerous electrolyte abnormality. It requires preoperative treatment by ion exchange resins or, if necessary, by hemo- or peritoneal dialysis. Metabolic acidosis, which potentiates the cardiac effects of hyperkalemia, does not require full correction, but the serum bicarbonate levels should be maintained above 20 meq/l. If the risk of volume overload prevents this from being achieved by the administration of sodium bicarbonate, the patient may still require dialysis (KASIKE and KJELLSTRAND 1983). Patients with renal insufficiency are usually well adapted to their anemia, but packed red cells should be transfused immediately preoperatively to raise the hematocrit above 25% (CZER and SHOEMAKER 1978). Despite a normal prothrombin time, partial thromboplastin time and platelet count, patients with advanced renal failure often have a prolonged bleeding time. Although the cause of this phenomenon is obscure, the prolongation of bleeding time correlates well with the blood urea nitrogen level. Preoperative hemodialysis has therefore been recommended for cases with a BUN above 100 mg%, although this maneuver does not always correct the clotting defect (KASIKE and KJELLSTRAND 1983). Clotting must then be corrected immediately preoperatively by giving Standard Red Cross Cryoprecipitate (JANSON et al. 1980).

Once normal electrolyte levels and circulating volume have been restored it is advisable to administer mannitol and/or frusemide prophylactically prior to surgery to maintain diuresis (DAWSON et al. 1965; NUUTINEN et al. 1978; MARBERGER 1979; OOSTERLINCK and DESY 1983). Giving mannitol, however, presupposes that diuresis has not already ceased, since oliguria rapidly results in mannitol toxicity (BORGES et al. 1982). Unless dialysis was required preoperatively it is exceptionally rare for hemodialysis to be required after technically satisfactory surgery (WITHEROW et al. 1980; MEBEL et al. 1982). It is therefore not advisable to prepare for this rather rare complication with a prophylactic arteriovenous shunt: unused shunts frequently obliterate, destroying valuable vessels that might be required for shunts in the future. For emergencies a central venous catheter will suffice until a suitable shunt can be established.

The anesthesia of patients with renal failure is beyond the scope of this article, yet express attention should be drawn to the hazards of methoxyflurane, ether, cyclopropane and muscle relaxants, as well as to the importance of careful volume replacement throughout the procedure and of proper postoperative analgesia (SIROTZKY and LEWIS 1978; WITHEROW et al. 1982; KASIKE and KJELLSTRAND 1983).

Properly prepared, patients on longterm hemodialysis survive routine surgical procedures with a mortality only slightly above that of normal patients (GIACCHINO et al. 1981; WIEHLE et al. 1981). The main problem lies in the danger of a peri-operative fluid overload and of hemorrhage from heparinisation during hemodialysis. The operation must therefore be timed to fit between dialysis sessions in an optimal fashion, dialysis being avoided for the first 48 hours postoperatively. Minimal heparinisation during perioperative dialysis is associated with less bleeding complications than regional heparinisation with simultaneous infusion of heparin and protamine (KJELLSTRAND and BUSELMEIER 1972; KASIKE and KJELLSTRAND 1983). Wound healing problems may be significantly reduced by atraumatic technique, intraoperative irrigation of the wound cavity with an antibiotic solution (WIEHLE et al. 1981) and an adequate calory intake by nasogastric tube or intravenously (GIACCHINO et al. 1981).

Transplanted kidneys may form stones, especially if hypercalcemia persists because secondary hyperparathyroidism has resolved incompletely after transplantation (LEAPMAN et al. 1976). Since these are essentially immunosuppressed patients with solitary kidneys, the hazards of obstruction and infection exceed those for normal kidneys (SCHWEIZER et al. 1977). Untreated stones are frequently the eventual cause of death (WALSH 1969; ROSENBERG et al. 1975). Any stone unable to pass spontaneously therefore requires operative removal. The most important preoperative maneuver is reversal of the biochemical cause, which may well involve parathyroidectomy (LEAPMAN et al. 1976). Even if the urine is sterile, prophylactic perioperative antibiotic cover may be important. The exact operative procedure will depend chiefly on whether the implanted organ is a left or a right kidney. If the reanl vessels lie anterior to the renal pelvis primary dissection of the hilar region through the scarred retroperitoneal tissue is so hazardous that a retrograde approach along the ureter is to be preferred (SCHWEIZER et al. 1977).

V. Surgical Access to the Kidney

In any one case the best incision will be an optimal compromise between adequate exposure of the kidney for removal of all known stones and the minimum insult to the soft tissues and perirenal structures. The requirements of stone surgery differ from those of surgery for other indications because of the variability in shape and size of the stones, the possible need of pyeloscopy, intraoperative radiology or sonography for intraoperative stone localization and the high recurrence rate, which frequently necessitates re-operations in the same region. In view of the variability of renal calculous disease one single incision can not satisfy all demands (SIGEL 1963). Although choice of the incision depends to a large part on the training and operative habits of the surgeon he should nevertheless be equally conversant with the dorsal, supracostal and ventral approach to the kidney. A lumbotomy below the twelfth rib is usually too low and therefore unsuited for renal stone surgery. Because calculi are frequently infected the transthoracic approach is also rarely used.

The endoscopic approach to kidney stones via a percutaneous nephrostomy is dealt with in the chapter on "Percutaneous Manipulation of Renal Calculi" (pp. 181).

1. The Modified Posterior Lumbotomy Incision

The hilar region of the kidney, the proximal ureter and the lower pole can be reached through the thoracolumbar fascia lateral to the sacrospinalis and quadratus lumborum muscles without the need to divide muscle. In terms of postoperative pain and morbidity this incision is superior to all others. Renal pelvis and proximal ureter lie in a convenient horizontal plain in the centre of the exposure (SIGEL 1963; LUTZEYER and LYMBEROPOLOUS 1970) and the collecting system can be reached without the need to mobilize the kidney. This modified lumbotomy approach was first described by SIMON (1871) and has been popularized in two versions by LURZ (1956) and by GIL-VERNET (1965).

The patient is placed in the lateral position, healthy side down and with approx. 15° anterior rotation, such that the table breaks at the tip of the twelfth rib (Fig. 8). Simultaneous bilateral surgery may be undertaken with the patient prone (WARD et al. 1976; NOVICK 1980).

According to GIL-VERNET (GIL-VERNET 1965, 1972; WICKHAM 1979) the skin incision is made parallel and 3 cm lateral to the erector spinae and carried from the 12th rib down to the iliac crest (Fig. 9a). Fat and subcutaneous tissue are divided until the lateral fibres of the latissimus dorsi are exposed. The muscle is split parallel to the fibres to expose the subjacent twelfth rib. The posterior leaf of the thoracolumbar fascia is divided in the line of the skin incision and the lateral margin of the sacrospinalis muscle so exposed is retracted medially. The middle layer of the thoracolumbar fascia is then seen and incised somewhat lateral to the fleshy belly of the sacrospinalis muscle. The lateral border of the quadratus lumborum now comes into view and may be retracted with

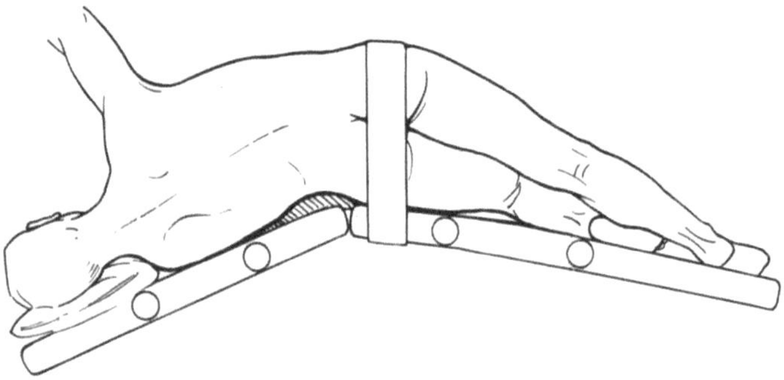

Fig. 8. Positioning the patient for the modified posterior lumbotomy

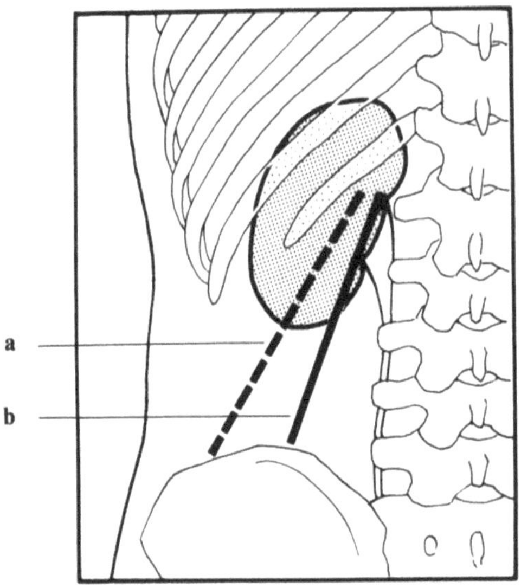

Fig. 9. Incision according to (**a**) GIL-VERNET and (**b**) LURZ

a hook toward the vertebral column. The deep layer of the thoracolumbar fascia is exposed and opened, care being exercised to spare the twelfth subcostal nerve and the iliohypogastric nerve coursing obliquely and laterally on its deep aspect. The perirenal fat is divided by blunt dissection to expose the renal pelvis and the hilum. Exposure may be improved by transecting the costovertebral ligament (BENSIMON 1974) or resecting a segment of the twelfth rib (WICKHAM 1979), which can then be swung upwards. Special selfretaining retractors with deep blades improve exposure considerably (GIL-VERNET 1965, 1972; WICKHAM 1979).

In the LURZ version (LURZ 1956; LURZ and LURZ 1961; LUTZEYER 1975) the incision runs obliquely from a point three fingers breadth lateral to the dorsal spines to the junction of the middle and anterior third of the iliac crest (Fig. 9b). The lower parts of the latissimus dorsi and the serratus posterior inferior and of the costovertebral ligament are divided and the middle and deep leaves of the thoracolumbar fascia split. A Finochietto rib retractor is inserted. The oblique course of the incision provides a wider field and therefore renders a rib resection unnecessary.

The wound drain is brought out through a separate stab incision. The wound is closed in two layers: the deep and the middle leaf of the thoracolumbar fascia as the first and the superfiscial leaf as the second layer. The quadratus lumborum acts as a shutter between the layers of the closure and thus butresses the closure.

The incision has a low morbidity, even for revisions or synchronous bilateral surgery (BRANDSTETTER 1975; WARD et al. 1976; LUTZEYER and LYMBEROPOLOUS 1970; NOVICK 1980). GARDINER et al. (1979) have compared pyelolithotomies performed through modified posterior lumbotomies and through loin incisions. Patients with the former incision were mobilized in an average of 3.3 days and had a mean hospital stay of 9 days, whereas the figures for loin incisions were 4.3 and 11.2 days respectively. The non-muscle-splitting incision also resulted in a significantly reduced analgesic intake, an observation also confirmed by DAS et al. (1983). Careful preservation of the iliohypogastric nerve and proper closure of the fascia effectively prevent incisional hernias and loin bulges.

The disadvantages of the incision are the limits imposed on exposure by the twelfth rib above and the iliac crest below. Operations on the upper pole or on the middle third of the ureter are difficult and complete mobilization of the kidney or dissection of the renal pedicle are virtually impossible without a T-shaped extension of the wound (LYTTON 1979). GIL-VERNET has developed special film holding forceps to permit in-situ renal radiology through this incision (GIL-VERNET and CULLA 1981). Without this instrument accurate intraoperative contact radiology is almost impossible. Although GIL-VERNET, the grand master of the modified posterior lumbotomy, routinely operates on difficult calculi by this approach with excellent results (GIL-VERNET 1972; GIL-VERNET and CARRALPS 1979), the general teaching view is that only immobile stones in the renal pelvis or proximal ureter should be approached in this fashion, which do not require intraoperative radiology (LUTZEYER 1975; LYTTON 1979; WICKHAM 1979).

2. The Supracostal Approach

Compared to the conventional flank approach incisions in the eleventh intercostal space provide excellent access to the kidney with little muscle injury. The oblique and transverse abdominal muscles need only be cut over a distance of a few centimeters and the subcostal and iliohypogastric nerves are easily avoided. Since there is no need for rib resection the wound is easily displayed by a rib retractor: postoperatively the wound is supported by the ribs and herniation is thus exceedingly rare. The length of the incision can be modified to suit the specific surgical problem and a frugal incision for simple pyelolithotomy is easily extended to allow complete mobilization of the kidney. The upper ⅔ of the ureter or the renal pedicle can be reached by extending medially into a transverse upper abdominal or pararectal incision. Lesions in the upper pole or highlying kidneys may be reached by an extrapleural approach through the tenth intercostal space (MARBERGER 1979). Although the supracostal approach was first described over 60 years ago, the rather high incidence of pleura lesions prevented it from becoming popular until the advent of routine endotracheal intubation and positive pressure ventilation (PRESMAN 1955; TURNER-WARWICK 1965; DETTMAR and SCHMITZ 1970; HOHENFELLNER 1977). Because of its universal usefulness it is today the incision of choice for all difficult renal calculi (BARRY and HODGES 1975; BOYCE 1975; WICKHAM 1979; HOHENFELLNER 1980).

The patient is placed in a lateral jack-knife position (Fig. 10). The skin incision runs parallel to the upper margin of the twelfth rib and distally in the line of the rib. Its length depends on the precise nature of the procedure. For simpler operations on the renal pelvis an incision along the distal half of the rib extending 5 cm into the abdominal muscles suffices. For more difficult procedures involving complete mobilization of the kidney and intraoperative radiology the incision should start three fingers' breadth lateral to the dorsal spines and be extended as far anteriorly as needed. After the subcutaneous fat has been divided, the fringes of the transverse abdominal musculature are incised immediately beyond the tip of the twelfth rib with cutting diathermy. The transversus abdominis muscle blends here with the deep leaf of the thoracolumbar fascia, which should be divided along the same line (Fig. 11). The second and third finger of each hand are now used to sweep the peritoneum off the underside of the abdominal wall muscles, prior to extending the muscle incision medially with cutting diathermy as required. The incision should be kept strictly in line with the extension of the twelfth rib, so as to keep well clear of subcostal vessels and nerves. Once the incision has been carried as far medially as needed, dissection can proceed in the opposite direction along the twelfth rib. The latissimus dorsi and intercostal muscles are divided by diathermy from before backwards along the upper margin of the rib. As the rib is progressively mobilized the insertion of the diaphragm and the pleural reflection come into view. The subcostal nerve is carefully preserved as the diaphragm is divided flush with its insertion into the abdominal wall and the pleura is pushed away by blunt finger dissection. Depending on the degree of exposure needed, dissection of the twelfth rib may proceed up to the vertebral column. After dividing the costovertebral ligament and complete elevation of the crus of the diaphragm, the twelfth rib can be swung outwards like a door. Opening the fascia of Gerota in the line of the skin incision allows direct access to the entire kidney and adrenal gland. A rib retractor (HOHENFELLNER 1977) or a special ring retractor (WICKHAM 1979) is used to define the optimal field, the blades also controlling the perirenal fat.

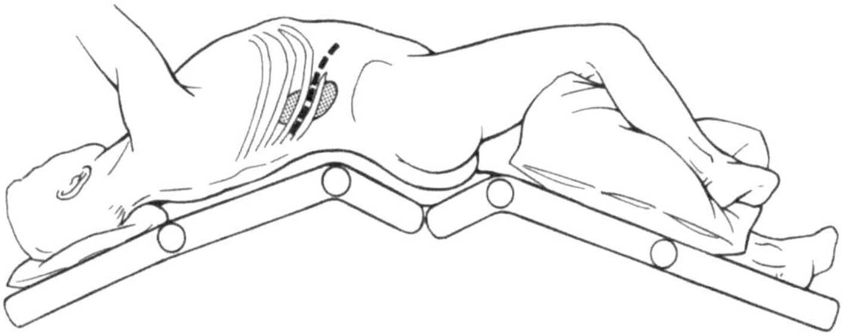

Fig. 10. Positioning the patient for a supracostal approach to the kidney

a b c

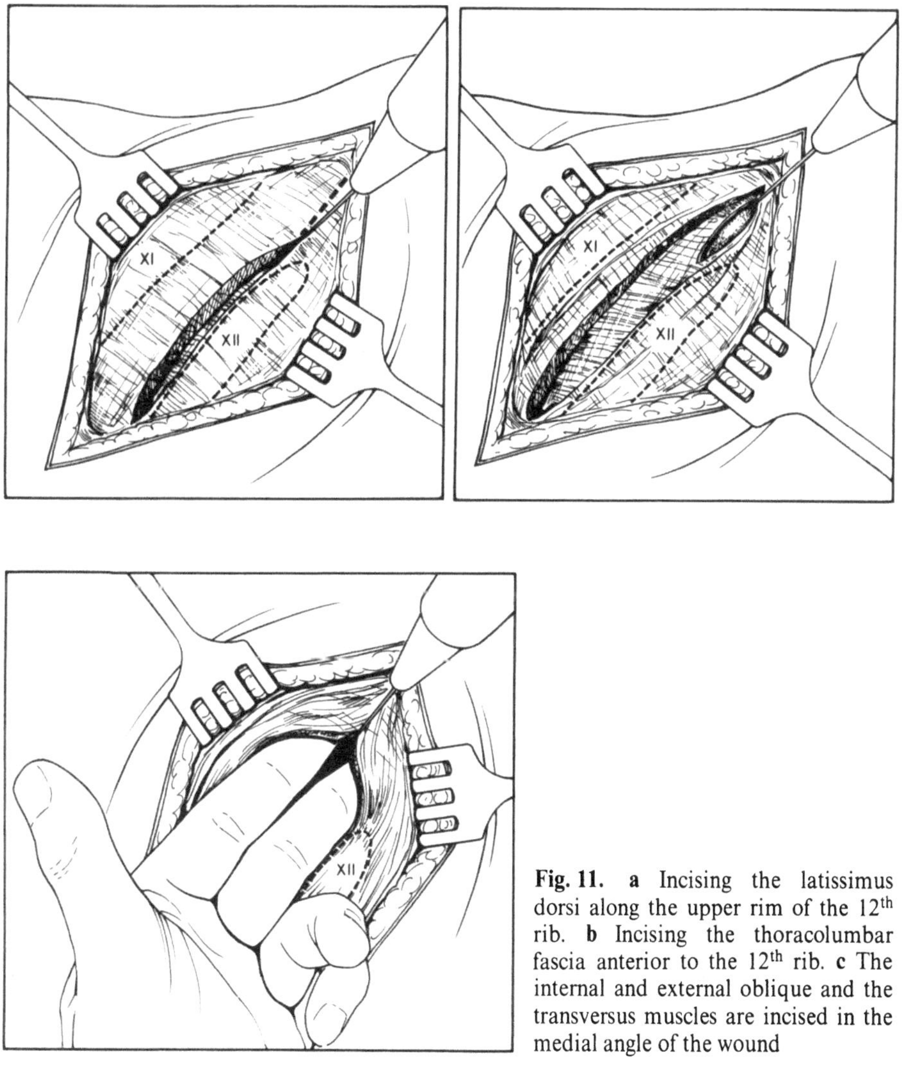

Fig. 11. **a** Incising the latissimus dorsi along the upper rim of the 12th rib. **b** Incising the thoracolumbar fascia anterior to the 12th rib. **c** The internal and external oblique and the transversus muscles are incised in the medial angle of the wound

The wound drain is brought out through all layers of the abdominal wall and Gerota's fascia via a separate stab incision lateral to the lower end of the main incision. The wound is closed with interrupted through and through 2-0 polyglycolic acid sutures including all intercostal and abdominal muscles, but avoiding lateral displacement of the layers. The sutures are preplaced and only tied after relieving the hyperextension, following which they are reinforced by a continuous suture or some interrupted sutures of the superficial muscles and associated deep fascia. Infiltration of the 10th, 11th and 12th intercostal nerves with 6 ml each 0.75% bupivicaine provides an initial postoperative period substantially free of pain, thus facilitating early mobilization (CRAWFORD et al. 1978). TURNER-WARWICK (1965) has recommended reattaching the diaphragmatic crus, but since this frequently leads to fraying of the muscle, it is generally omitted. This does not lead to negative effects on diaphragmatic activity or respiration (BARRY and HITCH 1975; MARBERGER 1979; SCHRAMM 1980).

The advantage of the supracostal approach lies in its universal applicability, as it provides excellent access in virtually any situation of renal calculous disease.

As long as the incision has not been carried too far medially beyond the tip of the rib, incisional hernias will not occur (BARRY and HUTCH 1975; HOHENFELLNER 1975; GARDINER et al. 1979). BARRY and HUTCH (1975) found persistant neuralgia or abdominal wall weakness after 4% of all procedures: nerve lesions were commoner after secondary procedures. Although adjacent organs are rarely damaged the pleura is opened quite frequently. In the series of BARRY and HUTCH (1975) this occurred in 18% of supra-12th rib and 67% of supra-11th rib incisions. SCHRAMM (1980) records a pleural injury in 17% of 300 cases. With correct intraoperative repair of the pleura with continuous 5-0 chromic catgut following expansion of the lung by positive pressure ventilation, this mishap remains without serious consequence. Intercostal drainage is not required. In six out of 50 patients whose pleura was inadvertantly opened, SCHRAMM (1980) found a peripheral pneumothorax immediately postoperatively, accompanied in four cases by a pleural effusion and in two patients by plate atelectasis. All cases were successfully treated conservatively without a chest tube.

More serious effects on lung function result from the hyperextended lateral position. The contralateral hemithorax is compressed and its respiratory movements impeded, with a consequent fall in vital and functional residual capacities (FAULCONER et al. 1946; SVANBERG 1957; POTGIETER 1959). Reduced venous return in the affected part of the lung (ROMMELSHEIM 1978) further promotes the onset of atelectasis and effusion, chiefly on the contralateral side (FAULCONER et al. 1946; ROMMELSHEIM 1976). In his prospective study SCHRAMM (1980) was able to show radiologic abnormalities on chest radiographs of 7.7% of patients on the side of the operation but in 38.4% on the contralateral side. The respiratory rate was elevated by a mean 35% on the first postoperative day, and vital capacity and FEV1 were reduced to 50% and 48% of the preoperative value respectively. Young patients with healthy lungs were easily able to compensate for these changes. The more elderly and those with previously impaired lung function may, however, be placed at considerable risk, especially after lengthy procedures involving hypothermia. BIRCH and MIMS (1975) recorded clinical and/or radiologic evidence of impaired lung function in 37% of 113 patients undergoing nephrolithotomy with regional cooling in the lateral position. Careful correction of intraoperative fluid and temperature alterations, early mobilization and chest physiotherapy reduce these complications. Since hypoventilation due to pain in the early postoperative phase also substantially increases the incidence of respiratory complications, all extensive procedures should routinely also have infiltration of the subcostal nerves passing the wound with a long-acting local anesthetic agent (CRAWFORD et al. 1978).

3. The Anterior Approach

Where extensive scar tissue from previous operations or from suppurative episodes impedes a flank access the anterior approach offers a convenient alternative (POUTASSE 1961; LINCKE et al. 1978). The vessels of the renal pedicle can be exposed directly and without any dissection of the kidney. Since previous operations will in general not have interfered with the great vessels of the abdomen, the planes of dissection are nearly always well preserved. Severe thoracic deformities and curvatures of the spine prevent effective hyperextension in the lateral position but will not interfere with an anterior approach. Furthermore, the ventilatory and circulatory changes induced in the lung by supine positioning are substantially less than for the lateral position, so that the anterior approach is safer for patients with impaired lung function. Surgery for bilateral kidney stones can be performed through an extended incision without the need to reposition the patient (DEMLER et al. 1983).

The patient is positioned supine in slight hyperextension. The incision may be performed parallel to the costal arch, but an upper tranverse incision, falling slightly laterally is more helpful (Fig. 12). If the normal tissue planes have not

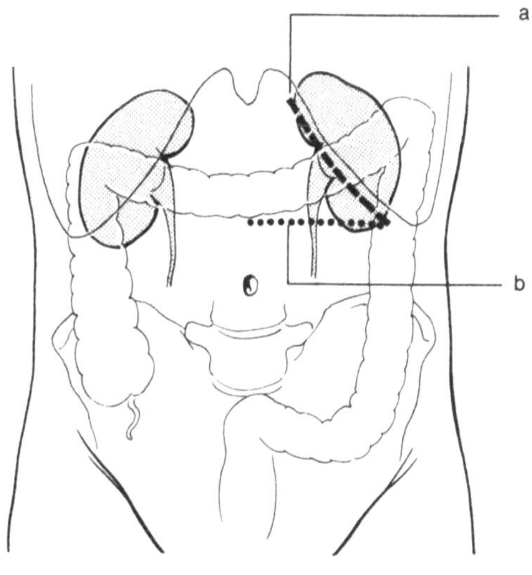

Fig. 12. Alternative incisions for the anterior approach

been obliterated by perirenal scarring the peritoneum can be swept medially by blunt dissection to expose the anterior aspect of the kidney. This approach is particularly suitable for procedures to the collecting system, renal pedicle and lower pole of children (ECKSTEIN 1975) but has little place in adult stone surgery. Since scarring from previous surgery and inflammatory processes prevents blunt dissection, the transperitoneal approach is preferable. BOSE and SHAW (1975) and LINCKE et al. (1978) were able to show that with proper wound drainage the complication rate from wound infection or extravasation of urine was no greater than for the traditional retroperitoneal approach. The peritoneum is therefore routinely opened after dividing the abdominal muscles and the ipsilateral rectus. The posterior peritoneum is then incised and dissected off medially. On the left the spleen and on the right the duodenum must both be swept away and carefully protected. The anterior aspect of the kidney and the renal vessels are now easily identified, usually quite free of scar tissue. The renal vessels may now be elevated with a hilar retractor, division of the spermatic vessels aiding mobilization on the left. This maneuver exposes the subjacent renal pelvis, and since the kidney is usually rotated somewhat posteriorly out of the coronal plane the hilar region is easily demonstrated.

The wound drain runs extraperitoneally through a separate retroperitoneal stab incision. The incisions in the posterior and anterior peritoneum are closed with a continuous absorbable suture and the abdominal muscles closed in layers in the usual way. The anterior and posterior rectus sheath need to be closed separately with interrupted sutures.

4. Access for Recurrent Disease

In secondary cases no hard and fast rules can be laid down and account must be taken of the individual situation and requirements. Nonetheless, a systematic approach and careful but concerted dissection to locate surgical landmarks will substantially reduce the complication rate of such procedures (HOHENFELLNER 1980).

The skin incision should be so placed as to give the best possible exposure whilst seeking to avoid regions of previous dissection. Cosmetic considerations will have a relatively low priority. The approach of choice is usually a supra-11-th rib or supra-12th rib incision, if necessary with rib resection (HOHENFELLNER 1980) or alternatively the transperitoneal route (LINCKE 1978). Although the modified lumbotomy approach may avoid the scar tissue of previous loin incisions, the almost inevitable need for intraoperative radiology usually renders this incision unsuitable.

If a supracostal approach is chosen, the dissection should begin as high as possible in the costovertebral angle, aiming to sweep off the pleura and divide the crus of the diaphragm. Pleural injuries are only dealt with once the kidney has been completely mobilized. Since the perirenal fat is nearly always fused with the psoas fascia, the subfascial plane of the psoas suggests itself as a primary plane of dissection, easily developed caudally in a few minutes to reach the lower pole by blunt dissection (Fig. 13). The abdominal wall incision is now

Fig. 13. Mobilizing a previously operated kidney by blunt dissection along the subfascial plane of the psoas

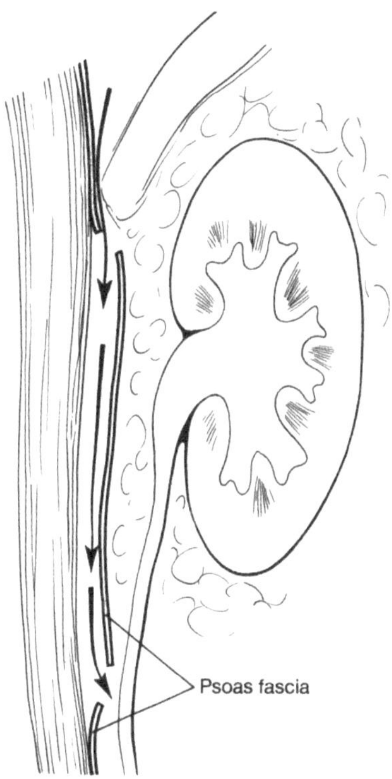

gradually carried medially to what ever extent allows adequate retraction – dividing the rectus if need be. If possible the peritoneum is swept medially, otherwise it is opened medially and as remotely from the colon as practicable. Once the wound can be adequately opened with hand retractors, the ureter is identified and snared within the unscarred connective tissue distal to the lower pole. Since intubated ureters are easier to identify a ureteric catheter should routinely be passed prior to any reexploration. With the ureter exposed there are no further important structures to be spared in the direction of the lateral abdominal wall and psoas, so that the scar and connective tissue in the region of the lower pole may be divided sharply to extend the exposure. The colon and, on the right, the duodenum are then dissected off. Under difficult circumstances it may only be posible to do this transperitoneally and under direct vision.

With the transperitoneal approach dissecting off the colon, mesocolon and duodenum medially is the first step before the renal vessels can be identified and snared. All important anatomical landmarks are now identified and secured.

Now the kidney is exposed step by step by sharp dissecting off of the adipose capsule in a plane just above the fibrous capsule of the kidney. In the course of this process substantial blood loss may occur from the severed scar tissue (WICKHAM et al. 1974). Damage to the capsule, and above all subcapsular dissection, should be avoided at all cost, since the renal capsule is essential for an atraumatic closure of nephrotomies (BOYCE and ELKINS 1974; BOYCE 1975; WICKHAM 1979). The ureter can usually be mobilized up into the sinus quite easily with a curved hemostat, so that the lower pole can be exposed by sharp dissection without a problem.

Accessory vessels are common in the region of the upper pole and along the medial border of the kidney: in difficult cases stepwise examination of the territory with a Doppler stethoscope may be helpful (BOYCE 1976, 1983). Large vessels always produce an audible signal and can be dissected to facilitate sharp division of the remaining scar tissue closely adhering to the renal capsule. This technique also safely avoids injuring the adrenal. The kidney must be so mobilized that a hand can be passed right round the organ and that it can be suspended in a Netelast sling (WICKHAM et al. 1979) or on tapes (BOYCE et al. 1974). Good intraoperative radiology usually requires dissection of the renal vessels to their point of union with the main abdominal vessels (MARBERGER and HRUBY 1984). Next, the hilar structures are dissected (see chapter on "Radial Nephrolithotomy Under Ultrasound and Doppler Probe Control", pp. 141), or a nephrolithotomy is performed.

VI. Pyelolithotomy

Renal arteries are end arteries (SIGEL 1961; GRAVES 1971; BOYCE et al. 1979) and any incision of the renal parenchyma therefore leads to infarction of the parenchyma supplied by the divided vessels. Although vessel-sparing techniques of incision (see chapter on "Radial Nephrolithotomy Under Ultrasound and Doppler Probe Control") have led to a marked reduction in parenchymal loss, every nephrotomy will of necessity have some negative effect on overall renal function (EISEN et al. 1974; MAY 1974; MARBERGER 1979; FITZPATRICK et al. 1980; MARBERGER and EISENBERGER 1980). On the other hand, removing stones through an incision into the collecting system avoids direct parenchymal damage, so that even extensive surgery of this kind does not cause any loss of renal function (GIL-VERNET 1965, 1972, 1979; EISEN et al. 1974; MAY 1974; FITZPATRICK et al. 1980; KAWAMURA et al. 1983). The only limitation of this approach to the collecting system is a disproportion between the size and shape of the intrarenal portion of the stone and the narrowest diameter of the collecting system through which it is to be extracted (HINMAN and CATTOLICA 1983). The systematic development of the concept of intrasinusal pyeloinfundibulotomy has opened up this approach even for complicated intrarenal calculi and led to an important change in stone surgery over the past two decades.

1. Simple Pyelolithotomy

Stones in the extrarenal part of the renal pelvis (C 1 – 2) are usually easy to extract through an incision in this part of the collecting system without any need to mobilize the kidney. The renal pelvis may be opened from the anterior or posterior side (LINCKE et al. 1978). Since the majority of the renal vessels, however, cross anteriorly posterior pyelotomy tends to be simpler (PYTEL et al. 1971; BOYCE 1975; PYRAH 1979; HOHENFELLNER and MARBERGER 1977; WICKHAM 1979). After incising the fascia of Gerota the perirenal fat is cleared from the hilar region by blunt dissection until the renal pelvis comes into view. At this point the kidney can be steadied by a sinus retractor and the calculus is palpated. Dissecting or snaring the proximal ureter is superfluous and should not be indulged in as it leads only to unnecessary scarring (PYTEL et al. 1971). Care is taken to spare the pelviureteric junction with a high incision of the pelvis parallel to the hilar margin. Transverse incisions reduce the danger of a tear extending into the pelviureteric junction and possibly resulting in late stricture, and correspond to the direction of the smooth muscle fibers in the renal pelvis (GIL-VERNET 1970). Once the stone has been extracted with stone hooks, the entire collecting system is carefully flushed with saline. A malleable metal catheter (GIL-VERNET 1965; MAHMOOD 1973) or a semirigid open-ended PVC catheter and a bladder syringe or pressure cuff and infusion bag (WICKHAM 1974, 1979) have proved helpful for this purpose. The patency of the ureter should always be controlled by passing a soft ureteral catheter. The collecting system is closed in a watertight fashion whenever possible, a continuous suture of 5-0 chromic catgut or coated polyglycolic acid usually being suitable for uncomplicated cases. Because of the hazard of encrustation, non-absorbable material is strictly to be avoided (HEALY and WARREN 1979). An inflamed and edematous pelvis can often only be approximated with interrupted sutures, care being taken not to evert the mucosa. Since the incision lies close to the hilum, renal sinus fat generally comes to overlie the suture line and provides an additional seal.

Previous surgery or extensive inflammation may make the dissection quite difficult, even if the pelvis is extrarenal and the stone simple. In this case it is best to identify the ureter as it passes the lower pole outside the scar tissue and dissect it in the retrograde direction. A good plane of cleavage can nearly always be found subadventitially, along the immediate surface of the ureteric musculature, and this provides a safe route up to the pelvis.

A drainage tube should be inserted via a separate stab incision through all layers of the abdominal wall and the fascia of Gerota to provide dependent drainage of the lowest point in the space opened up by the dissection within Gerota's fascia. If the drain lies outside this fascial space, urinoma may result (SCHREITER et al. 1975). WICKHAM (1980) has described prolonged urinary extravasation from tube drains and recommends the use of Penrose drains. Separately placed tube drains, however, permit clean collection of drainage fluid well away from the wound (MAYOR and ZINGG 1973) and in the experience of the authors are associated neither with an increased rate of fistula nor with added complications of wound infections. The perirenal fat and Gerota's fascia are closed with a running suture to restore the perirenal fascial space and to reduce penrenal scarring.

Simple pyelotomy correctly performed on sound indications has a minimal morbidity (PYTEL et al. 1971; WILLIAMS 1972; ZOEDLER 1974; RUMMELHARDT and DOBROVITS 1974; BOYCE 1975). The most common problem is prolonged leakage of urine from the drain. Frequently the tip of the drain has come to lie immediately adjacent to the pyelotomy, and careful withdrawal of the tube by about a centimeter leads to cessation of drainage within hours. Temporary intubation of the ureter is another simple way of drying up the wound, provided distal obstruction such as a calculus has not been overlooked (HILDRETH and CASS 1976). Internal ureteric stents are less prone to infection and are less unpleasant for the patient. Semirigid pigtail or double-J stents are easy to insert and have little tendency to migrate (FINNEY et al. 1978; CAMACHO et al. 1979; MARDIS et al. 1979). We therefore prefer them to simple silicone rubber tubes (ZIMSKIND et al. 1967; PAIS et al. 1975) or stents with retaining barbs (GIBBON et al. 1976; SINGH et al. 1979).

Correctly placed drains will nearly always prevent urinoma formation. Nonetheless, unexplained fever or pain in the wound should bring this possibility to mind. Large urinomas are easily detected by sonography, smaller extravasations may require an IVP with delayed films. With distal obstruction urinomas may also form delayed and virtually devoid of clinical symptoms, only to be diagnosed by chance as urinary pseudocysts (SCHREITER et al. 1975).

Inadequate exposure of the renal pelvis, especially through small incisions and in secondary procedures, may result in injuries to segmental arteries, especially the posterior segmental artery which crosses the dorsal aspect of the renal pelvis (ANDERSON 1976). The mishap is usually immediately apparent by the profuse hemorrhage that ensues and is difficult to control without loss of the vessel and its corresponding parenchymal segment. Careful dissection in the region where the vessel is to be expected, i.e. around the upper third of the renal pelvis near the hilar rim, will safely prevent this injury. With marked rotation of the kidney to expose the sinus the renal vein may erroneously be incised instead of the renal pelvis (HOHENFELLNER and MARBERGER 1977), a mistake hardly possible with correct dissection closely adhering to the renal pelvis. Injuries to the duodenum have also been described after pyelotomy (KUSS et al. 1972; HOHENFELLNER 1980), but occur almost exclusively in difficult recurrent cases requiring extensive mobilization of the kidney. It is therefore of fundamental importance not to incise the collecting system until the stone has been palpated or the pelvis unequivocally identified.

2. Coagulum Pyelolithotomy

Frequently one or more stones lie relatively mobile (C 1 – 3) within the intrarenal portion of the collecting system, where they are difficult to palpate or visualize despite excellent extrarenal access to the collecting system as a whole. Many of these calculi can be extracted with the pyeloscope, but from time to time a nephrotomy may seem unavoidable. With the proviso that the ratio stone diameter/infundibulum permits transhilar extraction, a coagulum pyelotomy may help to avoid incising the parenchyma.

As early as 1943, DEES and FOX were able to show that a coagulum of fibrin and thrombin dissolves in urine within 6 – 24 hours, whereas a whole blood clot would take at least 72 hours. If fibrinogen and thrombin are introduced into the collecting system, a solid coagulum forms within minutes throughout the entire pelvicalyceal lumen and encases any calculi, which may then be extracted in toto with the coagulum (DEES 1943). The complicated technique for preparing the coagulum led to a high technical failure rate and the procedure never gained a foothold. In a 1974 review of the literature, PATEL was able to find only 167 published cases.

KLOSTERHALFEN and his colleagues had tried as early as 1969 to improve the coagulation properties and tensile strength of the fibrin mixture. Utilizing thrombelastograms they were able to achieve an optimum clot if a human fibrinogen solution was mixed with fresh plasma and a solution of thrombin and $CaCl_2$. Although equally good results were obtained with platelet rich freezedried plasma, the former mixture was more convenient to prepare and the group decided to use these substrates for their clinical work. The components were mixed within the collecting system by means of a double lumen cannula.

PATEL (1973, 1974) further simplified the system and thus achieved a clinical breakthrough. One gram of pooled human fibrinogen is dissolved in 20 ml physiologic saline. 200 units of thrombin are dissolved in 4 ml physiologic saline and both solutions are kept at 37 °C for at least 15 minutes in a water bath. They are then rapidly mixed in a porcelaine crucible and injected within 30 seconds down a conical catheter into the collecting system. The ureter must first be occluded with a rubber sling and urine evacuated from the pelvis. The amount of solution injected must not exceed the aspirated urine volume, if over filling of the collecting system and the consequent hazard of intravenous injection are to be avoided. Within 5 minutes, the coagulum has so far solidified that it can be removed with the stones it encases, via a standard pyelotomy.

In PATEL's hands (1974) this technique has been extraordinarily successful. In only 7 of 224 cases was he unable to achieve a satisfactory clot and he observed no significant complications. The value of the procedure seems further underlined by the observation that in 33% of cases additional stones were extracted which had not been seen on the preoperative films. It is important, however, when preparing the mixture to adhere strictly to the technical details. SMITH (1978) recorded 19 failures out of a total of 25 attempts and it emerged that the chief source of problems was inadequate warming of the component solutions prior to mixing, too rapid coagulation of the mixture before it could be instilled into the collecting system and leakage from the pyelotomy site. The two components of the mixture must be kept at 37 °C for at least 15 minutes before they are mixed. Warming to over 37 °C causes denaturation and equally inadequate coagulation (SMITH et al. 1978; FISCHER et al. 1981).

Despite scrupulously careful preparation, commercially available pooled fibrinogen may be contaminated with hepatitis virus, and there have been increasing restrictions on product licenses for this type of material, chiefly in the United States. By 1977 a number of individual states (RATHORE and HARRISON 1976) had prohibited its sale and at this point the Food and Drug Administration deemed the hepatitis risk to warrant prohibition throughout the United States. Experimental attempts at producing fibrinogen coagula from autologous blood were substantially successful (RATHORE and HARRISON 1976; SEDDON and BONIN 1977), but the clots were too fragile for any wider clinical application. The tensile strength of a coagulum is directly proportional to its fibrinogen content, which is 50 times higher in pooled human fibrinogen than in normal human plasma. By cryoprecipitation of human plasma the fibrinogen concentration can be enriched by a factor of 10 to about 2000 mg/100 ml, resulting in a breaking strain of 100 g/cm^2 for the derived clots (MARSHALL 1978). MARSHALL (MARSHALL and LYON 1978) recommends a mixture of a 4% fibrinogen solution from cryoprecipitate plasma with 5 ml of a 50 units/ml thrombin solution and 1 ml 10% $CaCl_2$, injecting the mixture into the renal pelvis by the twin catheter technique. Within 7 minutes a tough coagulum has formed which is well suited for coagulum pyelolithotomy (BROECKER and HACKER 1979; SHERER 1980). FISCHER et al. (1979, 1980) were able to demonstrate that the tensile strength of the coagulum may be doubled by warming the fibrinogen solution to 37 °C – a maneuver not required for the other components because of their small volume. The same authors found that mixing the components prior to rapid instillation through a single catheter gave more consistent results, chiefly because coagulation within the collecting system tended to be more uniform. They also recommend adding methylene blue to make the coagulum easier to distinguish from the pelvicalyceal wall and surrounding renal tissue, especially where combined with a nephrotomy in ischemia (FISCHER et al. 1980; UEDA and MOMOSE 1982).

In properly selected cases there can be no doubt as to the value of coagulum pyelolithotomy, especially for multiple multilocular calyceal stones in a dilated system. Since the coagulum dissolves even in infected urine of chronic stone formers before encrustation has had time to occur, no side effects are to be anticipated from a retained clot (KLOSTERHALFEN 1969). If one excludes hepatitis contracted from commercial fibrinogen, the only serious mishap so far reported is a report on fatal pulmonary embolism (PENCE 1981) following coagulum pyelolithotomy. In experiments on the dog PENCE and colleagues found multiple peripheral pulmonary emboli, even if only small quantities of mixture were instilled into the collecting system. FISCHER et al. (1983), however, pointed out that both the human fatality and the animal experiments involved a fibrinogen-thrombin mixture 80 times stronger than that recommended by them. Since the tensile strength of the coagulum is greater, the less thrombin is added, the very lowest thrombin concentration adequate to convert all the fibrinogen to fibrin should be sufficient (MARSHALL 1978). The danger of accidental intravenous infusion of thrombin is further reduced by mixing the two components of the mixture outside the renal pelvis prior to instillation (PATEL 1973, 1974; FISCHER et al. 1980). In over 400 cases FISCHER et al. (1983) have seen not a single pulmonary complication with their technique. Nevertheless attempts are being made to avoid the use of thrombin altogether. Since fibrinogen cryoprecipitate is preserved either with EDTA or citrate-phosphate dextrose, addition of their antagonist, $CaCl_2$, leads to clot formation even in the absence of thrombin. KALASH et al. (1982) have reported on the clinical use of such a mixture.

3. Extended Pyelolithotomy (Intrasinusal Pyeloinfundibulotomy)

Stones in an intrarenal pelvis (E_i), calculi of which large proportions are within the intrarenal part of the collecting system or reaching into the calyces (C3, C4) or calyceal stones primarily do not appear to be amenable to a transhilar approach. To avoid nephrotomy and its high complication rate already HANDLEY (1923) and later BERESNEGOVSKY (1925) and SURRACO (1939) proposed an intracapsular approach to the intrarenal collecting system. The capsule is incised along the dorsal aspect of the kidney, parallel to the hilar margin, and swept off the parenchyma by blunt dissection to approach the sinus intracapsularly, through the inner leaf of the fibrous capsule. Despite the popularity of this approach in the '50s and early '60s it was limited in its applicability by the segmental arteries and veins, which cross the hilar region and seriously inhibit intrahilar exposure. Furthermore, traction on the decapsulated parenchyma with sinus retractors tended to cause annoying parenchymal tears (BUESCHER and GACA 1963; MAUERMAYER 1969; PYRAH 1979). The technique of extracapsular, intrasinusal pyeloinfundibulotomy as presented by GIL-VERNET in 1965 was the first transhilar approach to avoid these problems. Through its wide applicability and low morbidity the procedure has today become the standard technique for removing difficult renal calculi.

Under normal anatomical circumstances the renal sinus is sealed by a thin diaphragm of connective tissue radiating from the fibrous capsule of the kidney to fuse with the pelvis and enclose the renal pedicle (GIL-VERNET 1965). Behind this structure the intrarenal collecting system and the segmental vessels lie embedded in the loose fatty connective tissue of the renal sinus. Once the diaphragm has been opened along the dorsal aspect of the renal pelvis, the perihilar structures may be lifted off the intrarenal collecting system by blunt dissection. Although the renal sinus varies considerably in its dimensions, it is usually possible to expose the entire pelvis and the infundibula of the main calyces by this procedure. As long as dissection proceeds along a plane close to the collecting system, the segmental vessels are retracted away in the perihilar fat where they are neither easily injured nor hinder access (Fig. 14), GIL-VERNET (1965) has described special retractors which facilitate this maneuver considerably. In a modified form with malleable blades and available in various sizes they can be adapted to any individual situation (Fig. 15), providing not only retraction of the perihilar structures but also protection of the retracted vessels from inadvertant injury during intrarenal dissection. The latter may be carried out either with a Lahey dab or, most effectively, with wet ribbon gauze which is gradually packed into the cavity as it develops and is held under the retractors (GIL-VERNET 1972).

Severe perihilar inflammation or previous surgery may obliterate the usual planes of dissection. Despite this, it is usually possible to develop the renal sinus as long as dissection proceeds along the muscular layer of the collecting system. The scarred connective tissue is thus lifted away with the peripelvic adventitia. Sharp dissection may be needed, but since all the major vessels lie outside the adventitia and are protected by the retractors, a vascular injury is most unlikely. As dissection proceeds more deeply into the pelvis, small veins may be

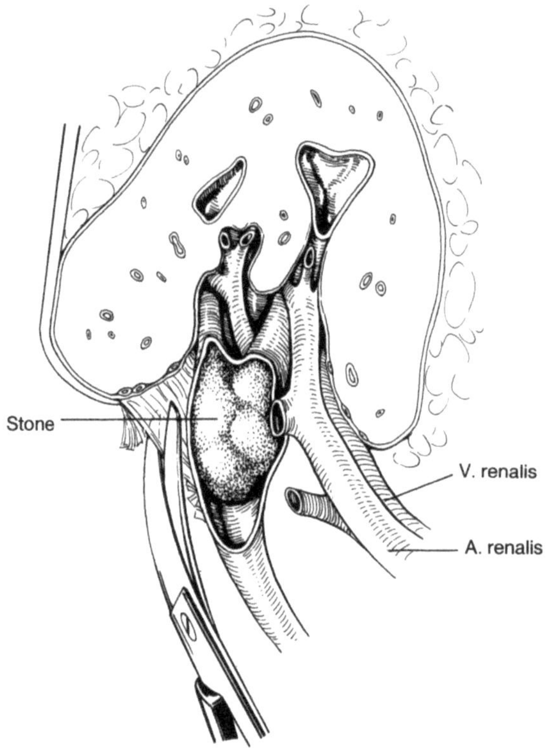

Fig. 14. Intrasinusal dissection: the sinus is opened in a plane just over the musculature of the collecting system and the intrahilar fat and vessels are deflected from the intrasinusal collecting system with sinus retractors

opened, but venous hemorrhage is easily controlled by pressure with the retractors. By packing neurosurgical patties under the retractors, the renal parenchyma is protected from retractor pressure and the surgical field cleared as oozing blood is absorbed.

The muscle fibers of the renal pelvis take a circulo-spiral course (GIL-VERNET 1970) with a very small angle of inclination. A transverse incision parallel to the transverse diameter of the kidney and roughly at right angles to the course of the ureter will cause the least muscle damage. At the same time the danger of a tear extending into the pelviureteric junction to cause late stricture is reduced. Naturally, this basic incision must be adapted to the individual shape and position of the stone: for very large staghorns the incision should be U-shaped with its convexity toward the ureter and it may extend up into the calyceal necks to allow the extraction of calyceal calculi. The renal collecting system is so well vascularized that even the division of multiple vessels will not impair healing (SPORER and SEEBODE 1981), but because of the risk of stricture the pelviureteric junction must always be spared (GIL-VERNET 1972). The further intrarenally the incision into the collecting system is placed, the less likely is extravasation of urine from a poor closure, the incision being covered

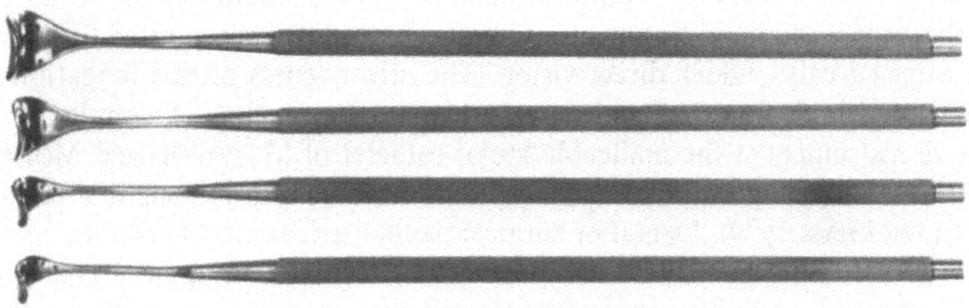

Fig. 15. Sinus retractors of various sizes and with malleable blades

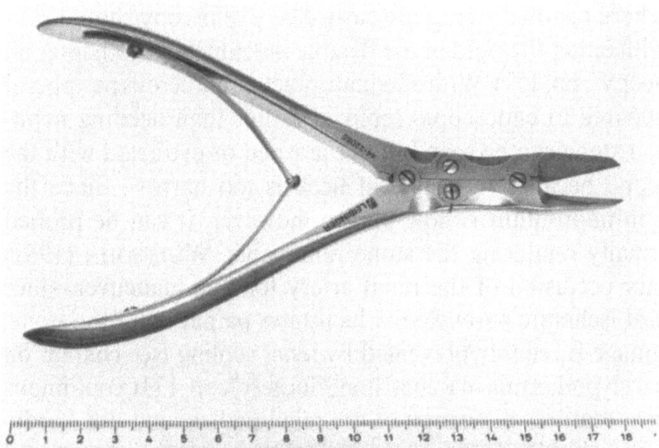

Fig. 16. Stone cutter designed to give a clean cut across branching calculi

by parenchyma once the retractors are released (HOHENFELLNER and MARBERGER 1977).

The stone is extracted with stone hooks or atraumatic stone forceps. Branching staghorns are first mobilized by luxation of the pelvic portion of the stone out of the renal pelvis and the shorter calyceal extensions are then developed through generous incisions in the affected infundibula. Finally the entire stone is lifted out by gentle rotation along the axis of the remaining calyceal extensions (GIL-VERNET 1972). Ideally the stone should not be broken: if the stone is too branched for extraction in one piece, it is best divided under direct vision with a special stone cutter (Fig. 16). Because of the poor irrigating conditions in an open wound, ultrasound drills tend to generate a slurry which is difficult to clear and with the osteotomy technique of GRAVES (1977), one slip is enough to inflict serious parenchymal injury. Correct intrasinusal dissection will expose the infundibula of the main calyces of the upper and lower poles and of the anterior calyces. Residual stones can then be retrieved under direct vision with fine forceps. Peripheral fragments are best removed by concentrated flushing of the affected calyx under direct vision. The effectiveness of this irrigation depends on a high flow rate and on an adequate jet of saline. A simple and effective instrument is the malleable metal catheter of MAHMOOD and MORALES (1973), saline being supplied under pressure from an infusion bag in a pressure cuff (WICKHAM 1979). Dental or surgical wound irrigators (MOYA-PRATS 1970; BOYCE 1975; WICKHAM 1979) are even more effective. During intrarenal flushing the wound around the pyelotomy should be protected, to prevent stone fragments being lost in the wound: on later radiographs they would be indistinguishable from residual stones.

An expert will be able to locate and remove residual calculi in secondary calyces by palpation with a malleable probe (LUTZEYER et al. 1970; GIL-VERNET 1972), but this technique is unreliable in routine use and frequently provokes hemorrhage. Where residual stones are suspected pyeloscopy should routinely be performed, with either the rigid or the flexible instrument (see chapter on "Intraoperative Pyeloscopy", pp. 157). With adequate practice numerous peripheral stones will prove amenable to endoscopic removal rather than needing nephrotomy. Occasionally, a stone can be seen but not grasped or extracted with the forceps of the renoscope because the calyceal neck is too narrow. Since the exact position of the infundibulum is now known, however, it can be probed and gently dilated, usually rendering the stone removable. WULFSOHN (1981) recommends temporary occlusion of the renal artery for this maneuver, since the reduced turgidity of ischemic parenchyma facilitates palpation of the stone. Although ischemic damage is reliably prevented by renal cooling (see chapter on "Ischemia and Regional Hypothermia in Renal Stone Surgery", pp. 133), continuous surface cooling, at least, requires dissection of the renal pedicle and this hardly appears justified by the slight advantage gained. As even the most careful pyeloscopist will be unable to see about one third of secondary calyces (ZINGG and FUTTERLIEB 1980), intraoperative sonography and/or radiology are always needed to confirm complete stone removal in technically difficult cases.

Intrasinusal dissection can proceed in situ, i.e. without the whole kidney being mobilized (GIL-VERNET 1966; LUTZEYER et al. 1970). If the stones are restricted to a localized part of the calyceal system it may be adequate to expose only the related parenchyma for sonographic examination (RIEDMILLER et al. 1983). With the need for intraoperative radiology exposure of the entire kidney becomes mandatory (WICKHAM 1979; ZINGG and FUTTERLIEB 1980; MARBERGER and HRUBY 1983). Adequate contact films of the entire organ can only be obtained if a sterile plate can be placed behind the kidney and exposed without the interposition of the abdominal wall, ideally with exposures in two planes (GIL-VERNET and CULLA 1981). Even if a radiological unit with a finger-shaped anode (Renodor) specially designed for intraoperative kidney roentgenography is used, good exposures require a film–focus distance of at least 7 cm (LEUSCH 1970; ALBRECHT and MONCADA 1979; BAUR 1982). If intraoperative radiology is likely to be needed it is therefore worth exposing the entire kidney at the outset, even if the stone appears to be removable by the transhilar route. Where this proves unsuccessful multiple radial nephrotomies are the logical extension of the procedure (GIL-VERNET 1965, 1972, 1979; WICKHAM 1974, 1979; see chapter on "Radial Nephrolithotomy Under Ultrasound and Doppler Probe Control", pp. 141). If technical difficulties are to be expected it is also worth dissecting the renal pedicle at the beginning of the operation.

Watertight closure of the renal pelvis with fine, absolute suture material should always be attempted. In the hands of the authors 2 running sutures of 5-0 polyglycolic acid or chromic catgut have proven very effective. Both sutures start at the point of maximum convexity of the posterior pelvic flap and run in opposite directions toward the upper and lower ends of the incision. Because space under the retractor blades is often restricted, incisions in the calyceal necks may not be closable by this technique, in which case a few interrupted 6-0 sutures should be inserted with a 5/8 circular needle. Even if such a loose approximation cannot be achieved a massive extravasation of urine is unlikely, since the incision will be well covered by fat and parenchyma once the retractor is removed. Occasionally inflammatory change has rendered the pelvic wall so brittle that only a loose approximation with some interrupted sutures can be achieved. In these cases, and whenever poor drainage is anticipated, e.g. because of problems with blood clots, an internal ureteric splint should be left in situ (see page 114; BOYCE 1975).

In recurrent cases intrasinusal dissection occasionally leaves a defect in the pelvic wall. Because of the risk of iatrogenic stricture of the pelviureteric junction, the temptation to close it under tension must be resisted. The defect is usually easily covered by a free graft of peritoneum loosely tacked on the defect with the shiny side inwards (THUEROFF et al. 1980; HOHENFELLNER 1980). Peritoneum shrinks less than flaps raised from the posterior aspect of the renal capsule and swung over the defect (MAUERMAYER 1969; THOMPSON et al. 1969; ENGBERG et al. 1976; HUTSCHENREITER et al. 1978). If closure of Gerota's fascia is impossible, the kidney may be enveloped in well vascularised fatty tissue swung in from the greater omentum (TURNER-WARWICK 1976). It is particularly important to interpose healthy fatty tissue between the ureter and the lower pole (HOHENFELLNER 1980).

The extended sinus approach has stood the test of time as a safe routine procedure for the majority of renal calculi not manageable by simple pyelotomy. Even in large series of staghorn calculi, the most challenging stones to be treated this way, there has been no mortality and minimal morbidity (GIL-VERNET and CARALPS 1979; WOODHOUSE et al. 1981). Branched renal calculi usually develop in a funnel shaped intrarenal pelvis and initially only fill the pelvis and infundibula (HINMAN and CATTOLICA 1981). Transpelvic removal is then almost always practicable because no part of the stone is bigger than the surrounding collecting system. As stone formation approaches the junction with the calyx, infundibular obstruction occurs and clubbed calyceal extensions requiring nephrotomy begin to form. GIL-VERNET (GIL-VERNET and CARALPS 1979), the master of extended pyelotomy, successfully removed 236 of 328 staghorn calculi by this technique, i.e. only 26% advanced type stones needed additional nephrotomies. In the authors' experience about 23% of all kidney stones coming to surgery need a parenchymal incision of some kind, a figure which rises to 42% for recurrent staghorns (MARBERGER and ALKEN 1979).

Table 1. Complications occuring after intrasinusal pyelotomy

Author	n	Residual stones	Hemor-rhage	Wound infection	Secondary nephrectomy	Mortality
LUTZEYER (1970)	86	0	?	?	0	0
SINGH (1971)	54	12	0	0	0	0
BENNET (1972)	8	0	?	?	?	0
MAHMOOD (1973)	25	2	?	?	?	0
STEPHENSON (1975)	10	2	1	?	?	1
BLANDY (1976)	152	30	0	?	0	0
GIL-VERNET (1979)	328	26	?	?	?	0
BROWN (1981)	20	0	?	?	?	0
WOODHOUSE (1981)	189	18	?	?	?	0
WULFSOHN (1981)	5	0	?	?	?	0
	877	90 (10.5%)	1 (0.5%)	0	0	1 (0.1%)

However, even with these most daunting stones the major portion or all of the pelvic extension can usually be removed via the sinus, reducing the need for parenchymal surgery to small nephrotomies.

As long as nephrotomies can be avoided, postoperative complications are few (Table 1) and easily controlled. Intraoperative hemorrhage results almost exclusively from lacerated intrahilar veins, which can usually be controlled by pressure or suture-ligation. In recurrent cases too generous a resection of fibrotic hilar fat may result in a lesion of the posterior segmental artery. Since re-anastomosis is only possible in favorable cases and with the availability of the operating microscope and regional hypothermia (ROCCO 1982), it is of the greatest importance to avoid this injury in the first place by remaining in the correct anatomical plane (i.e. subadventitial on the surface of the collecting system musculature). Rarely, spasm of the vessel masks the injury at the time of surgery and severe secondary hemorrhage ensues (BLANDY and SINGH 1976). Urinoma and fistula formation can be largely avoided by proper closure of the collecting system, unimpeded outflow of urine from the kidney and proper drainage. The treatment of these complications is as for simple pyelotomy (see page 114).

As calculous residuals considerably promote renewed stone growth or stone recurrence, the residual stone rate significantly affects the recurrence rate. In a series of 152 staghorn calculi BLANDY and SINGH (1976) recorded a recurrence or growth of residual calculi in 53% of patients whose stones has been incompletely cleared, as against 4.1% for patients known to have been left completely clear. The number of cases in which stones are left behind depends largely on meticulous technique and perseverence in removing all stones at the time of surgery.

Naturally there is also some risk of scarring and late stricture of the pelviureteric junction, but in the series described in Table 1 the incidence of this has been no higher than for other procedures requiring dissection of the hilar region. The most decisive advantage, however, of limiting the incision to the collecting system comes from the fact that renal function is not compromised by transecting parenchyma or interrupting renal circulation. Neither in experimental studies (FITZPATRICK et al. 1980) nor in large clinical series has extended pyeloinfundibulotomy been shown to have any deleterious effect on renal function. If obstructing stones are removed renal function may even improve (GIL-VERNET and CARALPS 1979; MAY 1974; SINGH et al. 1971; WOODHOUSE et al. 1981).

References

Albrecht KF, Moncada J (1979) Probleme der intraoperativen Röntgenuntersuchung bei Nierenausgußsteinen. In: Propaczy P (ed) Int Symp on Staghorn Calculi. Egerman, Vienna, p 161

Allo M, Simmon RL (1983) Surgical infections disease and the urologist. Urol Clin North Am 10:131

Alter AJ, Peterson DT, Plautz AC Jr (1979) Non-opaque calculus demonstrated by computerized tomography. J Urol 122:699

Andaloro VA Jr, Schor M, Marangola JP (1976) Intraoperative localization of a renal calculus using ultrasound. J Urol 116:92

Anderson J (1976) Renal artery lesions after pyelolithotomy. Acta Radiol [Diagn] (Stockh) 17:685

Ball TP Jr (1979) Intrarenal stone manipulation: Summary of recent experience. Trans Am Ass Gen Urin Surg 70:16

Ball TP Jr, Bobroff LM (1975) Selective caliceal catheterization for stone manipulation. J Urol 114:172

Barbaric ZL, Davis RS, Frank IN, Linke CA, Lipchick EO, Cockett ATK (1976) Percutaneous nephropyelostomy in the management of acute pyohydronephrosis. Radiology 118:567

Barry JM, Hodges CV (1975) The supracostal approach to the kidney and adrenal. J Urol 114:666

Baur HH (1982) Zehn Jahre Renodor. Urologe [Ausg A] 21:358

Bennett AH, Harrison JH (1972) Results of surgery on branched renal calculi. J Urol 107:174

Bensimon H (1974) Muscle protective incisions in renal surgery. Urology 4:476

Beresnegowsky N (1925) Zur Pyelolithotomiefrage. Zentralbl Chir 34:1882

Birch AA, Mims GR (1975) Anesthesia considerations during nephrolithotomy with slush. J Urol 113:433

Bischoff PF (1969) The surgical treatment of the solitary kidney. Urol Int 24:527

Blandy JP, Marshall VR (1976) Size of renal calculi, recurrence rate and follow-up. Br J Urol 48:525

Blandy JP, Singh M (1976) The case for a more aggressive approach to staghorn stones. J Urol 115:505

Blandy JP, Tressider GC (1967) Extended pyelolithotomy for renal calculi. Br J Urol 39:121

Borger HF, Hocks J, Kjellstrand CM (1982) Mannitol intoxication in patients with renal failure. Arch Intern Med 142:63

Bose TK, Shaw R (1975) Transperitoneal ureterolithotomy. Br J Urol 47:613

Boyarski S, Labay PC (1979) Glucagon, ureteral colic and ureteral peristalsis. Trans Am Ass Gen Urin Surg 70:22

Boyce WH (1975) Surgery of renal calculi. In: Glenn JF, Boyce WH (eds) Urologic surgery (2nd ed). Harper & Row, Hagerstown-New York Evanston San Franzisco London

Boyce WH (1977) The localisation of intrarenal calculi during surgery. J Urol 118:152

Boyce WH (1983) Personal Communication ct by Resnick MI Editorial comment. J Urol 130:224

Boyce WH, Elkins S (1974) Reconstructive renal surgery following anatrophic nephrolithotomy: Follow-up of 100 consecutive cases. J Urol 111:307
Boyce WH, Stubbs AJ, Resnick MI (1978) Intrarenal nephrolithotomy and reconstructive of the solitary kidney. Trans Am Ass Gen Urin Surg 69:118
Boyce WH, Russel JM, Webb R (1979) Management of the papillae during intrarenal surgery. Trans Am Ass Gen Urin Surg 71:76
Brandstetter LH, Schwentker FN (1975) Comparison of Gil-Vernet and classic flank approaches to pyelo- and ureterolithotomy. Urology 5:37
Britton KE, Brown NJG (1968) The clinical use of CABBS renography. Br J Radiol 41:570
Broecker BH, Hackler RH (1979) Simplified coagulum pyelolithotomy using cryoprecipitate. Urology 14:143
Brown RB (1981) A five-year follow-up of 57 staghorn calculus operations. In: Brockis JG (ed) Urinary calculus. PSG Publishing Company Inc Littleton Massachusetts
Buck AC, Mac Leod MA, Blacklock NJ (1980) The advantage of 99m DTPA (Sn) in dynamic renal scintigraphy and measurement of renal function. Br J Urol 52:174
Bueschen AJ, Lloyd LK, Dubovsky EV, Tanxe WN (1978) Radionuclide kidney function evaluation in the management of urolithiasis. J Urol 120:16
Büscher HK, Gaca A (1961) Therapie der Nieren- und Harnleitersteine. In: Alken CE, Dix VW, Weyrauch HM, Wildbolz E (Hrsg) Handbuch der Urologie. Die Steinerkrankungen. Springer, Berlin Göttingen Heidelberg
Buttermann G, Wolf IH, Heidenreich P, Oberdorfer M, Kuhlmann H, Czempiel H, Hör G, Pabst HW (1978) Comparison of different methods of clearance determination. In: Bianchi C, Blaufox MD (eds) Unilateral renal function studies. Contributions to Nephrology. Vol 11. Karger, Basel
Camacho MF, Pereiras R, Carrion H, Bondhus M, Politano VA (1979) Double-ended pigtail ureteral stent: Useful modification to single-end ureteral stent. Urology 13:516
Carl P, Schmiedt E (1974) Urolithiasis and Urosepsis in der Urologischen Universitätsklinik München, 1960–1973. Helv Chir Acta 41:389
Cibert J, Massoumi J, Mohadjer R (1972) Symptomatologie bruyante de certains calculs caliciels. J Urol Nephrol 78:197
Constantinople NL, Bedford Waters W, Yalla SV (1979) Operative versus non-operative management of patients with staghorn calculi and neurogenic bladder. J Urol 121:716
Corriere JN, Sandler CM (1982) The diagnosis and immediate therapy of acute renal and perirenal infections. Urol Clin North Am 9:219
Cox CE (1974) Urinary tract infection and renal lithiasis. Urol Clin North Am 2:283
Crawford ED, Skinner DG, Capparel DB (1978) Intercostal nerve block with the thoracoabdominal incision. J Urol 121:290
Czer LSC, Shoemaker WC (1978) Optimal hematocrit value in critically ill postoperative patients. Surg Gynecol Obstet 147:363
Daly MJ, Jones W, Rudd TG, Tremann J (1979) Differential renal function using technetium-99m dimercaptosuccinic acid (DMSA): in vitro correlation. J Nucl Med 20:63
Das S, Harris CJ, Amar D, Egan RM (1983) Dorsovertical lumbotomy approach for surgery of upper urinary tract calculi. J Urol 129:266
Davidson AJ, Talner LB (1973) Urographic and angiographic abnormalities in adult-onset acute bacterial nephritis. Radiology 106:249
Davidson AJ, Talner LB (1978) Late sequelae of adult-onset bacterial nephritis. Radiology 127:367
Dawson JL (1965) Post-operative renal function in obstructive jaundice: effect of a mannitol diuresis. Br Med J 1:82
Dees JE (1943) The use of an intrapelvic coagulum in pyelolithotomy. South Med J 36:167
Dees JE, Fox H (1943) The properities of human fibrinogen coagulum. J Urol 49:503
Demler JW, Dennis WA, Finlayson B (1983) Bilateral nephrolithiasis. Simultaneous operative management. J Urol 129:263
Dettmar H, Schmitz W (1970) Der Intercostalschnitt als Zugang zur Niere. Urologe [Ausg A] 9:329
Diffay BL, Hall FM, Corfield JR (1976) The 99m Tc-DTPA dynamic renal scan with deconvolution analysis. J Nucl Med 17:352

Djurhuus JC, Stage P (1976) Percutaneous intrapelvic pressure registration in hydronephrosis during diuresis. Acta Chir Scand 472:43
Doppelfeld EL, Weißbach L (1979) Untersuchungen zum Einfluß von Harnabflußstörungen auf die Ergebnisse der katheterlosen seitengetrennten Bestimmung der renalen Hippuran-Clearance. Akt Urol 10:85
Drach GW (1974) Perioperative aspects of renal stone surgery. Urol Clin North Am 1:299
Eckstein HB (1977) Anterior approach. In: Eckstein HB, Hohenfellner R, Williams DI (eds) Surgical Pediatric Urology. Thieme, Stuttgart
Edell S, Zegel H (1978) Ultrasonic evaluation of renal calculi. Am J Roentgenol 130:261
Eisen M, Altrock K, Pixberg HU, Pfannenstiel P (1974) Nierenfunktion nach Ausgußsteinoperation. Helv Chir Acta 41:309
Eisenberg RL, Bank WO, Hedgock MW (1981) Renal failure after angiography can be avoided with hydration. Am J Roentgenol 136:859
Elliot JA (1954) Spontaneous dissolution of renal calculi. J Urol 72:331
Engberg A, Lönnerholm T, Norlén BJ (1976) Repair of renal pelvic defects with a capsular flap. Scand J Urol Nephrol 11:301
Engberg A, Norlén BJ, Källskog Ö, Wollgast M (1983) Pathophysiology of renal ischemia. In: Marberger M, Dreikorn K (eds) Renal Preservation. Williams & Wilkins, Baltimore London
Enlander D, Weber RM, Remedios LV (1974) Renal cortical imaging in 35 patients: superior quality with 99m-Tc-DMSA. J Nucl Med 15:743
Faulconer A, Gaines TR, Grove JS (1946) Atelectasis during operations on the upper urinary tract. Anesthesiology 7:637
Faure G, Sarramons JP (1982) Rapport: La lithiase coralliforme. J Urol Nephrol 88:415
Federle MP, McAninch JW, Kaiser JA, Goodman P, Roberts J, Mall JC (1981) Computed tomography of urinary calculi. Am J Radiol 136:255
Fingerhut A, Marichez PH, Fendler JP, Terville JP, Lesaget F, Pourcher J, Nouailhat F, Ronat R (1982) Les lithiases rénourétérales compliquées de septicémie. J Chir (Paris) 119:23
Finney R (1978) Experience with new double-J ureteral catheter stent. J Urol 120:678
Fischer CP, Sponda LP (1979) Cryoprecipitate, its use and effects in canine coagulum pyelolithotomy. Invest Urol 16:266
Fischer CP, Sonda LP III, Diokno AC (1980) Use of cryoprecipitate coagulum in extracting renal calculi. Urology 15:6
Fischer CP, Sonda LP III, Diokno (1981) Further experience with cryoprecipitate coagulum in renal calculus surgery. A review of 60 cases. J Urol 126:432
Fitzpatrick JM, Sleight MW, Marberger M, Wickham JEA (1980) Intrarenal access: Effects on renal function and morphology. Br J Urol 52:409
Gardiner RA, Naunton-Morgan TC, Whitfield HN, Hendry WF, Wickham JEA (1979) The modified lumbotomy versus the oblique loin incision for renal surgery. Br J Urol 51:256
Gates GF, Green GS (1983) Transient reduction in renal function following arteriography: a radionuclide study. J Urol 129:1107
Georgi M, Marberger M (1976) Möglichkeiten der Stereoangiographie in der Urologie. 27 Verh Ber Dtsch Ges Urol. Springer, Berlin Heidelberg New York, p 299
Georgi P (1982) Nuklearmedizin. In: Hohenfellner R, Zingg EJ (Hrsg) Urologie in Klinik und Praxis Vol I. Thieme, Stuttgart New York
Giacchino JL, Geis WP, Wittenstein BH (1981) Surgery, nutritional support and survival in patients with end-stage renal disease. Arch Surg 116:634
Gibbons RP, Correa RJ, Cummings KB, Mason JT (1976) Experience with indwelling ureteral stent catheters. J Urol 115:22
Gillenwater JY (1979) Hydronephrosis induced changes in renal hemodynamics and function. Cardiovasc Med 4:701
Gil-Vernet JM (1965) New surgical concepts in removing renal calculi. Urol Int 20:255
Gil-Vernet JM (1970) Les voies d'abord du bassient et des calices dans la chirurgie de la lithiase rénale. Editions Medicales Flammarion, Paris
Gil-Vernet JM (1972) Extended pyelolithotomy of staghorn calculus. In: Scott R (ed) Current controversies in urologic management. WB Saunders Co, Philadelphia
Gil-Vernet JM (1977) Minimum nephrostomy. Urology 6:620

Gil-Vernet JM, Caralps A (1979) Indications, surgical techniques, postoperative control and later results of staghorn calculi. In: Porpaczy (ed) Internat Symp Wien 1979. Egermann, Vienna
Gil-Vernet JM, Culla A (1981) Advances in intraoperative renal radiography: 3-dimensional radiography of the kidney. J Urol 125:614
Goldstein AE, Goldstein RB (1968) Management of the diseased solitary kidney. J Urol 90:361
Graves FT (1977) An osteotomy technique in the treatment of staghorn calculus. Eur Urol 3:116
Graves MS (1971) The arterial anatomy of the kidney. The basis of surgical technique. John Wright & Sons LTD. Bristol
Greenberg M, Falkowski WS, Sakowicz BA, Neiman HL, Schaeffer AJ (1982) Use of computerized tomography in evaluation of filling defects of the renal pelvis. J Urol 127:1172
Gregoir W (1975) The avascular nephrotomy. Eur Urol 1:57
Griffith DP, Gibson JR, Clinton C, Musher DM (1978) Acetohydroxamic acid: clinical studies of a urease inhibitor in patients with staghorn renal calculi. J Urol 119:9
Hamburger JG, Richet G, Crosnier J, Funck-Brentano J, Antoine B, Ducrot H, Mery J, De Montera (1966) Nephrologie. Flamarion, Paris
Handley WS (1923) Subcapsular pyelotomy with remarks on the origin and treatment of renal calculi. Proc Soc Med 16:21
Haschek H, Porpaczy P, Schmidt W (1974) Urosepsis bei Urolithiasis. Helv Chir Acta 41:385
Healey GB, Warren MM (1979) Stone formation on polypropylene suture. J Urol 121:836
Heidenreich PB, Egger G, Hör K, Kempken K, Oberdorfer M, Huber H (1976) Klinische Anwendung nuklearmedizinischer Nierenclearance-Meßtechnik: Bestimmung der tubulären, glomerulären und seitengetrennten Nierenclearance im Verlauf von Nierenoperationen. In: Höfer R (ed) Radioaktive Isotope in Klinik und Forschung Bd XII. Urban und Schwarzenberg, München
Heinze HG, Eisenberger F, Pfeifer KJ, Zimmer JM (1977) Wertigkeit der quantitativen Funktionsszintigraphie der Nieren in der Urologie. Fortschr Roe-Str 126:241
Hildreth T, Cass AS (1976) Management of postoperative fistula of upper urinary tract. Urology 7:264
Hinman F, Cattolica EV (1983) Branched calculi: Shapes and operative approaches. J Urol 126:291
Hohenfellner R (1977) The supracostal approach to the kidney. In: Eckstein HB, Hohenfellner R, Williams DI (eds) Surgical Pediatric Urology. Thieme, Stuttgart
Hohenfellner R (1980) Sekundär- und Mehrfacheingriffe an der Niere. Akt Urol 11:123
Hohenfellner R, Marberger M (1977) Renal stones. In: Eckstein HB, Hohenfellner R, Williams DI (eds) Surgical Pediatric Urology. Thieme, Stuttgart
Holm-Nielsen A, Jorgensen T, Mogensen P, Fogh J (1981) The prognostic value of probe renography in ureteric stone obstruction. Br J Urol 53:504
Huland H (1983) Protection of the kidney against temporary ischemia with renin antagonists. In: Marberger M, Dreikorn K (eds) Renal Preservation. Williams & Wilkins, Baltimore London
Hutschenreiter G, Rumpelt HJ, Klippel KF, Hohenfellner R (1978) The free peritoneal transplant as a substitute for the urinary bladder wall. Invest Urol 15:375
James R, Novick AC, Straffon RA, Stewart BH (1980) Anatrophic nephrolithotomy for removal of staghorn or branched renal calculi. Urology 15:108
Janson PA, Jubelirer SJ, Weinstein MJ (1980) Treatment of the bleeding tendency in uremia with cryoprecipitate. N Engl J Med 303:1318
Jeffs RD (1981) Editorial comment: Functional evaluation of the obstructed kidney. J Urol 126:512
Johnston JH (1969) The pathogenesis of hydronephrosis in children. Br J Urol 41:725
Joost J, Skoluda D (1977) Zur Klinik der septischen Niere. 28. Verh Ber Dtsch Ges Urol. Springer, Berlin Heidelberg New York
Kaden W, Born U (1975) Pyelolithotomy using coagulation. Urol Nephrol 68:415
Kalash SS, Young JD, Harne G (1982) Modifications of cryoprecipitate coagulum pyelolithotomy technique. Urology 19:467
Kasike BL, Kjellstrand CM (1983) Perioperative management of patients with chronic renal failure and postoperative acute renal failure. Urol Clin North Am 10:35

Kawamura J, Itoh H, Okada Y, Higashi Y, Yoshida O, Fujita T, Torizuka K (1983) Preoperative and postoperative cortical function of the kidney with staghorn calculi assessed by 99m-technetium-dismercaptosuccinic acid renal scintigraphy. J Urol 130:430

Kerr WS (1954) Effect of complete ureteral obstruction for one week on kidney function. J Appl Physiol 6:762

Kerr WS Jr (1970) Surgical management of renal stones with emphasis on infundibulotomy. J Urol 103:130

Kjellstrand CM, Buselmeier TJ (1972) A simple method for anticoagulation during pre- and postoperative hemodialysis, avoiding rebound phenomena. Surgery 72:630

Klosterhalfen H (1969) Experimentelle Untersuchungen zur Fibrinpyelotomie. Urologe [Ausg A] 8:167

Kofler K, Pum H, Schmidt W (1977) Der septische Schock. 28. Verh Ber Dtsch Ges Urol. Springer, Berlin Heidelberg New York

Kuss R, Camay M, Lassau JP (1970) The evolution of renal function in 166 cases of coralliform calculi in adults. J Urol Nephrol 76:185

Kuss R, Truelle A, Jardin A (1972) Pyelo duodenal fistula. J Urol Nephrol 78:906

Leapman SB, Vidne BA, Butt KMH, Waterhouse K, Kountz SL (1976) Nephrolithiasis and nephrocalcinosis after renal transplantation: A case report and review of the literature. J Urol 115:129

Leusch G (1970) A new radiological technique in renal stone surgery. Urologe [Ausg A] 9:182

Linke CA, Linke CL, Davis RS, Barbaric ZL, Khuri FJ (1978) Anterior transperitoneal approach for treatment of urolithiasis. J Urol 119:453

Lurz H (1956) Ein muskelschonender Lumbalschnitt zur Freilegung der Niere. Chirurg 27:125

Lurz L, Lurz H (1961) Die Eingriffe an den Harnorganen, Nebennieren und männlichen Geschlechtsorganen. In: Guleke N, Zenker R (eds) Allgemeine und spezielle chirurgische Operationslehre. Springer, Berlin Heidelberg New York

Lutzeyer W (1975) Lumbodorsal exploration. In: Glenn JF (ed) Urologic Surgery. Harper & Row, Hagerstown Maryland New York Evanston San Francisco London

Lutzeyer W, Lymberopoulos S, Terhorst B (1979) Operative treatment of renal pelvic calculous casts by dorsal intrasinusal pyelocalicolithotomy in situ. Urol Int 25:224

Lytton B (1979) Surgery of the kidney. In: Campbell (ed) Urology. WB Saunders, Philadelphia London Toronto

Mahmood P, Morales PA (1973) Extended pyelolithotomy (Gil Vernet's pyelotomy). J Urol 109:772

Marberger M (1978) Ischämie und regionale Hypothermie bei Operationen am Nierenparenchym. Steinkopff, Darmstadt

Marberger M (1979) Regionale Kühlung der Niere bei Nierensteinoperationen: wann und weshalb? Akt Urol 10:313

Marberger M (1983) Klinik und operative Therapie der Steinerkrankungen. In: Hohenfellner R, Zingg EJ (eds) Urologie in Klinik und Praxis. Thieme, Stuttgart

Marberger M, Alken P (1979) Fortschritte in der Therapie des Nierenausgußsteines. In: Porpaczy (ed) Internat Symp Wien 1979. Egermann, Vienna

Marberger M, Eisenberger F (1980) Regional hypothermia of the kidney: Surface or transarterial perfusion cooling? J Urol 124:175

Marberger M, Hruby W (1984) Intraoperative roentgenology: The place of the film. In: Wickham JEA (ed) Intrarenal surgery. Churchill, Livingstone Edinburgh London New York

Marberger M, Stackl W (1981) Renal hypothermia in situ. In: Resnick MI (ed) Current Trends in Urology. Williams & Wilkins. Baltimore London

Mardis HK, Hepperlen TW, Kammandel H (1979) Double pigtail ureteral stent. Urology 14:23

Marshall S (1978) Commercial fibrinogen, autogenous plasma, whole blood and cryoprecipitate for coagulum pyelolithotomy: a comparative study. J Urol 119:310

Marshall S, Lyon RP, Scott MP Jr (1978) Further simplifications for coagulum pyelolithotomy. J Urol 119:588

Marx FJ, Hofstetter A, Schilling A (1977) Urosepsis bis septischer Schock: II. Pathophysiologie der Hämostasestörungen. Urologe [Ausg A] 16:241

Mauermeyer W (1969) Nierensteinchirurgie. Habil Schrift TH München

May P (1974) Nierenbeckenkelchausgußsteine. Grenzen der Operabilität. Urologe [Ausg A] 13:244
Mayor G, Zingg E (1973) Urologische Operationen. Thieme, Stuttgart
Mebel M, Brien G, Bick C, Gremske D, Fahlenkamp D, Eger E (1982) Results of surgical and conservative therapy on patients with nephrolithiasis and chronic renal insufficiency. Eur Urol 8:150
Meridies R (1973) Der „Sektionsschnitt" der Niere unter besonderer Berücksichtigung des Einflusses auf die Nierenfunktion und im Vergleich mit anderen Operationsverfahren. Habil Düsseldorf
Metzner PJ, Boyce WH (1971) The staghorn calculus. An immediate indication for nephrolithotomy. Med J Aust 2:1062
Michaelson G (1974) Percutaneous puncture of the renal pelvis, intrapelvic pressure and the concentrating capacity of the kidney in hydronephrosis. Acta Med Scand [Suppl] 559:1
Michalowski E, Modelski W, Kowalski A (1970) The operative treatment of bilateral urinary stones. Urol Nephrol 63:495
Mitcheson HD, Zamenhof RG, Bankoff MS, Prien EL (1983) Determination of the chemical composition of urinary calculi by computerized tomography. J Urol 130:814
Mogensen P, Bay-Niesen H, Egerblad M, Munck O (1976) 131-J-hippuran renography for control of patients with ureterolithiasis. Scand J Urol Nephrol 10:253
Moody TE, Vaughan ED Jr, Gillenwater JY (1975) Relationship between renal blood flow and ureteral pressure during 18 hours of total unilateral ureteral occlusion. Implications for charging sites of increased renal resistance. Invest Urol 13:246
Moores WK, O'Boyle PJ (1976) Staghorn calculi of the kidney. Eur Urol 2:216
Moya-Prats A (1970) Cirugia de los calculos coraliformes. XV. Congrès de la société internationale d'urologie. Tokio
Novick AC (1980) Posterior surgical approach to the kidney and ureter. J Urol 124:192
Nuutinen LS, Kairaluoma M, Tuononen S (1978) The effect of furosemide on renal function in open heart surgery. J Cardiovasc Surg (Torino) 19:471
Oberhausen E (1971) Messung der getrenntseitigen Nierenclearance und der intrarenalen Transportzeit. NUC-Compact 3:51
Ofstad J, Nordahl EH, Gjersvik T (1973) Renal function in patients with unilateral staghorn calculi. Acta Med Scand 194:65
Oosterlinck W, De Sy WA (1983) The value of mannitol volume expansion and diuretics for renal protection during in situ renal surgery. In: Marberger M, Dreikorn K (eds) Renal Preservation. Williams & Wilkins, Baltimore London
Otnes B, Rootwelt K, Mathisen W (1975) A comparison between urography and radioisotope renography in the follow up of surgery for hydronephrosis. Scand J Urol Nephrol 9:50
Pais VM, Spellman RM, Stiles RE, Mahoney SA (1975) Internal ureteral splints. Urology 5:32
Pansadoro V (1983) The posterior lumbotomy. Urol Clin North Am 10:573
Parker RM, Rudd THG, Wonderly RK, Ansell JS (1981) Ureteropelvic junction obstruction in infants and children: Functional evaluation of the obstructed kidney preoperatively and postoperatively. J Urol 126:509
Patel VJ (1973) The coagulum pyelolithotomy. Br J Surg 60:230
Patel VJ (1974) Die Koagulum-Pyelolithotomie. Urologe [Ausg A] 13:168
Pence JR, Airhart RA, Novicki DE, Williams JL, Ehler WJ (1982) Pulmonary emboli associated with coagulum pyelolithotomy. J Urol 127:572
Perry NM, Wickham JEA, Whitfield HN (1980) Hypothermic nephrolithotomy in solitary kidneys. Br J Urol 52:415
Potgieter SV (1959) Atelectasis: Its evolution during upper urinary tract surgery. Br J Anaesth 31:472
Poutasse EF (1961) Anterior approach to upper urinary tract surgery. J Urol 85:199
Presman D (1955) Eleventh intercostal space incision for renal surgery. J Urol 74:578
Proca E (1970) The treatment of bilateral nephrolithiasis associated with chronic renal insufficiency. Chirurgia 19:617
Pyrah LN (1979) Renal calculus. Springer, Berlin Heidelberg New York
Pytel YA, Aslamazov EG, Gogichaev EK (1971) Posterior superotransverse subcortical pyelolithotomy. Khirurgiia (Mosk) 47:144

Rathert P, Lutzeyer W, Durben G, Laval KU (1977) Die septische Niere – eine "Surgical Kidney"? 28. Verh Ber Dtsch Ges Urol. Springer, Berlin Heidelberg New York
Rathore A, Harrison JH (1976) Coagulum pyelolithotomy using autogenous plasma and bovine thrombin. J Urol 116:8
Redman JF, Bissada NK (1976) Extensive nephrolithotomy in previously operated solitary kidneys. J Urol 115:502
Redman JF, Scriber LJ, Bissada NK (1975) The surgical management of the symptomatic solitary caliceal calculus. J Urol 114:175
Rees AJ (1976) Acute renal failure. In: Williams DI, Chisholm GD (eds) Scientific Foundations of Urology. Heinemann, London
Resnick MI, Boyce WH (1980) Bilateral staghorn calculi – patient evaluation and management. J Urol 123:338
Resnick MI, Grayhack JT (1974) Simple and extended pyelolithotomy. Urol Clin North Am 1:319
Resnick MI, Pounds D, Boyce WH (1981) Surgical anatomy of the kidney and its application. Urology 17:367
Riedmiller H, Thüroff J, Alken P, Hutschenreiter G, Hohenfellner R (1981) Gefäß- und Steinlokalisation durch Ultraschall – das Ende von Ischämie und Kühlung in der Nierensteinchirurgie? Akt Urol 12:210
Riedmiller H, Thüroff J, Alken P, Hohenfellner R (1983) Doppler and B-mode ultrasound for avascular nephrotomy. J Urol 130:224
Rocco F (1982) Reanastomosis of the posterior segmental artery. Presentation 7th Meeting European Society of Intrarenal Surgeons. Ghent
Rocco F, Mandressi A, Larcher P (1984) Surgical classification of renal calculi. Eur Urol 10:121
Rommelsheim K, Thelen M, Hack G, Siedeck M (1976) Röntgenologische Lungenveränderungen nach thorakoabdominalen Eingriffen in Seitenlage. Prakt Anästh Wiederbel Intensivmed 11:165
Rommelsheim K, Schäfer R, Biersack HJ (1978) Verteilung der Lungendurchblutung bei Operationen in Seitenlage. Computerszintigraphische Untersuchungen. Prakt Anästh Wiederbel Intensivmed 13:283
Rosenberg JC, Arnstein AR, Ing TS, Pierce JM Jr, Rosenberg B, Silva Y, Walt AJ (1975) Calculi complicating a renal transplant. Am J Surg 129:326
Rous SN, Turner WR (1977) Retrospective study of 95 patients with staghorn calculus disease. J Urol 118:902
Rummelhardt S, Dobrovits G (1974) Fatal complications of renal and ureteral stones. Helv Chir Acta 41:321
Schilling A, Bassermann R, Pratschke E, Rindfleisch GE, Zirkelbach U (1980) Lessening of post ischaemic damage of the microcirculation and protection of nephron structures by blockade of renin-angiotensin system (RAS) Urol Res 8:228
Schlegel JU (1977) Radionuclides in Urology. In: Andersson L, Gittes RF, Goodwin WE, Lutzeyer W, Zingg E (eds) Encyclopedia of Urology. Vol V/1. Suppl Diagnostic Radiology. Springer, Berlin Heidelberg New York
Schneider HJ, Hienzsch E (1975) Welche Bedeutung hat die operative Therapie der Urolithiasis heute? Z Urol 68:547
Schramm M (1980) Lungenkomplikationen nach Nierenoperationen in extremer Seitenlagerung. Inauguraldissertation, Universität Mainz FRG
Schreiter F, Marberger M, Wörsdörfer O (1975) Das chronische pseudozystische Urinextravasat. Akt Urol 6:157
Schweitzer FAW (1973) Intrapelvic pressure and renal function studies in experimental chronic partial ureteric obstruction. Br J Urol 45:2
Schweizer RT, Bartus SA, Graydon RJ, Berlin BB (1977) Pyelolithotomy of a renal transplant. J Urol 117:665
Seddon JM, Bonin RE (1977) Coagulum pyelolithotomy. Urology 9:564
Segal AJ, Spataro RF, Linke CA, Franf IN, Rabinowitz R (1978) Diagnosis of nonopaque calculi by computed tomography. Radiology 129:447
Seidenfeld SM, Luby JP (1982) Urologic sepsis. Urol Clin North Am 9:259

Semb C, Hoeg K, Vogt A (1963) Die Teilresektion der Niere und die Nierenfunktion. Urologe [Ausg A] 2:131
Sherer JF Jr (1980) Cryoprecipitate coagulum pyelolithotomy. J Urol 123:621
Sigel A (1961) Die anatomische Grundlage der partiellen Nephrektomie. Urol Int 11:154
Sigel A (1965) Was ist das renale Minimum? 20. Verh Dtsch Ges Urol. Springer, Berlin Heidelberg New York
Sigel A (1973) Grenzen der Operabilität – Nephrolithiasis. 25. Verh Ber Dtsch Ges Urol. Springer, Berlin Heidelberg New York
Simon G (1870) Exstirpation einer Niere am Menschen. Dtsch Klin 22:137
Singh B, Kim H, Wax SH (1979) Stent versus nephrostomy. J Urol 121:268
Sirotzky L, Lewis EJ (1978) Anaesthesia related muscle paralysis in renal failure. Clin Nephrol 10:38
Smith PJB, Roberts JBM, Dunn M (1978) Coagulum pyelolithotomy. Br J Urol 50:298
Sporer A, Seebode JJ (1981) Study of renal blood supply and its implication in renal pelvis surgery. Urology 17:18
Stackl W, Hofmann E, Marberger M (1983) Is the solitary kidney a privileged kidney? Br J Urol 55:460
Staude G, Stoll W, Schneider H (1980) Nuklearmedizinische Funktionskontrollen nach Quer- und Längsnephrotomie bei Korallenausgußsteinen der Niere. Urol Nephrol 73:865
Stecker JF Jr (1978) Functional and metabolic alternatives in the hydronephrotic kidney. In: Devine CH Jr, Stecker JF Jr (eds) Urology in Practice. Little, Brown & Co, Boston USA
Stephenson TP, Bauer S, Hargreave TB, Warwick RT (1975) The technique and results of pyelocalycotomy for staghorn calculi. Br J Urol 47:751
Streenevasan G (1974) Bilateral renal calculi. Ann R Coll Surg Engl 55:13
Sutherland JW (1982) Recurrence following operative treatment of upper urinary tract stone. J Urol 127:472
Surraco L (1939) L'extraction des gros calculus du rein: pyélotomie postérieure étendue pelvicaliculaire. J Urol (Paris) 48:217
Svanberg L (1957) Influence of posture on the lung volumes and circulation in normals. Scand J Clin Lab Invest 9:25
Swartz RD, Rubin JE, Leeming BW, Silva P (1978) Renal failure following major angiography. Am J Med 65:31
Tasker PRN, Mac Gregor GA, De-Wardener HE (1974) Prophylactic use of intravenous saline in patients with chronic renal failure undergoing major surgery. Lancet II:912
Thompson IM, Baker J, Robbards WL Jr, Kovacsi L, Ross G Jr (1969) Clinical experience with renal capsula flappyeloplasty. J Urol 101:487
Thüroff JW, Hutschenreiter G, Frohneberg D, Hohenfellner R (1980) Das freie Peritoneallappentransplantat in der Chirurgie des Nierenbeckens und Ureters. Akt Urol 11:189
Thüroff JW, Frohneberg D, Riedmiller R, Alken P, Hutschenreiter G, Hohenfellner R (1982) Localization of segmental arteries in renal surgery by Doppler sonography. J Urol 127:863
Truesdale BH, Rous SN, Nelson RP (1977) Perinephric abscess: A review of 26 cases. J Urol 118:910
Turner-Warwick RT (1963) The supracostal approach to the renal area. Br J Urol 37:671
Turner-Warwick R (1976) The use of the omental pedicle graft in urinary tract reconstruction. J Urol 116:341
Ueda T, Momose S (1982) Modified inferior pyelocalicotomy for staghorn calculi and multiple stones: The use of pedical clamp and fibrin coagulum. Urol Int 37:49
Ueno A, Kawamura T, Ogawa A, Takayasu H (1977) Relation of spontaneous passage of ureteric calculi to size. Urology 10:544
Vahlensieck W (1985) Diagnosis of urinary calculi. In: Schneider H-J (Ed) Urolithiasis: Etiology, Diagnosis. Springer, Berlin Heidelberg New York Tokyo (Handbook of urology, Vol. 17/II, p 335–424)
Vargas AD, Bragin SD, Mendez R (1982) Staghorn calculus: Its clinical presentation, complications, and management. J Urol 127:860
Vaughan ED Jr, Gillenwater JY (1971) Recovery following complete chronic unilateral occlusion: Functional radiographic and pathologic alterations. J Urol 106:27

Walker RD, Richard GA, Bueschen AJ, Retik AB (1980) Pathophysiology and recoveribility of function and structure in obstructed kidneys. Urol Clin North Am 7:291
Walsh A (1969) Néphrocalcinose sur rein greffé. J Urol Nephrol [Suppl] 12 75:244
Walz PH, Riedmiller H, Alken P, Hutschenreiter G (1981) Technik und Fehlermöglichkeiten der perkutanen Nephrostomie unter sonographischer Kontrolle. Akt Urol 12:232
Walz PH, Klose K, Goldmann F, Evers E, Alken P (1981) Kontrastmittelabhängige Dichteveränderungen gesunder und geschädigter Nieren in der Sequenz-Computertomographie. Akt Urol 13:33
Walz PH, Klose K, Weimer G, Alken P, Thelen M, Hohenfellner R (1982) Nachweis der normalen und geschädigten Tubulusfunktion mit o-Jod-Hippuran in der Sequenz-CT. Akt Urol 13:311
Ward JP, Smart CJ, O'Donoghue EPN, Wickham JEA (1976) Synchronous bilateral lumbotomy. Eur Urol 2:102
Whitfield HN, Britton KE, Nimmon CC, Hendry WF, Wallace DMA, Wickham JEA (1981) Renal transit time measurements in the diagnosis of ureteric obstruction. Br J Urol 53:500
Wickham JEA (1979) Urinary calculous disease. Churchill, Livingstone Edinburgh London New York
Wickham JEA (1980) Personal Communication
Wickham JEA, Coe N, Ward JP (1974) One hundred cases of nephrolithotomy under hypothermia. J Urol 112:702
Wickham JEA, Fry IK, Wallace DMA (1980) Computerized tomography location of intrarenal calculi prior to nephrolithotomy. Br J Urol 52:422
Wiehle SP, Banowsky LH, Nicastro-Lutton JJ, Radwin HM, Chauvenet PH (1981) Pretransplant bilateral nephrectomy and adjuvant operations. Urology 13:349
Williams RE (1963) Long term survey of 538 patients with upper urinary tract stone. Br J Urol 35:416
Williams R (1972) The results of conservative surgery for stone. Br J Urol 44:292
Wilson DR (1977) Renal function during and following obstruction. Am Rev Med 28:329
Wilson RT, Soullier G, Antonenko D (1979) Creatinine clearance in critically ill surgical patients. Arch Surg 114:461
Witherow RON, Wickham JEA (1980) Nephrolithotomy in chronic renal failure: Saved from dialysis. Br J Urol 52:419
Wojewski A, Zajaczovski T (1973) The treatment of bilateral staghornstones of the kidneys. Int Urol Nephrol 5:249
Woodhouse CRJ, Farrell CR, Paris AMI, Blandy JP (1981) The place of extended pyelolithotomy (Gil-Vernet operation) in the management of renal staghorn calculi. Br J Urol 53:520
Yokoyama M, Watanabe K, Inatsuki S, Ochi K, Takeuchi M (1982) Computerized tomography of the kidney: Tissue–plasma ratio of contrast enhancement with bolus injection and renal function. J Urol 127:721
Wulfsohn MA (1981) Extended pyelolithotomy: The use of renal artery clamping and regional hypothermia. J Urol 125:467
Young LS (1979) Gram-negative sepsis. In: Mandel G, Douglas RG, Bennet JE (eds) Principles and Practice of Infectious Diseases. John Wiley & Sons, New York
Young SW, Noon MA, Marincek B (1981) Dynamic computed tomography time density study of normal human tissue after intravenous contrast administration. Invest Radiol 16:36
Zimskind PD, Fetter TR, Wilkerson JL (1967) Clinical use of long-term indwelling silicone rubber ureteral splints inserted cystoscopically. J Urol 97:840
Zingg EJ, Futterlieb A (1980) Nephroscopy in stone surgery. Br J Urol 52:333
Zoedler D (1974) Intra- und posteropative Komplikationen der Nephrolithiasis. Helv Chir Acta 41:299

Ischemia and Regional Hypothermia in Renal Stone Surgery

H.-J. SCHNEIDER

I. Introduction

The aim of renal stone surgery must be the complete clerance of all calculous material. Residual stones grow, provoke the formation of new calculi and hinder the resolution of pyelonephritis. An attempt should always first be made to extract the stones through a pyelotomy or an extended intrasinusal pyelocalycotomy. Nevertheless, it is often impossible to avoid extensive or multiple incision of the parenchyma and this inevitably entails ischemia: a bloodless surgical field is the sine qua non for the complete retrieval and extraction of calculi. However, if ischemia is extended beyond 20 or maximally 30 minutes, there will be loss of renal function of varying severity postoperatively, occasionally even renal atrophy. Retarding renal metabolism, either by pharmacologically active substances or by hypothermia, is a safe way to prolong renal ischemia time.

An alternative and elegant technique of avascular transparenchymal approach is described in detail in the chapter on "Radial Nephrolithotomy Under Ultrasound and Doppler Probe Control". Stones are located by ultrasound examination of the exposed kidney and major vessels detected by Doppler probe. The nephrotomy may then so placed as to give direct access to the stone through tissue of low vascularity.

Because of its technical simplicity and guaranteed absence of bleeding renal ischemia with hypothermia has nowadays become the technique of choice.

If one assumes a future situation in which extracorporeal shockwave lithotripsy (ESWL) is available on demand (chapter "Extracorporeal Shockwave Lithotripsy (ESWL) in the Treatment of Kidney and Ureter Stones") and in which liberal use is made of percutaneous nephrolithotripsy, nephrolitholapaxy (chapter "Percutaneous Manipulation of Renal Calculi") and of ureterorenoscopy (chapter "The Instrumentation and Surgery of Ureteric Calculi"), only 10% of the renal and ureteric stones nowadays coming to surgery should still require an open approach. One may reasonably speculate that these will principally be complicated calculi. In the University Urological Clinic, Mainz (FRG), for example, the number of staghorn calculi coming to surgery has not yet been reduced by the advent of ESWL and of the percutaneous technique (HOHENFELLNER 1985).

II. Renal Ischemia

As a rule ischemia of the entire kidney is achieved by clamping the renal pedicle or the main renal artery. A variety of clamps may be used, any of which must meet the following requirements:
1. Secure occlusion of the vessel
2. No slipping during surgery
3. No hampering of the operator
4. Atraumatic action to spare the vessel wall

Occlusion of the renal artery alone results in better postoperative function than does clamping the entire pedicle. Even worse ischemia tolerance results from incomplete arterial occlusion and venous engorgement with hemorrhagic infarction of the parenchyma. It is thus of special importance that clamps be applied to the renal pedicle under meticulous direct visual control.

One problem of isolated arterial occlusion lies in venous bleeding if large vessels are opened in the hilus or if caval pressure is allowed to rise (e.g. during coughing). Even if suitable clamps are applied correctly, mechanical irritation of the vessel wall may still occur. Intraluminal balloon occlusion of the renal artery is less traumatic and may be achieved with a Swan-Ganz balloon-tip floatation catheter. The catheter is introduced through the femoral artery by the Seldinger technique and advanced up to the renal arterial orifice. Elastic occlusion of the artery is then brought about by inflating the balloon.

According to the clinical and experimental studies of MARBERGER (1978) substantially less vascular damage follows on balloon occlusion than on the use clamps or tourniquets with rubber slings. For solitary stones not requiring extensive nephrotomy there is much to be said for dissecting out and clamping individual segmental arteries.

III. Drug-Mediated Prolongation of Renal Ischemia Tolerance

However great the advantages of a bloodless field for the retrieval and clearance of calculi, there is nevertheless a price to be paid in loss of function after prolonged ischemia.

Short periods of ischemia are best tolerated if diuresis is maximal at the moment the circulation is interrupted. For this reason EISENBERGER et al. (1977) recommend giving 1500 ml of saline 12 hours preoperatively and maintaining full hydration throughout the procedure. Another valuable maneuver to cover short term ischemia is the infusion of hypertonic mannitol solution. 0.2 to 0.4 g mannitol per kg body weight should be given rapidly, immediately before and after ischemia. In this way ischemia times of up to 30 minutes are well tolerated. Once again, the beneficial effect rests on more rapid restoration of normal microperfusion after ischemia (MARBERGER 1978).

A detailed description of the mode of action and clinical administration of mannitol and diuretics for renal protection during in situ surgery may be found in OOSTERLINCK and DESY (1983).

Of the wide variety of pharmacological substances employed to extend renal ischemia time only inosine (FITZPATRICK and WICKHAM 1983; WICKHAM et al. 1981; FITZPATRICK et al. 1981; MARBERGER et al. 1978) has achieved some importance. After occlusion 30–60 mg of inosine are injected intraarterially distal to the clamp. Mean ischemia time was 52 minutes (25–94 minutes). With ischemia of less than 60 minutes duration there was no postoperative loss of renal function. Inosine is unable to protect the kidney for longer periods of ischemia than this.

In animal experiments a useful improvement in renal ischemia tolerance can be demonstrated after administration of an ATP-$MgCl_2$ complex (LYTTON and HERTER 1983). So far no clinical data are to hand.

IV. Increasing Ischemia Tolerance by Hypothermia

As the temperature of the kidney falls so does its metabolic activity and oxygen consumption. Numerous animal experiments have been conducted to establish optimal parameters for renal ischemia protection by hypothermia. By 1974 there were reports on over 1000 kidney operations conducted under hypothermia (MARBERGER 1978).

A wide variety of temperatures are quoted as giving the best protection from ischemia during in situ surgery to the renal parenchyma, ranging from 10 to 25 °C (WICKHAM 1979). A series of critical experiments by WARD (1975) established 15 °C as the ideal renal temperature: if the kidney was cooled either to 22 °C or to 10 °C, post-ischemic renal function was 20% poorer than after cooling to 15 °C. For ischemia times up to 2 hours renal cooling to 18–25 °C is adequate (MARBERGER et al. 1976). In the presence of previous parenchymal damage or active pyelonephritis the kidney exhibits increased sensitivity to ischemia.

The following cooling techniques are variously employed. Since regional cooling of the kidney is simpler, more effective and less invasive for the patient, *whole body hypothermia* is now rarely used.

The method most commonly adopted is *surface cooling* with soft ice by the technique of METZNER and BOYCE (1972). Electrolyte solutions are sterilized in double plastic bags and frozen down to so-called soft ice. Once the kidney is fully exposed, the sterile inner bags are so packed around the kidney as to leave only the site of the incision exposed. The temperature of the kidney falls gradually and takes about 30 minutes to reach 15 °C. Disadvantages of this method include the bags getting in the surgeon's way, differential cooling of cortex and medulla and the need to remove the ice packs during radiological procedures.

Immersion cooling according to GRAVES (1963) (Fig. 1) involves sliding a plastic sleeve over the kidney and securing it around the pedicle with a rubber band. The space between bag and kidney is perfused with acqueous glycerine solution at −10 °C to achieve a renal temperature around 17 °C within 5–8 minutes. One disadvantage of this technique is the rapid warming of the kidney once the system is removed.

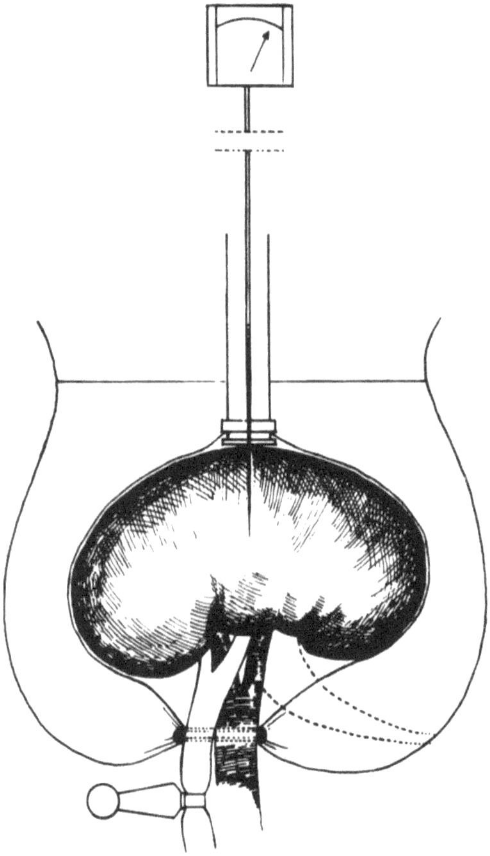

Fig. 1. Technique of immersion cooling of kidney with invaginated vinyl bag filled with liquid coolant (From MARBERGER 1983)

The application of *external cooling devices* in the form of cooling sleeves or coils (WICKHAM 1979) (Fig. 2) simplifies renal cooling, because the cooling medium remains within the system. The disadvantage of this technique is the requirement to interrupt the operation for further cooling as gradual warming of the kidney ensues during protracted surgery.

Perfusion cooling via the *pelvicalyceal system* is the simple technique devised by JONES and POLITANO in 1963. Following clamping of the renal artery a No. 7 PVC catheter is inserted into the renal pelvis, sealed and perfused under gravity with saline at 4 °C. Drainage is via the ureter and an indwelling bladder catheter. Depending on the thickness of the parenchyma and on the site of obstructing calyceal stones, however, cooling is extremely uneven and has anyway to be interrupted once the pelvicalyceal system has been opened.

More effective cooling can be achieved by *retrograde perfusion through the renal vein* (WILHELM et al. 1978). For this purpose the renal vein is intubated with a double lumen catheter and perfused under gravity with 140 cm water pressure.

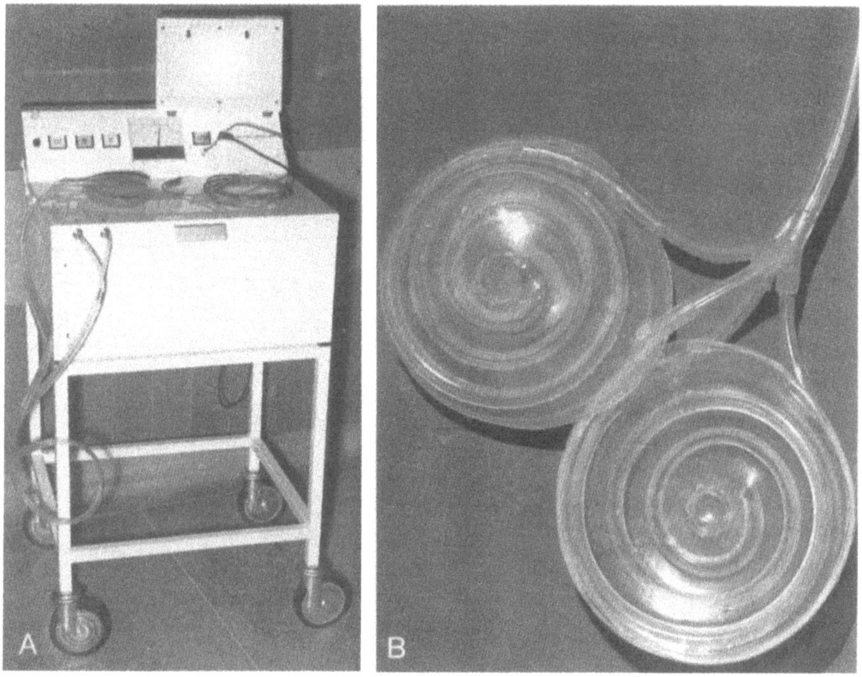

Fig. 2. Renal hypothermia unit for surface cooling after Wickham (From MARBERGER 1983)

The most effective technique is undoubtedly *transarterial perfusion cooling* of the kidney, especially since it gives very even cooling of the entire parenchyma (Fig. 3). The renal artery is punctured distal to the clamp with a thin catheter or a cranked needle (Fig. 4). The kidney is then perfused with Ringer-lactate or dextran solution at 4–8 °C, the correct temperature being achieved after about 10 minutes. Papaverine is added to prevent vasospasm. The principal problem of this technique lies in the need for frequently difficult arterial puncture. A *percutaneous approach* by the Seldinger technique avoids this difficulty (EISENBERGER et al. 1973). However, the renal vessels still need to be dissected out for application of an occlusive tourniquet. This can be avoided by balloon occlusion with simultaneous perfusion cooling after MARBERGER (1978) (Fig. 5).

The Swan-Ganz catheter already described provides secure occlusion of the renal artery whilst allowing perfusion at 40–50 ml/minute. After 7–10 minutes a uniform renal temperature is achieved of 15–20 °C. However, the technique cannot be used in kidneys with accessory arteries and the surgeon must therefore be conversant with a variety of cooling techniques.

The perfusion fluid drains via the veins into the rest of the body. For prolonged periods of ischemia (over 2 hours) external drainage should be provided via a puncture of the renal vein or, on the left, of the spermatic vein.

Since the introduction of regional renal hypothermia there has been a marked improvement in the recovery of renal function to be expected following surgery. The benefit is especially marked for the more complicated stones.

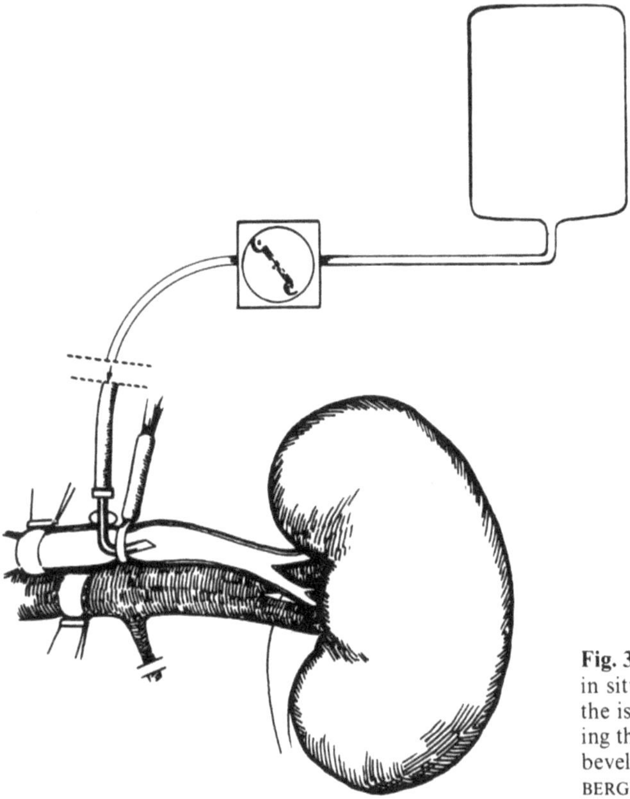

Fig. 3. Gil Vernet technique of in situ hypothermic perfusion of the ischemic kidney by cannulating the renal artery with a curved bevelled needle (From MARBERGER 1983)

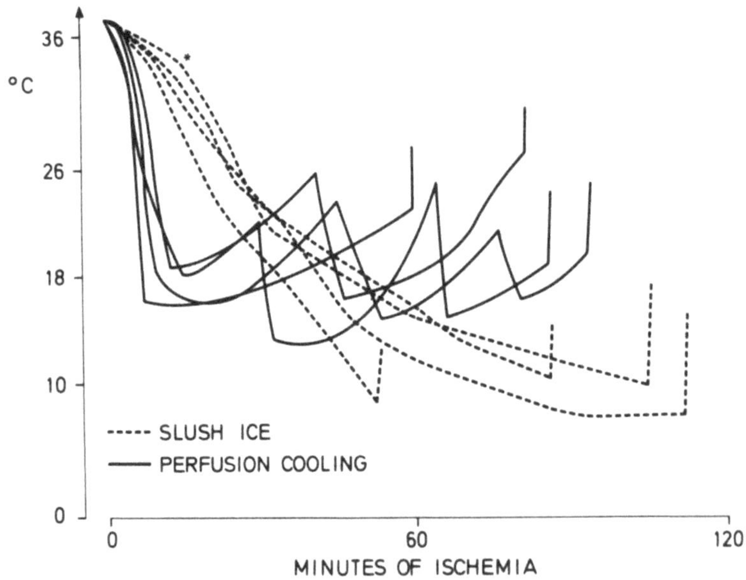

Fig. 4. Core temperature of kidneys during extended nephrolithotomies in ischemia and hypothermia by surface cooling with "soft" ice or transarterial perfusion cooling (From MARBERGER 1983)

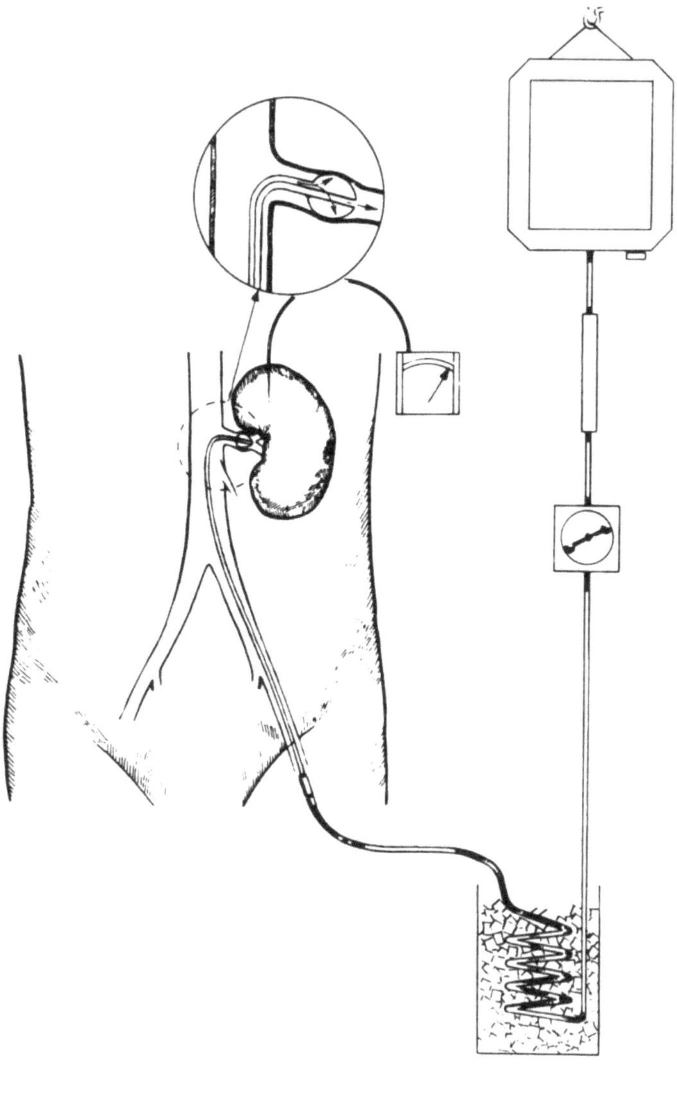

Fig. 5. Technique of simultaneous balloon occlusion of the renal artery and hypothermic perfusion of the ischemic kidney with a double-lumen catheter (From MARBERGER 1983)

References

Eisenberger F, Schmiedt E, Pfeifer KJ, Chaussy Ch, Rother R, Klein V, Riedl P (1973) In situ Perfusion und Kühlung der Niere bei Ausgußsteinen. MMW 115:404–408

Eisenberger F, Marx FJ, Schmiedt E (1977) Die transfemorale Kanülierung der Nierengefäße. Diagnostisch-therapeutische Anwendungsmöglichkeiten bei urologischen Erkrankungen. Urologe [Ausg A] 16:1–5

Fitzpatrik JM, Wickham JEA (1983) Protection of function by inosine during ischemic renal surgery. In: Marberger M, Dreikorn K (Hrsg) Renal preservation. Int Perspectives in Urology, Vol 8. Williams and Wilkins, Baltimore London, p 64–79

Fitzpatrick JM, Wallace DMA, Whitfield HN, Watkinson LE, Fernando AR, Wicktom JEA (1981) Inosine in ischaemic renal surgery: long-term follow-up. Br J Urol 53:524–527
Graves FT (1963) Regional hypothermia: an aid to partial nephrectomy. Brit J Surg 50:362–365
Hohenfellner R, Alken P, Thüroff J (1985) Derzeitige Strategie bei Ausgußstein-Therapie mit offenchirurgischen Methoden, perkutane Techniken, ESWL und deren Grenzen. 8. Internationales Symposium des Ludwig-Boltzmann-Instituts, Wien
Jones WR, Politano V (1957) The effects of renal artery occlusion on renal function under normothermic and regional hypothermia. J Urol 77:19–22
Lytton B, Herter GE (1983) The effects of ATP-$MgCl_2$ complex on ischemic renal injury. In: Marberger M, Dreikorn K (Hrsg) Renal preservation. Int Perspectives in Urology, Vol 8. Williams and Wilkins, Baltimore London, p 95–108
Marberger M (1978) Ischämie und regionale Hypothermie bei Operationen am Nierenparenchym. Fortschritte der Urologie und Nephrologie, Bd 10. Steinkopff, Darmstadt
Marberger M (1983) In situ cooling of the kidney. In: Marberger M, Dreikorn K (Hrsg) Renal preservation. Int Perspectives in Urology, Vol 8. Williams and Wilkins, Baltimore London, p 38–63
Marberger M, Günther R, Mayer EJ, Wiestler M (1976) A simple method for in situ preservation of the ischemic kidney during renal surgery. Invest Urol 14:191–196
Marberger M, Georgi M, Günther R, Hohenfellner R (1978) Simultaneous balloon occlusion of the renal artery and hypothermic perfusion in in situ surgery of the kidney. J Urol 119:463–466
Marberger M, Günther R, Alken P, Rumpf W, Ranc M (1980) Inosine: alternative or adjunct to regional hypothermia in the prevention of post-ischemic renal failure? Eur Urol 6:95–102
Metzner JP, Boyce WH (1972) Simplified renal hypothermia: an adjunct to conservative renal surgery. Br J Urol 44:76–80
Oosterlinck W, DeSy WA (1983) The value of mannitol volume expansion and diuretics for renal protection during in situ renal surgery. In: Marberger M, Dreikorn K (Hrsg) Renal preservation. Int Perspectives in Urology, Vol 8. Williams and Wilkins, Baltimore London, p 109–118
Ward JP (1975) Determination of optimum temperature for regional renal hypothermia during temporary renal ischaemia. Brit J Urol 47:17–22
Wickham JEA (1979) The surgical treatment of renal lithiasis. In: Wickham JEA (ed) Urinary calculous disease. Churchill, Livingston Edinburgh
Wickham JEA, Fernando AR, Hendry WF, Whitfield HN, Fitzpatrick JM (1979) Intravenous inosine for ischaemic renal surgery. Br J Urol 51:439–442
Wilhelm E, Schrott KM, Krönert E, Sigel A, Schwille PO (1978) Transvenous perfusion cooling of the kidney. A new technique of local renal hypothermia. Invest Urol 16:87–91
Zechner O (1985) Die anatrophen Nephrolithotomien: Indikationen, Technik und Komplikationen. 8. Internationales Symposium des Ludwig-Boltzmann-Instituts, Wien

Radial Nephrolithotomy Under Ultrasound and Doppler Probe Control

P. ALKEN

I. Introduction

The operative treatment of urolithiasis is undergoing a process of great change. A variety of invasive and noninvasive techniques such as ureterorenoscopy (REUTER and REUTER 1983), percutaneous nephrolithotomy (ALKEN 1984) and extracorporeal shock-wave lithotripsy (CHAUSSY et al. 1984) are currently displacing classical operation. However, neither of the two latter techniques in particular has so far become the treatment of choice for large staghorn calculi, the percutaneous approach being time consuming and associated with a high incidence of residual calculi. Despite extensive overall experience in some 1000 cases (CHAUSSY et al. 1984), shock-wave therapy has, similarly, not yet been applied to a sufficient number of staghorn stones to establish its role. It is nevertheless to be expected that some combination of shock-wave therapy and percutaneous nephrolithotomy will prove suitable for the treatment of at least part of these cases.

In the meantime, however, the classical staghorn (always a source of great operative difficulty) continues to require an open surgical approach. The same will be true of cases where an upper tract stenosis, either congenital or acquired through past surgery or inflammation, needs to be corrected at the same time as the calculi are removed.

The surgery of staghorn calculi has also undergone radical change. New techniques have been developed in pursuance of two principal aims: minimisation of residual stones and conservation of functioning parenchyma. These aims have been achieved by following anatomically preferred planes of section and by the introduction of a variety of technical aids, ranging from improving renal ischemia time to location of calculi by various radiologic techniques or by intraoperative endoscopy. The principal approaches through the exposed kidney were all described some time ago:

1. The approach of GIL-VERNET (pyelocalycotomy, 1965), of which the underlying principle is to dissect along the collecting system up to its junction with the renal parenchyma high in the renal sinus. Staghorn calculi may thus be removed without transparenchymal surgery (see chapter on "Surgical Treatment of Renal Calculi").

2. Longitudinal anatrophic nephrolithotomy (SMITH and BOYCE 1967), a technique involving a preferred approach along the hypovascular boundary between anterior and posterior segments of the kidney. Wide exposure of the collecting system is thus achieved.

Table 1. Outcome of various forms of operative treatment for staghorn calculi

Author	Year	n	Technique	Residual stone rate	post-operative nephrectomy	Late results free of infection	Late results nephrectomy	Late results function
WICKHAM	1982	250	radial nephrotomy and pyelocalycotomy	14% [a]	3	74%	3	no significant change
GIL-VERNET	1983	328	pyelolithotomy (236) + nephrolithotomy (86) extracorporeal surgery (6)	8%	0	81%	11	81% stable or improved
BOYCE	1983	1065	anatrophic nephrolithotomy	20.5% [b]	0	62%	0	?

[a] WICKHAM 1984
[b] papillary or parenchymal calcification

3. Radial nephrotomy (WICKHAM et al. 1974). Short incisions on the dorsal or ventral aspect of the kidney, parallel to the interlobular arteries, allow a transparenchymal approach to one calyx at a time. This procedure is usually combined with pyelocalycotomy.

A glance at publications from the protagonists of each technique (GIL-VERNET 1983; BOYCE 1983; WICKHAM 1982) would seem to suggest that their methods yield similar results (Table 1). It is worth remembering that each of these authors has accumulated many years of experience in his technique, one possible reason for this apparent equivalence. The less practiced surgeon will have to chose the technique he finds easiest and which yields the best results in his hands. There can be no doubt that pyelocalycotomy is the least traumatic procedure for the kidney, but a survey of 1,642 operations by surgeons using a variety of techniques shows that pyelocalycotomy had to be combined with nephrotomy (in 40%) for complete stone removal. Longitudinal nephrotomy was undertaken in only 16% of cases (Table 2). Our own experience of nephrolithotomy under ultrasound control suggests that the indications for anatrophic nephrotomy can be restricted still further.

II. Preoperative Investigation

No special preoperative investigations are required. Plain tomography or possibly CT will improve preoperative documentation of weakly opaque calculi.

Table 2. Frequency of different surgical techniques for removal of staghorn stones

Author	Year	n	Pyelocali-cotomy	Pyelocali-cotomy and Nephro-lithotomy	Nephro-lithotomy	Partial resection
Rous	1977	28	19 (68%)	4 (14%)	3 (11%)	2 (7%)
Constantinopel	1979	24	17 (70%)	4 (17%)	3 (13%)	–
Bueschen	1980	22	8 (36%)	7 (32%)	4 (18%)	3 (14%)
Beurton	1981	56	12 (21%)	26 (47%)	18 (32%)	–
Stage	1981	12	4 (33%)	2 (17%)	6 (50%)	–
Egger	1982	85	49 (58%)	30 (35%)	–	6 (7%)
Vargas	1982	52	21 (40%)	14 (27%)	12 (23%)	5 (10%)
Faure	1982	1363	470 (34%)	565 (42%)	219 (16%)	109 (8%)
		1642	600 (36%)	652 (40%)	265 (16%)	125 (8%)

Split isotope renal function studies also provide a useful preoperative baseline. Renal angiography is unnecessary, even for renal malformations or where there has been previous renal surgery.

III. Apparatus

A real time scanner and a Doppler ultrasound unit must be available for intraoperative use. The frequency range of the probes should be chosen to permit good imaging at distances of 0–6 cm on the real time scanner and to prevent penetration by the Doppler probe beyond 2–3 cm. The use of probes having these characteristics will ensure the most accurate detection of calculi and a proper identification of vessels within the area of the nephrotomy.

1. Doppler Probe

A simple nondirectional unit is quite adequate for intraoperative use, i.e. one without measurement of flow rate or direction. Waves emitted by the output transducer will be frequency shifted as they are reflected by blood flowing through the ultrasound beam. This frequency shifted signal will be picked up by the receiving transducer and the difference between transmitter and receiver frequencies rendered audible as a rushing noise. Since this difference is directly proportional to the rate of flow, arteries may be identified by a high pitched pulsatile signal, whereas veins will give rise to a steadier lower pitched rumble. The depth of penetration of the Doppler signal is inversely proportional to frequency. 7–10 MHz probes yield the best results in the kidney. There is of course no fundamental reason why directional Doppler units cannot be used, allowing measurement of the direction of flow. The combination of a pulse-modulated Doppler probe with a B-scanner allows Doppler confirmation that structures previously identified as vessels on the B-scan are just that. In view of the extremely high price of this equipment, however, its application to renal surgery is only justifiable where it is already available within the hospital or clinic.

2. The B-Scanner

Calculi can be detected within the collecting system even with relatively simple equipment, since the requirements of grey-scale separation or variable depth of penetration are not particularly stringent. It is of far greater importance that the actual scanning head be of small enough physical dimensions and contact surface to permit convenient application to the exposed kidney. Good imaging should be available to a depth of 5 cm. As with Doppler units, the depth of penetration is inversely proportional and resolving power and quality of near image are directly proportional to frequency. A unit operating at 8 MHz will thus provide the optimum results. In the immediate near field directly beneath the head itself the area of tissue imaged will correspond to the size of window in the tip of the head. Depending on the characteristics of the head used, deeper penetration is associated with a fanning out of the beam to include larger volumes of tissue. Current equipment, however, only permits examination of a fairly localized region of the kidney and, since the whole kidney can never be shown at any one time, is inherently incapable of proving the kidney entirely stone free.

At present a variety of instruments are commercially available for intraoperative applications. Some are specifically designed for this purpose, whilst others comprise special scanning heads for intraoperative use of equipment normally used for external scanning. The choice between linear array or sector scanning equipment is of no importance for intraoperative applications. The final decision is therefore likely to revolve around the equipment already available and the rate of use of individual instruments.

IV. Practical Application

1. Sterilization

Ultrasound probes and cables suitable for gas sterilization are to be preferred, because they are more convenient to use. It must, however, be born in mind that gas sterilization involves deaeration times of up to 24 hrs, depending on the equipment, and these must be adhered to. Thus an individual probe can only be used every other day. This problem is frequently got over by enclosing the entire probe and its cables in suitable sterile disposable plastic sleeves containg water or ultrasound coupling jelly.

2. Exposing the Kidney

In cases where nephrolithotomy was decided on preoperatively, e.g. of solitary calyceal stone, the kidney need only be exposed to permit adequate access to the affected area. Only where stone fragments are expected to pass down into the centre of the collecting system is it necessary to expose the renal pelvis and sling the ureter. The hilar vessels are left undissected and the pedicle is only defined to the extent required to permit mobilization of the kidney. Where the need for nephrolithomy first arises intraoperatively from the incomplete removal of a staghorn by pyelocalycotomy, the kidney usually needs to be completely mobilized.

3. Intraoperative Ultrasonography

If pyelocalycotomy yields a bulk of stone material clearly less than that seen on the preoperative plain film, the presence of residual calculi within the calyces must be suspected. An initial intraoperative X-ray film will give an overall view of the removability of further material via the collecting system and suggest ultrasonography of specific regions of the kidney. Particularly where numerous calculi remain in the collecting system, the area of parenchyma containing the largest stone should be selected for the first nephrotomy. The dilatation of the collecting system by this calculus may then permit further direct inspection of other stone bearing segments, perhaps obviating further nephrotomies. The ultrasound scanner is next applied to the chosen area. No special coupling media are required, blood and exsudate on the surface of the kidney ensuring adequate contact between probe and kidney. Submersion of the kidney in warm saline (SIGEL 1982) to provide improved coupling is unnecessary and indeed impedes subsequent exact siting of the nephrotomy.

Two characteristics of calculi identify them on the scan image (Figs. 1, 2): The highly echogenic surface of the stone appears as an area of white, depending on the dimensions of the stone, ranging from a small oval reflection (small calculi) to large white bands (large stones). The extensive reflection and ab-

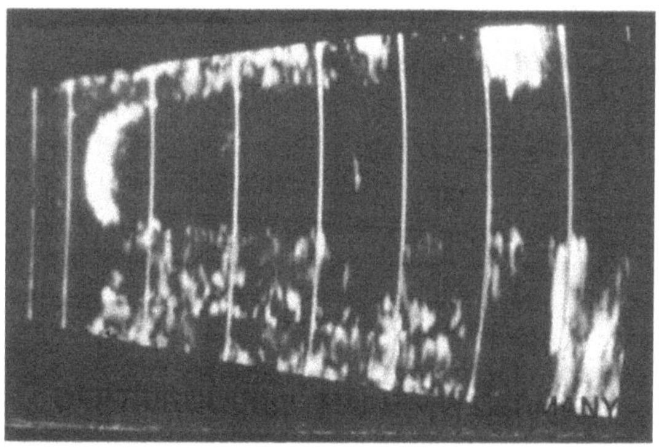

Fig. 1. B-scan image of a renal calculus. Kidney surface shown on the left. Scale divisions 5 mm

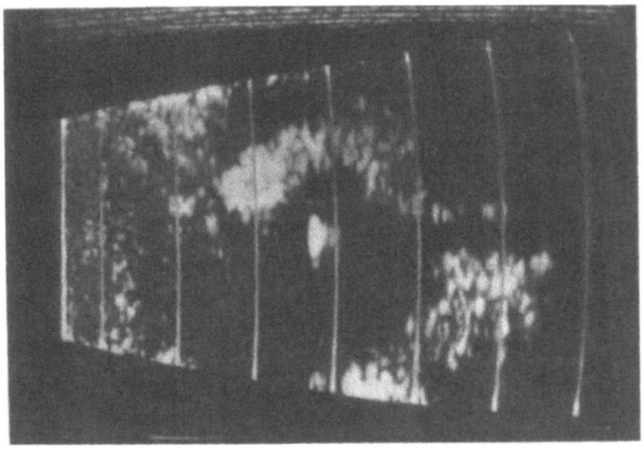

Fig. 2. B-scan image of a small calyceal stone. Stone appears as a bright spot with an acoustic shadow

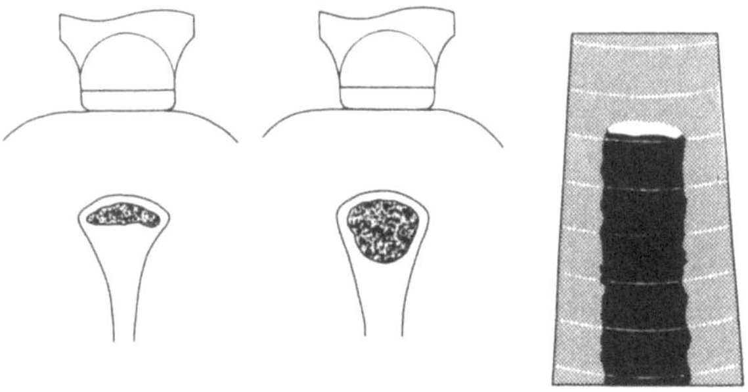

Fig. 3. Schematic drawing of both large and discoid calyceal stones, as seen by the B-scan

sorption of ultrasound waves by the stone gives rise to the second characteristic appearance, that of a dark shadow region beyond the calculus, in which no further structures can be detected. Since the image is derived mainly from the surface of the stone, its complete extent may not be shown. A flat discoid calculus may, depending on the direction of the beam, take on the same appearance as a large and bulky one (Fig. 3).

4. Limitations of B-Scanning

a) Stone Surface and Density

Smooth surfaced stones provide for optimal reflection of ultrasound waves with corresponding image quality. Stones of very small size or irregular surface scatter sound waves and the typical brilliant image becomes blurred, fewer waves being echoed straight back at the scanner to contribute to image build-up. In particular small loose nests of stones deep in the calyces are often not detected with the usual clarity and may be difficult to distinguish from surrounding tissue. A thickened calyceal wall may even yield more brilliant echoes than the calculous material itself. Two techniques can be employed to clarify doubtful

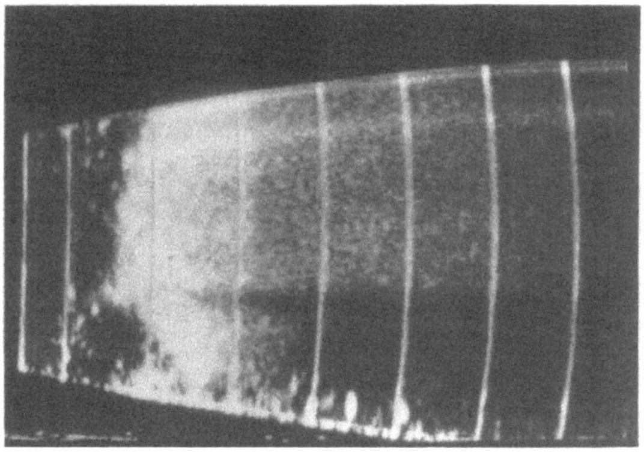

Fig. 4. B-scan appearance of an air-filled calyx, showing a diffuse echo pattern

cases: Reducing the sensitivity of the instrument decreases or even suppresses echoes from surrounding tissue, whereas the echo from the stone will persist. Fine needle puncture of the suspicuous area under ultrasound control will allow the needle tip to be observed along its track toward the putative stone. If the latter moves within the image as the needle tip reaches it, its nature is confirmed. In addition there will be the sensation of touching a calculus. However, very loose aggregates of calculi may still be misinterpreted by these techniques.

b) Air

Since air is a diffuse reflector of ultrasound (Fig. 4), air bubbles within the collecting system may impede proper orientation. The remedy is to fill the system with sterile saline.

c) Scars

Intraparenchymal scarring or fibrous change of the collecting system wall may appear on the scan as densely echogenic structures. However, the characteristic stone shadow will be absent. Distinction from small stones may nevertheless be problematic.

d) Urine, Clots

Liquid within the collecting system is homogeneously non-reflecting, thus appearing dark. The transition across the wall of the collecting system leads to signal amplification and the consequent appearance of bright echo bands. Obstructed calyces close to the surface of the kidney may be misinterpreted as stones. Careful observation of the echo from the far side wall of the collecting system and the underlying structures of the kidney will help to avoid this blun-

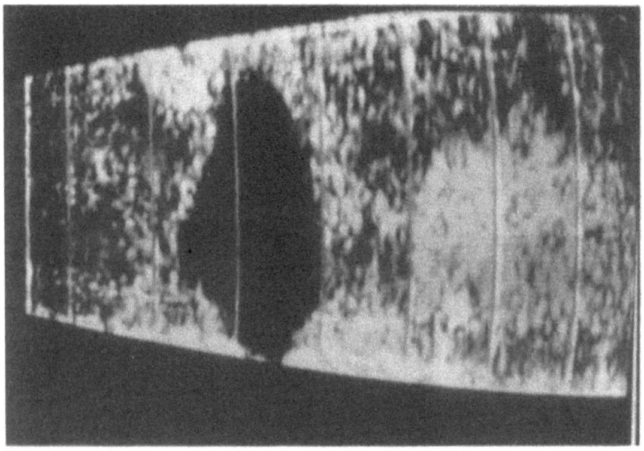

Fig. 5. B-scan appearance of a hydrocalyx. Cross section of the calyx shown in Fig. 4

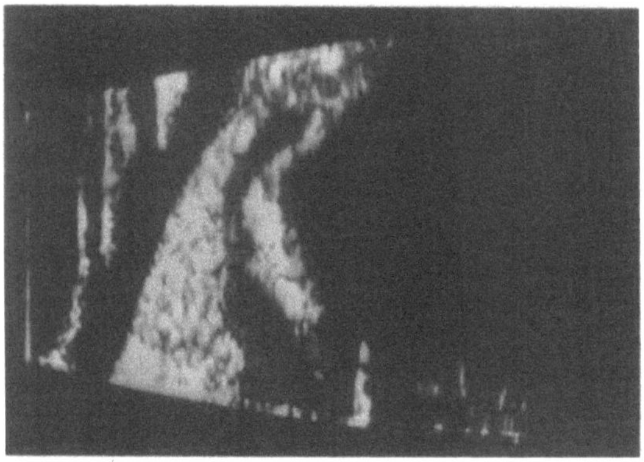

Fig. 6. B-scan image of an intraparenchymal vessel with two branches, running parallel to the renal surface (*at the left*). A large stone in a slightly dilated calyx is indicated by the sickle shaped echo with an acoustic shadow

der. Again the characteristic sonographic shadow behind a stone will be absent (Fig. 5). Clots which may occur within the collecting system in the wake of nephrotomy or pyelolithotomy are less of a problem, being of less echogenicity than either renal parenchyma or stones.

e) Vasculature

Arteries and veins may be imaged as circular, oval or linear dark zones within the parenchyma (Fig. 6), with clearly echogenic walls, depending on the angle at which they transsect the sonographic plane. It is rare to mistake them for echoes from calculi. The demonstration of vessels during a search for residual calculi is nevertheless of value in excluding vascular areas as sites of nephrotomy. Because such vessels take a variable course relative to the sonographic plane, however, a systematic search for vessels in the parenchyma overlying a calculus is too time consuming and is better accomplished by Doppler ultrasonography.

5. Doppler Ultrasonography

Doppler probes may also be suitable for gas sterilization or may be applied to the surface of the kidney in a sterile plastic wrapping. Coupling jelly is unnecessary. Wherever the sound waves meet a moving surface, e.g. blood corpuscles within the lumen of an artery or vein, a rushing sound will be audible. Arteries can be recognised by a high pitched pulsatile signal in time with the pulse, whereas veins produce a more continuous low frequency rumble.

a) Limitations of Doppler Ultrasonography

There are few sources of error in using the Doppler probe. As long as the correct frequency (and therefore a depth of penetration of not more than 3 cm) is employed, vessels outside the vicinty of the planned nephrotomy site will not be heard. Only in the region of the renal poles may the ever decreasing thickness of the parenchyma allow the ultrasound beam to reach distant vessels.

The Doppler probe should be passed across the surface of the kidney quite slowly, since, depending on the make of equipment used, there may be delay in signal reproduction. Rapid movements may then simulate the absence of vessels.

6. Siting the Nephrotomy

First the dorsal and ventral aspects of the kidney should be scanned to determine whether the stone lies in a dorsal or ventral group of calyces. Next the point on the surface of the kidney having the shortest distance from the stone should be determined and may conveniently be marked out with a suitable pen. The Doppler probe is now used to map out the course of arteries within this field. Beginners are recommended to use a pen for this also. The more ubiquitous venous network should, however, not be marked. Nevertheless one should attempt to avoid areas of definite venous noise with the ensuing incision. With increasing experience formal surface mapping may be dispensed with altogether. If the planned site of incision directly overlies a vessel the B-scanner may be used to search for an alternative site.

If the stone has been identified as filling more than half the screen of the scanner one can proceed directly to nephrotomy, since minor variations in the plane of dissection will still lead to the calculus. If the calculus, or rather its echo image, is substantially smaller, it is preferable to determine the direction of nephrotomy more precisely, so as not to miss the stone bearing sector of the collecting system altogether.

With this in mind the scanning head should be applied radially to the proposed site of nephrotomy and moved gradually toward the periphery of the kidney so as to demonstrate both the calculus and the more laterally placed parenchyma (Fig. 7). At this stage it is frequently necessary to gently press the scanning head into the parenchyma. Under continuing ultrasound observation a

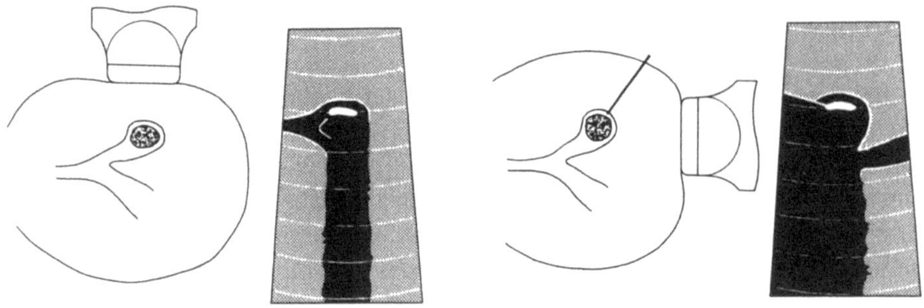

Fig. 7. Schematic drawing of a small calyceal stone as seen on the B-scan when scanned from two different positions and with a needle introduced under ultrasound guidance

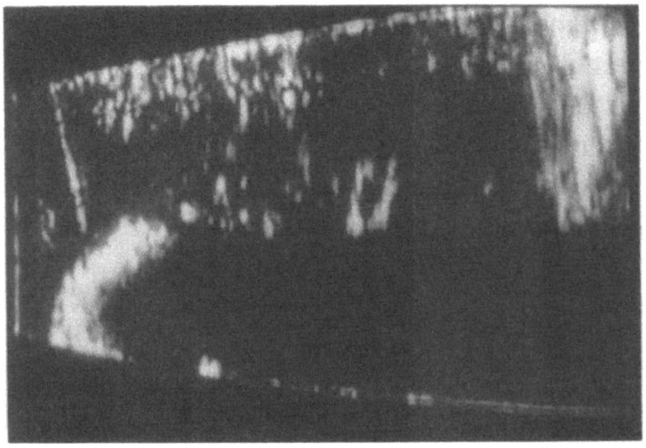

Fig. 8. B-scan image of a stone (*bottom left*). A needle (*top left*) has been advanced up to the stone. The use of a fine needle permits echos still to be obtained from the parenchyma beyond

fine needle may then be passed down the sonographic plane to make contact with the stone. By this procedure the needle remains visible throughout its track through the parenchyma and minor alterations of direction are made easily and under direct control (Fig. 8). A puncture perpendicular to the sonographic plane has proved of less value, since the needle is only seen as a dot where it transects the beam, rendering changes of direction less easy to control.

7. Making the Nephrotomy

An approximately 5 mm lang sharp incision is made into the renal capsule. The subjacent parenchyma is then parted by blunt dissection with neurosurgical dissectors, following the track of the guide needle if used. If the nephrotomy leads straight through a papilla into the collecting system, the latter will be entered by the dissector without marked resistance being encountered. A dissection through the calyceal side wall will involve overcoming the toughness of this tissue, and the wall of the calyceal neck may be perforated with the dissectors closed. If at this stage urine flows from the nephrotomy or if palpation indicates that the stone has been reached, a bivalve speculum with fiber light attachment should next be introduced into the nephrotomy and gently opened. If the stone is small or the collecting system not at all obstructed, blunt dissection may occasionally accidentally push the latter to one side rather than perforating it. If this mishap occurs the speculum should be introduced before opening the collecting system. Small angled scissors can then be used to open the calyx along the track of the guide needle. Parenchymal bleeding may obscure the view and should be dealt with by a fine sucker. Opening the speculum usually arrests this bleeding by tissue compression. If small vessels have been entered, the finest arterial twigs may be controlled by coagulating diathermy under direct vision. If the bleeding point is venous, the speculum should be rotated until its blades compress the bleeder. In the exceptionally rare event of an injury to an arterial branch or a large vein local suturing may be necessary. Most venous bleeding stops of its own accord. The speculum is now gradually opened further and blunt dissection continued until the nephrotomy is large enough to permit the introduction of further instruments. A three bladed speculum with a light attachment is available for larger nephrotomies.

Small or soft calculi may be extracted with stone forceps or are evacuated by a combined cold light and suction device. Calculi too large to be delivered through the nephrotomy in one piece are first reduced by stone crushing forceps, ultrasound lithotresis or by drilling and sawing. Once all visible stone material has been removed from the lumen the speculum is angulated to allow systematic inspection of the entire sector of the collecting system which has been opened. The whole collecting system is then irrigated with saline to remove stone residue and air bubbles.

If hemorrhage should at any point obscure the view the entire nephrotomy is carefully packed with small gauze pledgelets and these left in situ for several minutes. Further inspection then usually shows a marked reduction in bleeding. If additional nephrotomies are required for complete removal of all stones, the first incision may also be packed and left while the above ultrasound guided procedure is repeated elsewhere. When scanning for further calculi it should be remembered that the packs may produce stone-like echoes. Where real doubt persists the packs may need temporarily to be removed.

If further copious irrigation of the kidney both via the nephrotomies and via the pyelotomy is followed by a scan showing no further stones, a plane X-ray film should be taken to confirm this state of affairs.

The nephrotomies are closed with a continuous suture to the capsule only. The insertion of a Ch. 8–10 silastic nephrostomy catheter is optional.

V. Results

Since May 1980 we have applied these principles to 107 operations on 99 patients aged 4 to 76 years (Table 3). 15 operations consisted of nephrotomy alone. In 87 pyelocalycotomy was combined with radial nephrotomy.

Table 3. Position of renal stones in 107 operations

Solitary calyceal	multiple calyceal	pelvic and calyceal	complete staghorn stones
12	25	20	50

Table 4. Ultrasonically guided nephrotomy (n = 107)

	Median	Range
Nephrotomies per kidney	3,5	1– 12
Duration (minutes)	270	110– 610
Blood loss (ml)	1065	20–4500
Residual stone rate	7,5%	

Table 5. Ultrasonically guided nephrotomy (n = 107)

Complications		
Postop. hemorrhage	2	(reoperation 1)
Perirenal abszess	2	(reoperation 1)
Urinoma	1	
UPJ-stenosis	1	(reoperation)
Pneumonia	1	
Sepsis	1	
Mortality		
Myocardial infarction	1	

One case required 12 individual nephrotomies for complete stone clearance (Table 4). Blood loss was not related to the number of nephrotomy incisions and in a group of 6 patients with 8 to 12 nephrotomies averaged only 615 ml.

3 cases required temporary clamping of the renal artery. 3 of the 8 residual stone fragments failed to pass. Inadequate mobilization of the kidney had hidden them from both ultrasound and subsequent plain X-ray. Of the 9 postoperative complications only the 2 cases of hemorrhage are directly related to the surgical technique (Table 5).

Split ^{131}I-hippuran clearance studies revealed an average loss of function of 8% on the operated side 6–8 weeks following surgery. A group of 14 patients reinvestigated 1–3 years after surgery had had a mean improvement in function of 10%.

There are few comparable reports on ultrasound guidance of nephrolithotomy in the literature. BOYCE (1980) has used the Doppler probe to locate vessels in the hilum and aberrant renal arteries, as well as to demonstrate the return of normal blood flow following temporary crossclamping of the renal artery (BIRCH and BOYCE 1977). BRYNIAK and CHESLEY (1981) have used the Doppler probe to delineate the posterior segment boundary and in 13 cases were able to demonstrate an exact correspondence to the segmental boundary found by the classical methylene blue technique. On one occasion they successfully used the Doppler probe to determine a suitable avascular nephrotomy site. WOODHOUSE et al. (1981) have employed Doppler ultrasonography during radial nephrotomy but have not reported their experience in any detail. The experimental basis of our own technique resides in the animal work of THUEROFF et al. (1980), who demonstrated the strict correlation between the vascular map traced on the surface of the kidney by Doppler examination and the anatomy shown on subsequent angiography. First clinical results were reported in 1982 (THUEROFF et al. 1982).

Reports on intraoperative ultrasound scanning for renal calculi are rather more numerous. SCHLEGEL et al. (1961) used A-scanning to identify stones in the exposed kidney. HEINE and VOGEL (1972) and HEINE et al. (1973), also using A-scanning, were able to report the identical echogenicity of stones of varying mineral composition and the strict dependence of the image quality on the surface properties of the stone and the characteristics of the transducer – a finding subsequently confirmed by DEMPSEY et al. (1977). In 1977, COOK and LYTTON, using an instrument originally developed for ophthalmology, were able to describe the first use of a B-scanner for the detection of renal calculi. The great advantage of this technique over A-scanning consists in its ability to present a composite image of the tissue scanned. The technique has since become widespread and over 100 stone operations employing intraoperative ultrasonic B-scan have since been described in the literature (COOK and LYTTON 1977; LE DUC et al. 1973; DEMPSEY et al. 1977; LYTTON 1983; MARSHALL et al. 1981; RUBIN et al. 1983; SIGEL 1982; HARTUNG and MEYER-SCHWICKERATH 1983). As far as one can deduce from these authors' figures the false negative rate is of the order of 7%. The value of ultrasound examination was generally considered to lie not only in the demonstration of calculi but also in precise determination of the optimum nephrotomy site, in much reduced radiation exposure for the operator and in the availability of quasi-three-dimensional information on the position of the stone.

BOYCE (1983) has written: "The surgeon's ability to move about inside the kidney with preservation of renal function is directly related to the definition of the vascular segments and their relationship to other features of renal anatomy and to the pathologic process. This must be accomplished for each and every kidney at the time of surgery." Clearly this requirement is to date best fulfilled by nephrotomy under ultrasound guidance, permitting as it does direct assessment on the exposed kidney of anatomical variations in each individual case.

References

Alken P (1984) Perkutane Nephrolithotomie. Urologe [Ausg A] 23:20–24

Andaloro VA, Schor M, Marangola JP (1976) Intraoperative localization of a renal calculus using ultrasound. J Urol 116:92–93

Beurton D, Gonties D, Malloum M, Ngeh D, Daskalov J, Pascal B, Cukier J (1981) Evaluation du retentissement rénal en fonction de la technique opératoire dans la chirurgie de 190 calculs, coralliformes ou caliciels. J Urol (Paris) 87:131–138

Birch AA, Boyce WH (1977) Changing renal blood flow following sodium nitroprusside in patients undergoing nephrolithotomy. Anesth Analg 56:102–108

Boyce WH (1983) Surgery of urinary calculi in perspective. In: Resnik MI (ed) Surgery of stone disease. Urol Clin North Am 10:585–594

Boyce WH, Stubbs AJ, Resnick MI (1978) Intrarenal nephrolithotomy and reconstruction of the solitary kidney. Trans Am Ass Genitourin Surg 69:118–122

Bryniak SR, Chesley AE (1981) The use of the Doppler stethoscope in anatrophic nephrotomy. J Urol 126:295–296

Bueschen AJ, Zahm MJ, Lloyd LK (1980) Adjuvant surgical techniques in the removal of staghorn calculi. J Urol 123:342–344

Chaussy Ch, Schmiedt E, Jocham D, Schuller J, Brandl H (1984) Extracorporale Stoßwellenlithotripsie – Beginn einer Umstrukturierung in der Behandlung des Harnsteinleidens? Urologe [Ausg A] 23:25–29

Constantinople NL, Waters WB, Yalla SV (1979) Operative versus non-operative management of patients with staghorn calculi and neurogenic bladder. J Urol 121:716–718

Cook JH, Lytton B (1977) Intraoperative localization of renal calculi during nephrolithotomy by ultrasound scanning. J Urol 117:543–546

Dempsey PJ, Shoaf MD, Weinerth LJ, Paulson DF (1977) Experimental basis for intraoperative calculus localization by ultrasound. Invest Urol 14:380

Egger G, Joost J, Marberger M (1982) Langzeitergebnisse nach konservativen Ausgußsteinoperationen. Z Urol Nephrol 75:365–368

Faure G, Sarramon JP (1982) La lithiase coralliforme. J Urol (Paris) 88:496–500

Gil-Vernet JM (1965) New surgical concepts in removing renal calculi. Urol Int 20:255–288

Gil-Vernet JM (1983) Pyelolithotomy. In: Roth RA, Finlayson B (eds) Stones, clinical management of urolithiasis. Williams and Wilkins, Baltimore London, p 277

Hartung R, Meyer-Schwickerath (1984) Intraoperativer Ultraschall bei der Chirurgie des Ausgußsteines. Verh Dtsch Ges Urol 35

Heine G, Vogel S (1972) Ultraschalldiagnostische Verfahren zur Lagebestimmung von Konkrementen im Nierenbeckenkelchsystem an der freigelegten Niere. Z Urol Nephrol 65:375–382

Heine G, Magnus S, Braun E (1973) Transpelvine Lokalisation von Nierenbecken-, Nierenkelch- und adrenalen Harnleitersteinen an der isolierten Niere mit einer Ultraschallsonde. Z Urol Nephrol 66:337–340

Le Duc A, Cariou G, Jeaneau PJ, Lagadec D, Merran S, Michon J (1983) L'échotomographie ultra-sonore per-opératoire du'rein. J Urol (Paris) 89:15–19

Lytton B (1983) Intraoperative ultrasound for nephrolithotomy. J Urol 130:213–217

Marshall FF, Smith NA, Murphy JB, Menon M, Sanders RC (1981) A comparison of ultrasonography and radiography in the localization of renal calculi: experimental and operative experience. J Urol 126:576–580

Reuter MA, Reuter HJ (1983) Die diagnostische und operative Endoskopie von Ureter und Niere. Urologe [Ausg A] 22:103–107

Rous SN, Turner WR (1977) Retrospective study of 95 patients with staghorn calculus disease. J Urol 118:902–904

Rubin JM, Bagley DH, Lyon ES, Huffman JL, Schoenberg HW (1983) Intraoperative real time ultrasonic scanning for locating and recovering renal calculi. J Urol 130:434–437

Schlegel JU, Diggdon P, Cuellar J (1961) The use of ultrasound for localizing renal calculi. J Urol 86:367–369

Sigel B, Coelho JCU, Sharifi R, Waters WB, Spigos DG (1982) Ultrasonic scanning during operation for renal calculi. J Urol 127:421–424

Smith MJV, Boyce WH (1968) Anatrophic nephrotomy and plastic calyrhaphy. J Urol 99:521–527

Stage KH, Lewis M (1981) Pre- and postoperative evaluation of renal function in patients with staghorn calculi utilizing quantitative renal scanning. Urology 17:29–32

Thüroff JW, Thüroff S, Frohneberg D, Riedmiller H, Alken P, Hohenfellner R (1980) Intraoperative Gefäßlokalisation bei Eingriffen am Nierenparenchym mittels Dopplersonographie. Tierexperimentelle Ergebnisse. Akt Urol 11:287–293

Thüroff JW, Frohneberg D, Riedmiller H, Alken P, Hutschenreiter G, Thüroff S, Hohenfellner R (1982) Localization of segmental arteries in renal surgery by Doppler sonography. J Urol 127:863–866

Vargas AD, Bragin SD, Mendez R (1982) Staghorn calculus: its clinical presentation, complications and management. J Urol 127:860–862

Wickham JEA (1981) 250 cases of complicated nephrolithotomy under regional hypothermia. In: Vahlensieck W, Gasser G (eds) Pathogenese und Klinik der Harnsteine VIII. Steinkopff, Darmstadt 17:433–437

Wickham JEA (1984) The radial paravascular multiple nephrotomy. In: Wickham JEA (ed) Intra-renal surgery. Churchill Livingstone, Edinburgh London Melbourne New York, p 166

Wickham JEA, Coe N, Ward JP (1974) One hundred cases of nephrolithotomy under hypothermia. J Urol 112:702–705

Woodhouse CRJ, Farrel CR, Paris AMI, Blandy JP (1981) The place of extended pyelolithotomy (Gil-Vernet operation) in the management of renal staghorn calculi. Br J Urol 53:520–523

Intraoperative Pyeloscopy

P. ALKEN

I. Introduction

The problems that are still inherent in intraoperative pyeloscopy are best depicted by the course that the development of the instruments used for this technique took.

II. Rigid Nephroscopes

In 1948, TRATTNER presented a modified straight cystoscope for intraoperative pyeloscopy. ROLNICK (1948) who already had used cystoscopes with unfavorable results for the same purpose commented: "It seems to me that it will prove to be of very little practical value", because complete visualization of the irregular cavity of the renal collecting system was practically impossible.

Better adopted to the needs of intraoperative pyeloscopy was a pyeloscope with a right angle working arm that could be introduced into the calyces without major distortion of the kidney, presented by LEADBETTER in 1949.

Similar to this instrument was a modified coledochoscope with a 60 degree working arm used by GRIESSMANN in 1958. These two types of instruments represent the basic design of rigid nephroscopes still in use today (Figs. 1, 2) which of course have been improved in terms of handling, size and optical systems. In the routine flank approach to the kidney the 90 or 60 degree angulation of the working arm of these instruments usually allow for an easy inspection of the ventral calyces. But the dorsal calyces may be difficult to reach because their long axis nearly points towards the examiner during surgery and except in cases with a wide exposure and good mobility of the kidney especially the dorsal calyces or parts of them may prove to be inaccessible with rigid instruments (Fig. 3).

An adjustable angulation of the working arm was realized by flexible nephroscopes.

III. Flexible Nephroscopes

The principle of using flexible instruments with flexible glass fibers as illumination and imaging system was primarily used for endoscopy of the gastrointestinal tract (HIRSCHOWITZ et al. 1958). MARSHALL (1964) and TAKAGI et

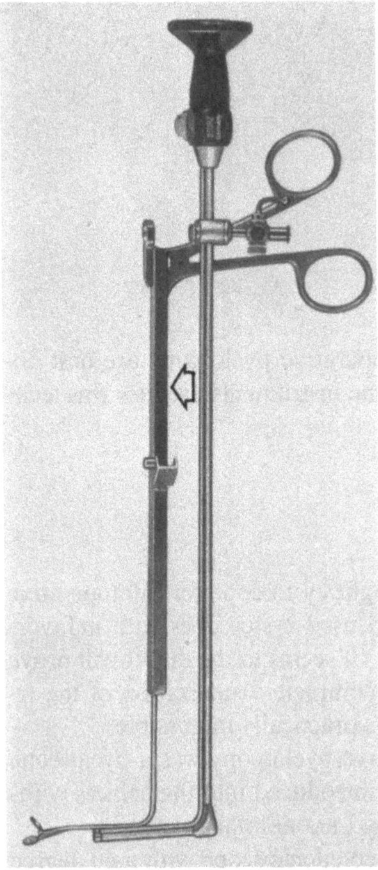
1

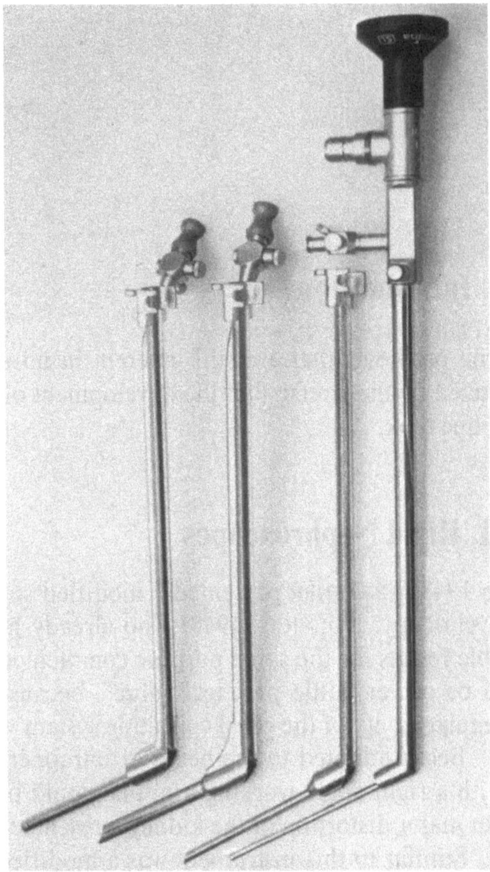
2

Fig. 1. Rigid nephroscope with 90 degree working arm (Karl Storz GmbH)

Fig. 2. Rigid nephroscope with 60 degree working arm (Richard Wolf GmbH)

al. (1968) first described the application of such flexible scopes for the inspection of the urinary tract. These instruments were ureteroscopes that had to be introduced via the urethra. Because of their small size they only allowed an inspection of the collecting system. STUART (1974) reported on intraoperative pyeloscopy by using a flexible bronchofiberscope and one year later TSUCHIDA (TSUCHIDA and TSUGAWARA 1975; TSUCHIDA 1977) presented an operative fiberpyeloscope with working and irrigation channel and a 6 cm long flexible tip of 8.5 mm diameter that could be bent 90 degrees up or down by remote control. This is the basic design of flexible pyeloscopes currently in use today (Figs. 4a, b). They have been improved in terms of quality of the optical system, size and flexibility of the tip. Although these flexible scopes are now available since nearly 10 years there are only few reports about their application in larger series. Flexibility, their main advantage, obviously did not outweight some draw-backs. Costs of these flexible instruments are rather high compared

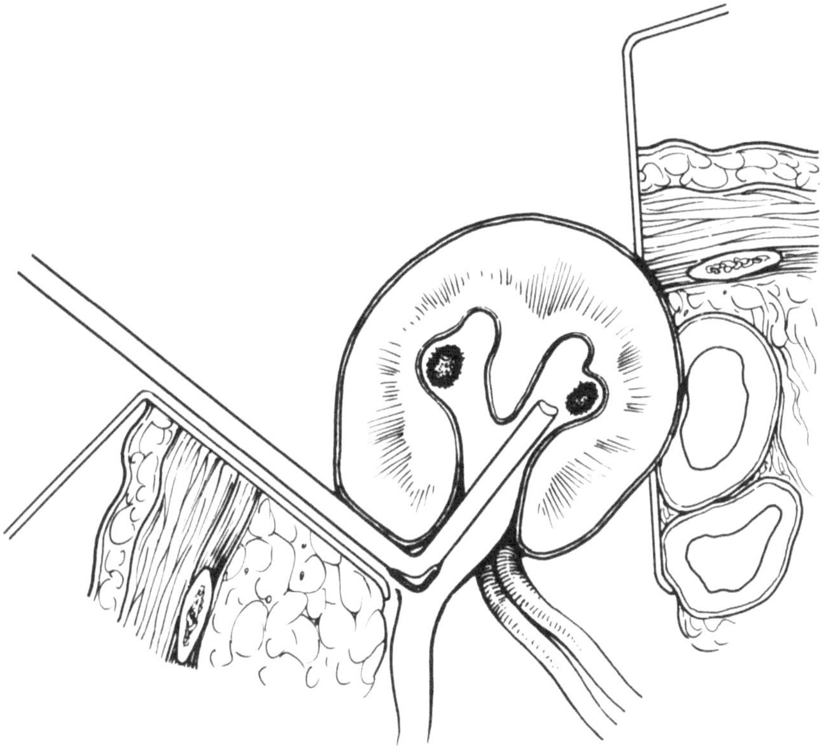

Fig. 3. The problem of reaching the ventral calyces in intraoperative pyeloscopy

to rigid instruments. The fiber bundles are delicate and if the instrument is not handled properly damage causing high repair costs is the result. The imaging quality of flexible scopes is somewhat inferior to that of rigid scopes although progress has been made in this area. Instruments that can be used through the working channel of the fiberscopes are small in size and have a limited power transmission that does for instance not allow the mechanical in situ disintegration of calyceal stones as it is possible with rigid instruments. In addition to this urologists do not seem to like to take the effort to get acquainted with the special instrumentation technique using fiberscopes.

A combination of rigid and flexible instrumental parts for intraoperative pyeloscopy has been realized by a prototype pyeloscope produced by ACMI (Fig. 5). It consists of different forceps with preshaped different angulations of 60-, 90-, and 160-degree which offer a strong grip on the stone. Either to these forceps or a malleable guide wire a small flexible scope with an irrigation channel can be attached for stone removal or inspection. The grip part of the scope containing the eye piece lense the light guide cable and the irrigation channel inlet is attached to a post affixed to the operating table. In this way the surgeon can look through the eye piece while his two hands are free to move the kidney and the stone forceps. Even though some of the flexibility of the scope is lost in this arrangement the fact that the surgeon has two hands on the kidney is favor-

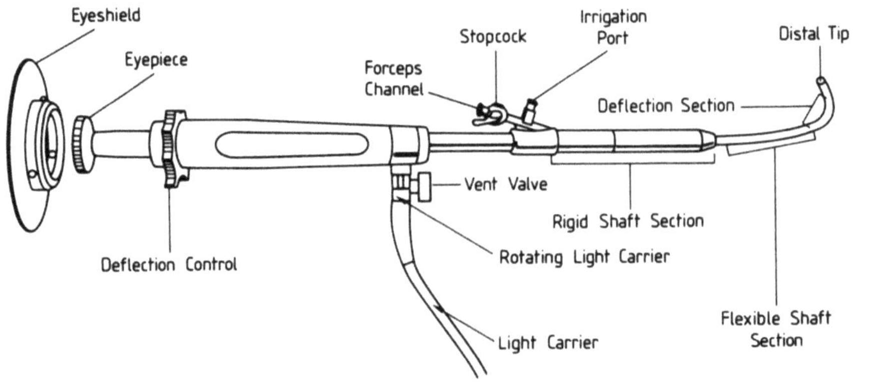

Fig. 4a. Schematic drawing of a flexible pyeloscope (ACMI)

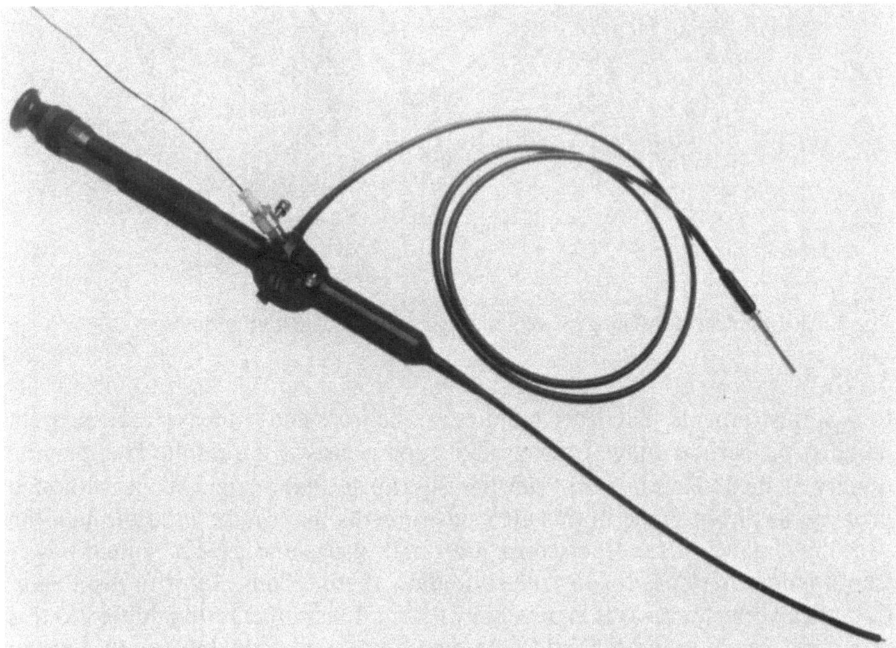

Fig. 4b. Flexible pyeloscope with electrohydraulic probe introduced (Karl Storz GmbH)

able compared to the pyeloscopy technique with ordinary flexible scopes. But the prototype instrument needs further improvement.

1. Equipment

Ordinary light fountains like for cystoscopy are used for illumination. Irrigation, using physiological saline, may be done by gravity flow or more ef-

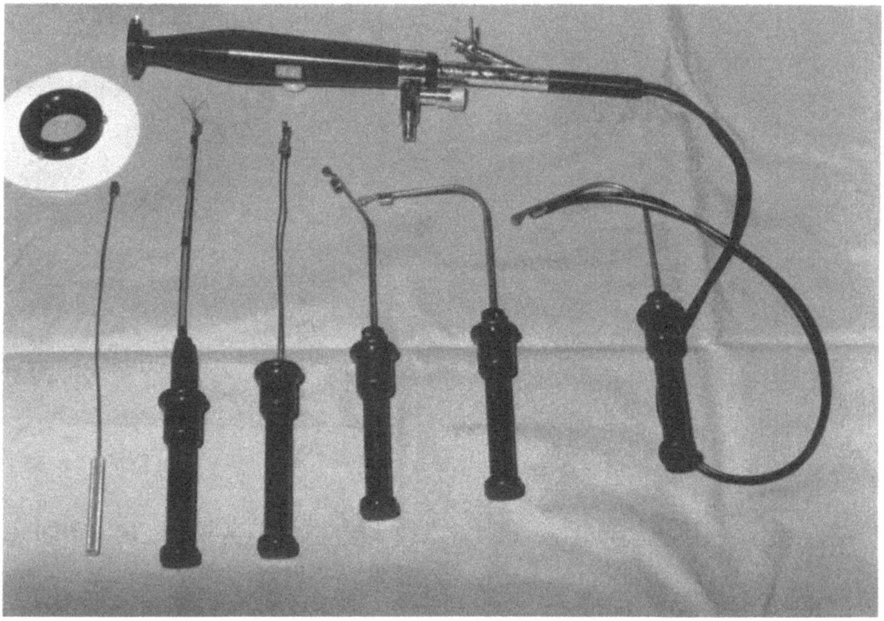

Fig. 5. Prototype version of intraoperative pyeloscope with flexible optical system and various forceps (ACMI)

fectively by using a fanwell pressure bag (Fig. 6) that is normally used for rapid blood transfusion. Soft plastic fluid containers of appropriate size fitting to the pressure bags are necessary. Also roler pumps with adjustable speed may be used for the same purpose. The use of a dental water pick that produces an adjustable pulsatile flow has been described for irrigation and flushing out of fragments (GIBBONS et al. 1974). Other authors have proposed the use of air (TSUCHIDA 1973; BURCHARDT 1982) whereby the visual field is increased by about 30% compared to water. Using air under pressure carries an uncalculable risk of air embolism. Also using fluid under pressure may cause disruption of the parenchyma with appearance of fluid under the renal capsule. All nephroscopes are delivered with an eye shield disk that can be attached to the eye piece to prevent wound contamination. Rigid and flexible forceps of different size attached to or introduced through the nephroscope (Figs. 7a, b) can be used with a rigid nephroscope. Flexible pyeloscopes go with small biopsy forceps which are of little value in stone surgery. Most widely applied are three hook graspers, dormia baskets or balloon catheters to dislodge calyceal stones (Fig. 8).

2. Technique

Extensive preoperative radiological studies to outline the anatomy of the collecting system are of little help for the intraoperative situation. The number of

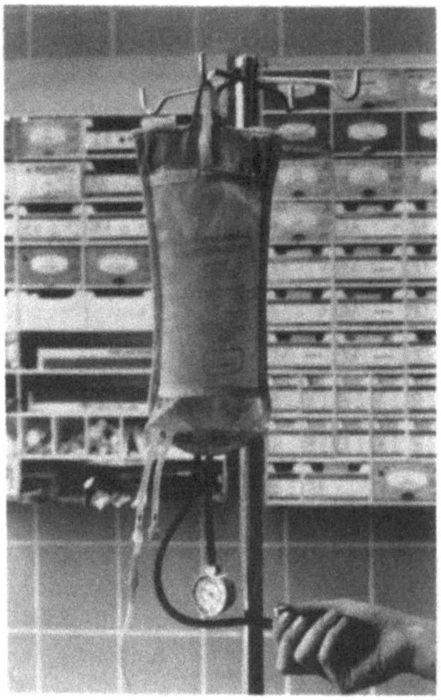

Fig. 6. Fanwell pressure bag

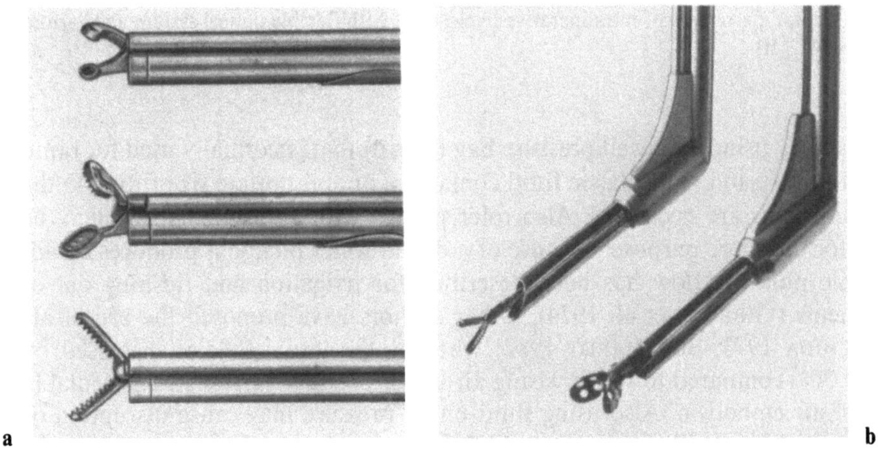

Fig. 7 a, b. Forceps used with the Storz (**a**) and Wolf (**b**) rigid nephroscopes

calyces that has to be inspected is usually determined by simple IVP and the plain film indicates the site of a calyceal stone. Intraoperative pyeloscopy can be used for three purposes:

1. Inspection
2. Stone extraction
3. Indication of a nephrotomy site.

An extrarenal pelvis and a dilated collecting system facilitate endoscopy. An intrarenal pelvis and sklerosis of the renal sinus with narrow infundibula render endoscopy difficult, or impossible. The spacial arrangement of the calyces determines their accessability for complete inspection. In complicated cases

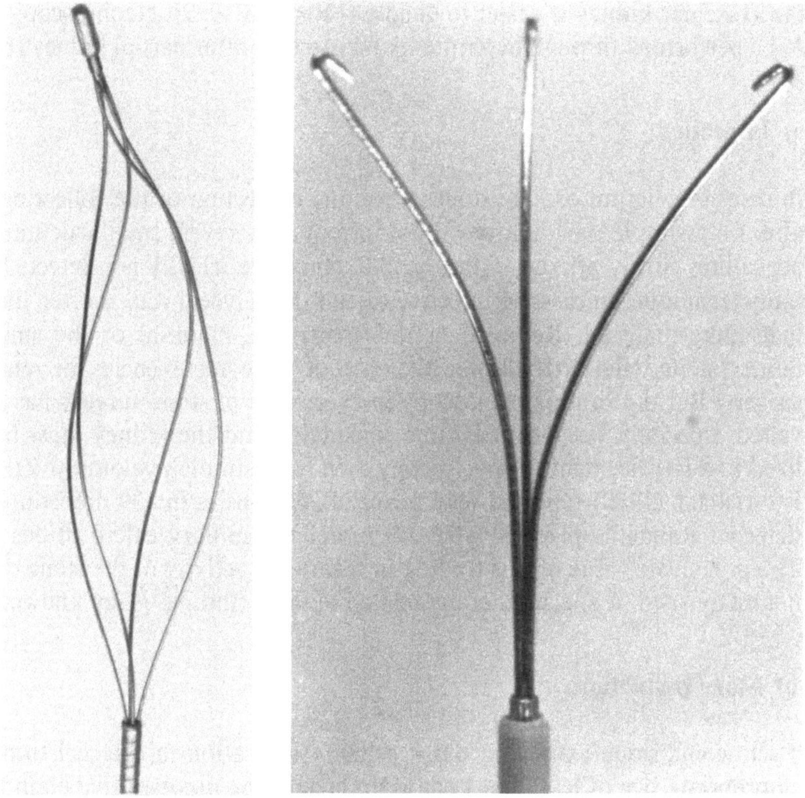

Fig. 8. Dormia basket and three prawn grasper used with flexible pyeloscopes

with staghorn stones or after previous surgery best results can only be achieved if the kidney is completely mobilized. In some cases a simple pyelotomy and an only partially mobilized kidney will offer a satisfying access. The kidney should be placed on white surgical cloths so that stone particles that are flushed out are easily detected. Especially when dealing with infective stones the irrigation fluid should be suctioned out continuously to reduce the risk of wound contamination. If the calyceal stones are mobile and small enough to be flushed out flushing of the collecting system may precede endoscopy. Whenever nephroscopy seems to be indicated it should be done before the blind introduction of other instruments for stone removal because they can cause bleeding which renders visibility and orientation difficult. Introduction of the instrument is facilitated if the renal hilus is exposed with parenchymal hooks which should be removed after the successful introduction. The introduction of the nephroscope through a small incision and a purse string suture which has been proposed by some authors may have its place when pyeloscopy is performed for a urothelial tumor to prevent tumor spillage. In stone surgery a wide opening of the renal pelvis will prevent an uncontrolled laceration of the pelvic wall during the manipulation. If the renal artery is clamped during endoscopy bleeding from the mucosa or the papilla is reduced, the visualization is improved and the avascular kidney is easier to handle (MOSTAFA 1979). Nephroscopy may also be performed through nephrotomy incisions or after partial kidney resection.

a) Inspection

In cases of calcium oxalate stones a routine inspection of the collecting system after f.i. a simple pyelotomy will not infrequently reveal small calcium oxalate crystallites firmly affixed to the papilla which are usually not detected by any x-ray technique. In cases of infective calculi the calyceal wall is often lined with matrixlike material. Removal of this matrixlike material or the small crystallites should definitely lower the rate of false recurrencies in renal stone surgery. But the routine pyeloscopy in every case of stone surgery has not prevailed especially because it is time consuming and the kidney must be mobilized to a larger extent for pyeloscopy then for a simple pyelotomy. ZINGG and FUTTERLIEB (1980) reported on a series of 32 biopsies in 139 procedures. They detected Randall's plaques type subepithelial papillary calcifications in 25%. The prognostic value of this finding in regards of activity of the stone disease is not established. A special therapy related to these findings is not known.

b) Stone Extraction

Pyeloscopic stone extraction has a primary indication in calyceal stones of an appropriate size of less than 1 cm in diameter. The preoperative plain film will indicate the route to the stone. A secondary indication is the extraction of residual stones in staghorn surgery. In these cases an intraoperative x-ray should be done before endoscopy to determine the sites of interest. In order not to miss the stone bearing calyx during the inspection it is necessary to inspect the wall of the collecting system in a circular clockwise fashion, when advancing the instrument until a calyx or a papilla is reached. If the stone containing area is not directly visualized the instrument should be removed in the same fashion, and instrument and kidney may be rotated and moved in order to get access to the different calyces. If the collecting system is not dilated inspection without an attached forceps should precede the stone extraction. But the subsequent introduction of the instrument with the forceps may prove difficult if the calyceal neck is narrow. In these cases the calyceal neck may be carefully dilated with the jaws of the stone grasper. If the instrument is simply pushed into the calyx visualization of the collecting system in this situation is usually poor. It may also happen that the forceps is perforating the wall of the collecting system during introduction of the instrument and once the stone becomes visible the forceps is not seen because it is lying underneath the calyceal wall. Soft stones too large to be extracted in one piece may be crushed with the forceps of the rigid nephroscopes. Using a flexible scope small stones can be extracted with a three hook grasper. Catching a stone with the dormia type soft basket may turn out to be difficult in a small calyx. Introducing a three French balloon catheter through the instrument into the calyx, blocking the balloon behind the stone and subsequent pulling of the balloon catheter is another way to remove stones with the flexible instruments.

c) Indication of a Nephrotomy Site

If the stone removal turns out to be impossible there are three techniques to determine the nephrotomy site. Pushing the instrument firmly against the stone it may be palpated from the outside as a resistance and the incision is carried onto the stone. In cases with reduced parenchymal thickness the light shining through the parenchyma can indicate the area of incision. A third technique is the introduction of small sharp wires through the instrument which are then pushed through the parenchyma and used as a guidance for the nephrotomy. Neither of these three techniques will guarantee, that the incision is not leading through an arterial branch within the parenchyma. This technique should therefore preferably only be applied in cases with thinned parenchymal covering of the stone bearing calyx.

IV. Results

The success rate in terms of complete visualization of the collecting system varies between 60 and 90%. VATS et al. (1972) who were the first to do systematic examinations of cadaver kidneys with a 90° working arm nephroscope were able to inspect 86% of all calyces. A similar study performed by HERTEL (1973) revealed a 91.6% success rate when a nephroscope with a 90° working arm was used and a 84.7% success rate with a 60° working arm nephroscope. In the clinical situation three authors who used a 90° working arm nephroscope reported on success rates of 60%, 80% and 90% respectively (ZINGG and FUTTERLIEB 1980; PEARSON 1975; SARRAMON et al. 1980). No larger series are reported in the literature concerning the use of flexible scopes. While KOSHIBA (1982) estimated the over-all success rate with flexible scopes to be less than 80% in skilled hands and less than 50% in the ordinary surgeon's hands, MCANINCH and FAY (1982) reported on a 100% success rate in 30 cases in which a flexible nephroscope was used which had a 16 French diameter working tip that could be bent 110° in two directions.

In terms of residual stone rate, the success rate of intraoperative pyeloscopy varies between 100 and 69%. The only series reporting about a 100% success rate is that of MCANINCH and FAY (1982) with a completely successful stone extraction in 18 cases. Unfortunately, there are no other reliable data in the literature confirming this high success rate. MIKI et al. (1978) reported about three successful procedures in four cases. Most statistics referred in the literature are concerning the use of the 90° working angle nephroscope (Table 1). Lowest success rates are achieved when the technique is applied in the removal of residual stones in staghorn surgery (GITTES 1975; MORELLE and FONTEYNE 1980). In a personal series of the author complete or partial success of

Table 1. Residual Stone Rate in Intraoperative Pyeloscopy

Author	Year	n	Instrument Type	Residual Stone Rate		Total
				Staghorn Stones	Other Stones	
HERTEL	1974	84	rigid			11%
GITTES	1975	49	rigid	5/16	1/33	12%
HERTEL and EGGER	1976	59	rigid			19%
MORELLE and FONTEYNE	1980	91	rigid	3/23	1/68	6,5%
SARRAMON et al.	1980	35	rigid			26%
MIKI et al.	1978	4	flexible			1/4
MCANINCH and FAY	1982	30	flexible			0%

Table 2. Effectivity of Intraoperative Pyeloscopy (Author's Series)

Result		Calyceal stones n=31	Staghorn stone residuals n=23
Complete removal	43%	16	7
Partial removal	30%	8	8
Stone not visualized	11%	4	2
Stone visualized but not extractable	16%	3	6

endoscopic stone removal obviated the needs for nephrotomies in 43% and reduced the number of necessary nephrotomies in an additional 23%. In a third of the cases the stone could not be visualized or despite its localization it could not be extracted (Table 2). The problems of stone extraction are also indicated in the series of SARRAMON et al. (1980) and HERTEL (1974). In their series, 37 respectively 51% of the stones were visualized but could not be extracted under endoscopic control. In these cases a blind extraction was performed after the stone was located by endoscopy.

A systematic clinical evaluation in which part of the kidney most stones are not detected by endoscopy is not available although most authors indicate that the posterior mid region calyces are most difficult to reach with the endoscope. In this regard a very interesting study has been performed by MANGIN (1982). An artificial staghorn calculus was created by injecting a solidifying mass into the collecting system of 50 human cadaver kidneys. Upon removal of most of this mass by an extended pyelocalicotomy residual calculi were removed either by endoscopy (n = 125) or by an endoscopically guided nephrotomy (n = 58). The residual stone rate was thereafter determined by complete dissection of the collecting system. Only 8 kidneys were completely stonefree. Residual stone particles were detected in 9 calyces of the polar regions, in 20 calyces of the ventral part of the kidney and in 43 dorsally located calyces. Thus clinical and experimental data clearly indicate that intraoperative pyeloscopy has its merits in reducing the number of transparenchymal approaches to renal stones but it can only be regarded as an additional technique for complete stone removal and it does not obviate the needs for other techniques to detect and remove residual calculi like intraoperative sonography and x-ray examinations.

V. Complications

Properly used intraoperative pyeloscopy carries a negligible risk of complications. Only a few cases of minor intraoperative bleeding have been reported and postoperative secondary wound healing which might be attributed to a contamination of the wound during endoscopy is observed infrequently (ZINGG and FUTTERLIEB 1980; PEARSON 1975; HERTEL 1974).

References

Burchardt P (1982) The flexible panendoscope. J Urol 127:479–481
Gibbons RP, Correa RJ, Cummings KB, Mason JT (1974) Use of water-pik and nephroscopy. Urology 4:605
Gittes RF (1975) Operative Nephroscopy. Trans Am Ass Genitourin Surg 67:49–53
Griessmann H (1958) Die Pyelo- und Ureteroskopie. Z Urol Nephrol 51:510–512
Hertel E (1973) Entwicklung der operativen Pyeloskopie. Urologe [Ausg A] 12:116–120
Hertel E (1974) Intraoperative nephroscopy. Urology 4:13–17
Hertel E, Egger B (1976) Die intraoperative Ureteropyeloskopie. Ein Routineverfahren. Akt Urol 7:343–348
Hirschowitz BI, Curtiss BS, Peters CW, Pollard HM (1958) Demonstration of a new gastroscope, the fiberscope. Gastroenterology 35:50
Koshiba K (1982) In: Symposium: Management of kidney and ureteral calculi. Contemp Surg 20:91–118
Leadbetter WF (1950) Instrumental visualization of the renal pelvis at operations as an aid to diagnosis. Presentation of a new instrument. J Urol 63:1006–1012
Mangin Ph (1982) Aide de l'endoscopie rénale dans la chirurgie du calcul coralliforme. J Urol (Paris) 88:681–682
Marshall VF (1964) Fiber optics in urology. J Urol 91:110–114
McAninch JW, Fay R (1982) Flexible nephroscope in calculus surgery. J Urol 128:5–7
Miki M, Yoshio I, Machida T (1978) Operative nephroscopy with fiberoptic scope: Preliminary report. J Urol 119:166–168
Morelle V, Fonteyne E (1980) Les indications de la pyéloscopie. J Urol (Paris) 86:751–752
Mostafa HM (1979) Technical aspects of nephroscopy (Letter to the editor). J Urol:258
Pearson B (1975) Discussion. Trans Am Ass Genitourin Surg 67:57
Rolnick HC (1948) Discussion. J Urol 60:836–837
Sarramon JP, Lhez JM, Soulie R, Lhez A (1980) Pyéloscopie et lithiase calicielle. A propos d'une experience de 51 cas. J Urol (Paris) 86:752–753
Stuart E (1974) Operative nephroscopy using bronchofiberscope. J Urol 111:9
Takagi T, Taigun G, Takayasu H, Aso Y, Mioki R (1968) Small-caliber fiberscope for visualization of the urinary tract, biliary tract, and spinal canal. Surgery 64:1033–1038
Trattner HR (1948) Instrumental visualisation of the renal pelvis and its communications: Proposal of a new method; preliminary report. J Urol 60:817–834
Tsuchida S (1977) A new operative fiberpyeloscope. J Urol 117:643–645
Tsuchida S, Tsugawara H (1975) A new operative fiberpyeloscope. Tohoku J Exp Med 116:362
Vats A, Berci G, Shore JM, Kudish H, Nemoy N (1972) Operative nephroscopy. J Urol 107:355–357
Zingg EJ, Futterlieb A (1980) Nephroscopy in stone surgery. Br J Urol 52:333–337

Intraoperative Radiology

P. ALKEN

I. Introduction

In renal stone surgery intraoperative radiology serves the dual purpose of locating the stone and of confirming complete clearance at the end of the procedure. The following technical requirements must be met:

1. Sensitivity adequate to detect very small and weakly opaque calculi.
2. The greatest possible three-dimensional information on the position of calculi within the collecting system.

II. X-Ray Equipment

Three different techniques are available, each involving its own equipment:

1. Stationary or mobile X-ray sets.
2. A special set with a beam source which can be lowered into the wound (Renodor).
3. A C-arm image intensifier.

A full range of exposure parameters (exposure time, voltage) can be set on all the modern equipment available from a variety of manufacturers.

1. Stationary or Mobile X-Ray Sets

This is the equipment most commonly employed. The radiation source is on a mobile mount, allowing the incident angle of the beam to be varied according to the individual intraoperative situation. A diaphragm lamp enables the beam to be pointed accurately at the kidney and a shutter allows the size of the radiation field to be tailored to the size of the kidney. This technique for centering the beam on the kidney obviates the use of sterile metal or plastic handles (ZAHM et al. 1981; BECK 1973) fitted to the tube for control by the surgeon. With good radiographic technique simple equipment can detect very small (Fig. 1) and poorly opacified stones. Multiple exposures give pseudo-three-dimensional information on the position of the stone in the collecting system. The basic requirements are thus already virtually met. Since the same equipment is also suitable for other operating room X-ray studies such as plain ab-

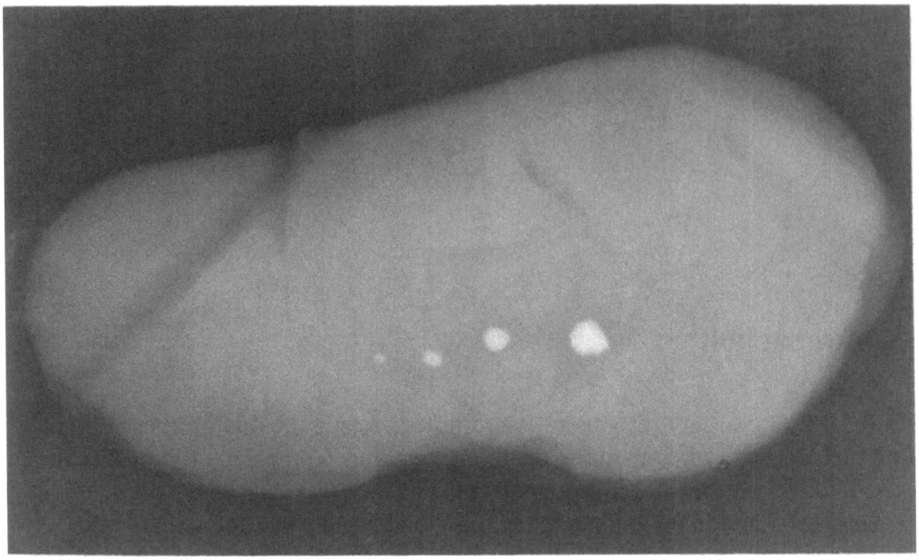

Fig. 1. X-ray of an animal kidney bearing oxalate calculi of 5-1 mm diameter

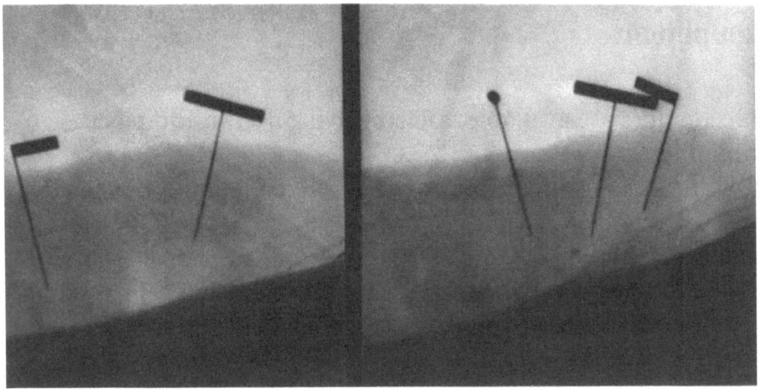

Fig. 2. Intraoperative film showing the kidney partially obscured by the 11th rib

dominal films and retrograde pyelography, this approach has become widespread. Adequate mobilization of the kidney will allow unimpeded views to be taken and is a prerequisite for optimal results. In obese patients or after previous surgery the kidney may not be brought fully into the beam so that some parts either cannot be shown or are always overlaid by soft tissue or ribs (Fig. 2). Residual calculi may then be missed, a problem only to be overcome by actually lowering the X-ray source into the wound.

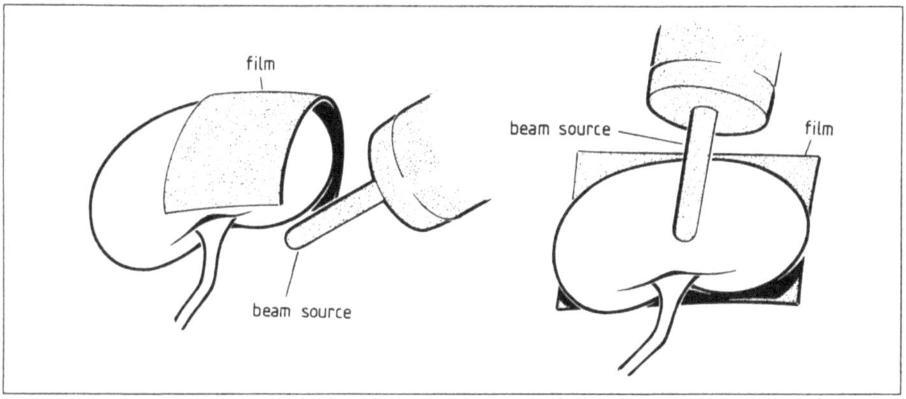

Fig. 3. Finger-shaped radiation source of the Renodor set

2. Renodor

LEUSCH (1970) was first to employ an instrument developed for maxillo-dental radiology in renal stone surgery, thus pioneering the idea that soft tissue shadows might be avoided by bringing the X-ray source to lie within the wound. The 12 × 9 cm rod-shaped anode of the generator easily fits alongside the kidney within the wound and allows views to be obtained even of poorly exposed organs (Fig. 3). With good mobilization the anode can be passed under the kidney or down to the lower pole. This apparatus allows multiple views which not only demonstrate calculi but give three-dimensional information on their position within the collecting system, fundamental advantages offset by a series of problems which have militated against its widespread use: Because the X-rays emanate from a point source there is a degree of image distortion: the closer a stone lies to the anode the larger it will appear on the film. For individual objects to be reproduced to scale the anode must be at least 15 cm from the film (BAUR 1972), conditions impossible to meet in renal stone surgery. A complete picture of the kidney usually requires two exposures, and for large kidneys three. Since the outline of the kidney is not always included in the view, the lack of anatomical landmarks may make orientation difficult. Views in various planes require a series of film holders. Despite the generally accepted superior quality of the individual pictures the chief drawback of this X-ray technique is the difficulty in learning to use the equipment and to interpret the plates. Satisfactory clinical results can only be obtained with experience (BAUER 1972; EISENBERGER 1984). One further obvious disadvantage of the system is its unsuitability for any other investigation.

3. The C-Arm Image Intensifier

The image intensifier differs from the other techniques, because the organs in its beam can be both continuously screened and shown on permanent plates. At first sight the use of a standard C-arm image intensifier would seem to be an attractive alternative: the equipment is available in most larger hospitals and provides a continuous control of the operative approach to the stone. A number of drawbacks have limited the popularity of the technique. Continuous screening results in a high radiation exposure (RUBINSTEIN et al. 1979). The use of modern equipment fitted with an image memory and a 100 mm hard copy camera reduces the dose and increases the capital cost considerably. Furthermore the use of the image intensifier suffers one great disadvantage compared to the other techniques, both for screening and for taking films. The tube and the camera are fixed in relation to one another by the C-arm and an unimpeded view of the kidney can only be obtained if the latter can be completely delivered from the wound. In the majority of cases the overlying soft tissues must be included in the view with a resulting significant deterioration in the detection rate of small and weakly opaque calculi. Attempts to introduce fluorescent screens into the wound (BASKIN et al. 1957) have not been actively pursued.

4. Film Stock and Intensifying Screens

In modern radiology, e.g. in intravenous urography, the use of intensifying screens is virtually universal. The screens contain a layer of metal salt which is excited by X-rays to emit visible light, to which X-ray film is more sensitive than it is to X-rays themselves. The immediate consequence of this practice is a reduction in the radiation dose by about 90% compared to conventional radiography. Various manufacturers offer screens with different characteristics, the amplification factor for X-rays or the photometric efficiency being inversely related to the quality of image produced. In other words, the lower the dose required, the less sharply the irradiated object will be depicted. Own experimental work on animal kidneys implanted with human kidney stones has shown so-called universal screens to provide an acceptable compromise between image detail and radiation exposure, allowing quite adequate intraoperative films to be taken. When choosing a combination of film and screen one should bear in mind that screens differ in their emission wavelength and this should correspond to the peak sensitivity of the film. As the quality of films produced will also depend both on technique and on the X-ray set employed, it is worth taking the advice of the equipment manufacturer when chosing films and screens. Our studies have shown special films, e.g. mammography film (FELDMANN et al. 1977; MARSHALL et al. 1981) or nuclear medical film (MARBERGER and HRUBY 1984) to yield no improvement in image content beyond increased definition of fine detail. In view of their added cost it is probably unnecessary to use these special film stocks and the same would appear to be true of the paired high and low sensitivity films offered by one manufacturer (KODAK X-Omat KS). Simultaneous exposure is intended to provide optimum imaging of both weakly and strongly opaque calculi, but the literature lends only tenuous support to the value of the twin film technique. The material is, however, particularly suitable for kidney stone surgery because it is provided with a notch, enabling it to be placed around the renal pedicle for views of the convexity of the kidney. For pediatric procedures the use of dental film has been advocated on the grounds that the smaller format more easily fits the wound (BRAREN 1982).

5. Polaroid Film

Any conventional X-ray film requires development in an automatic processor or a hand developing tank. In hospitals where the developing facilities are remote from the operating suite a considerable waste of operating time may result. The use of polaroid film (KOSHIBA et al. 1980; ROTH and GRIFFITH 1983) allows pictures to be developed in the operating department and within minutes. Standard intensifying screens can be used to reduce the radiation exposure (ZINK et al. 1984). So far, however, there is no literature containing detailed data on the picture quality for stones of varying density.

a) Packing and Sterilizing Film Material

Although it would in principle be feasible to add intensifying screens to individual sheets of film wrapped in light-proof paper in the darkroom, it is more convenient in practice to use twin plastic pouches with intensifying screens stuck in. Once the pouches are slid together the film is protected from light (Fig. 4). The reusable plastic pouches can be wrapped in plastic film, sealed into peal-packs and sterilized by ethylene oxide, where the manufacturer's data for a given film/screen combination so permits. Otherwise the film has to be welded into a plastic sleeve and decontaminated in a suitable solution prior to use. Some authors recommend plastic bags with an additional lead-coated metal backing plate to absorb secondary radiation and facilitate manipulation of the film within the confines of the wound. These bags are not available commercially and in our own practice we have found them to be unnecessary.

III. Aids to Intraoperative Radiology

Once the kidney has been adequately mobilized it is best secured with gauze tapes or in elastic netting and delivered as far as possible from the wound. GIL-VERNET (GIL-VERNET and CULLA 1981) has warned that excessive traction on the renal pedicle may lead to local vasospasm and subsequent functional impairment of the kidney. If adequately wide access has been gained to the kidney it may not be necessary to remove the wound retractors prior to radiography. The netting or slings are passed around the kidney and are fixed on the film

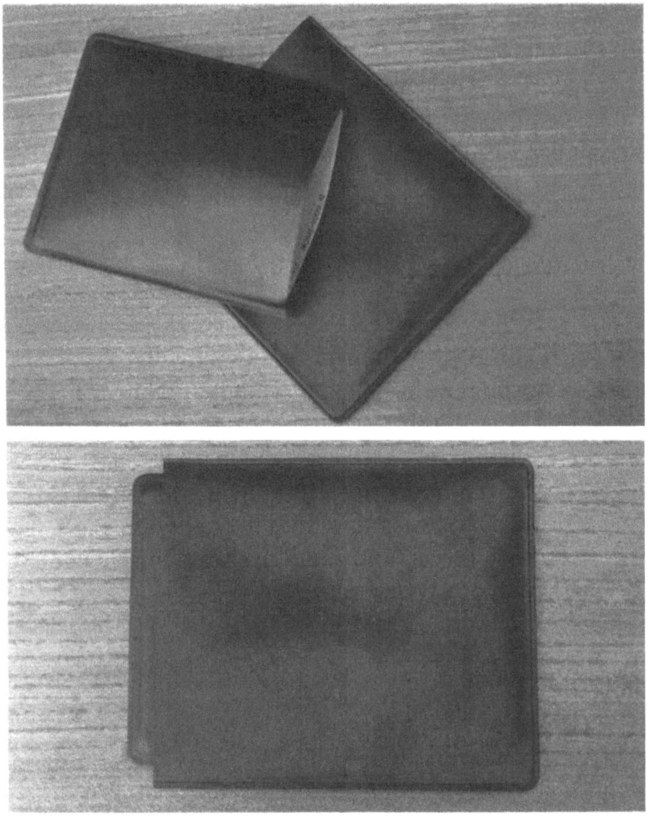

Fig. 4. Telescoping plastic film-wallets made of light-proof plastic and fitted with intensifying screens

pack thus securing close contact between the two (Fig. 5). The exactly perpendicular orientation of the film to the beam stressed by some authors is often made impossible by the geometry of the wound, but bending the film may introduce only trivial distortion. If the operating light is switched off, the crossed lines of the light diaphragm lamp are usually all that is needed to ensure that the whole kidney is properly in the field.

Various reference systems have been proposed to relate stones seen on X-ray to their site in the collecting system. Most frequently injection needles are pushed into the kidney at a series of points. The use of various shaped needles (Fig. 6) conveniently ensures optically accurate correlation of stones with specific areas of the kidney. Other authors use metal clips attached either to the surface of the kidney or to the netting in which it is suspended. Because clips occasionally migrate from their original position or are pulled by the netting out of the position shown on the X-ray plate, the quality of orientation deteriorates during long procedures. The same problem arises with foils marked out with dots or with reference grids laid between kidney and film (ROTH 1978; HANLEY 1967). Both BOYCE (1977) and GIL-VERNET (GIL-VERNET and CULLA

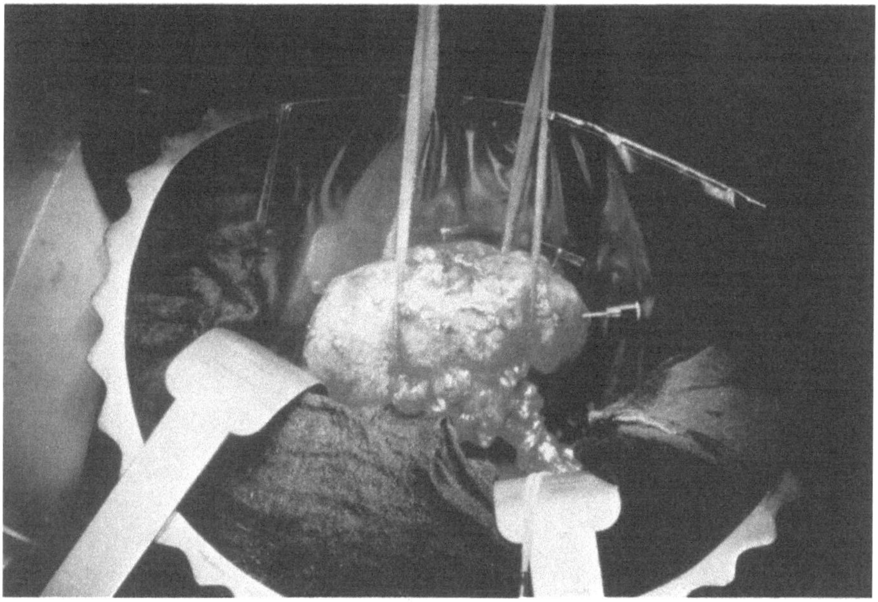

Fig. 5. Film packed in a sterile film wallet is introduced into the wound. The kidney has been delivered on tapes and is drawn against the film-wallet. Metal markers have been inserted into the kidney

1981) have immense experience of intraoperative radiology and these authors recommend preceding any pyelotomy or nephrotomy with a baseline film once the kidney has been mobilized. This allows the exposure to be optimized for subsequent films and may also detect small stones not seen on the preoperative plain film. A fracture seen in the stone at this stage may alter the course of the transrenal procedure (BOYCE 1977). IZQUIERDO (IZQUIERDO et al. 1982) has recommended pneumopyelography. Fine needle insufflation of air into the closed collecting system may demonstrate the distensibility of the calyceal necks, a finding said to be significant in assessing whether stones can be removed by pyelocalycotomy or whether nephrotomy will be called for. In addition BOYCE has suggested intraoperative pyelography for staghorn calculi, the ureter being cross-clamped and contrast injected by direct puncture of the collecting system. In his view this technique demonstrates papillary calcification which need not be removed at operation and also reveals calyceal neck stenosis requiring plastic reconstruction. When following the BOYCE technique of anatrophic nephrolithotomy it is worth-while permanently marking the anteroposterior segmental boundary of the kidney with the contrast thread from a gauze swab.

With proper exposure of the kidney there is usually little difficulty in taking a good lateral view of the whole kidney, but such a film is unable to distinguish whether stones or stone fragments are in the ventral or dorsal calyces. Irrespective of the approach chosen – pyelocalycotomy with radial nephrotomy or anatrophic nephrolithotomy – this information remains essential for correct

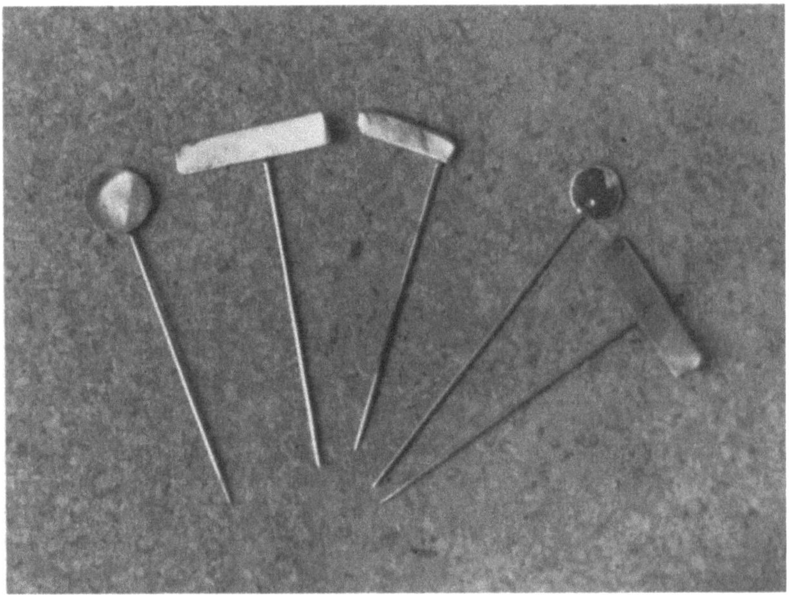

Fig. 6. Variously shaped needles for marking areas of the kidney

surgical orientation. Only rarely does perfect mobilization of an inherently mobile kidney enable a longitudinal view of the kidney to be achieved (Figs. 7a, b).

Two separate techniques of pseudo-three-dimensional kidney stone localization are described in the literature:

1. Multiple exposures of the kidney on a single film at various angles.
2. Multiple exposures in different planes.

Double exposure of one film at various beam angles permits the dorsal or ventral location of the calculus to be detected from its apparent movement in relation to radio-opaque markers, even if the beam path is exclusively anteroposterior (HEINE 1980; MATOUSCHEK 1978; MELCHIOR and LANG 1981). The information given in the literature is not adequate for any firm statement to be made about the practical aspects of this technique. Theoretically the position of the stone could be determined with millimetric precision, but it is unclear how easily the appropriate calculations are incorporated into a real surgical procedure. Apart from its requirement for multiple exposures the method has the distinct advantage of allowing three-dimensional localization by the simplest available X-ray techniques.

Kodak-X-Omat KS film has been designed specifically for views of the convexity of the kidney and incorparates a slot for the renal pedicle. If two such films are placed under the kidney and around the pedicle the bulk of the kidney can be brought into view. The only part of the kidney not seen on these views is that directly overlying the pedicle, for which an oblique beam may be needed. The fundamental difficulty of positioning film under the kidney has been satis-

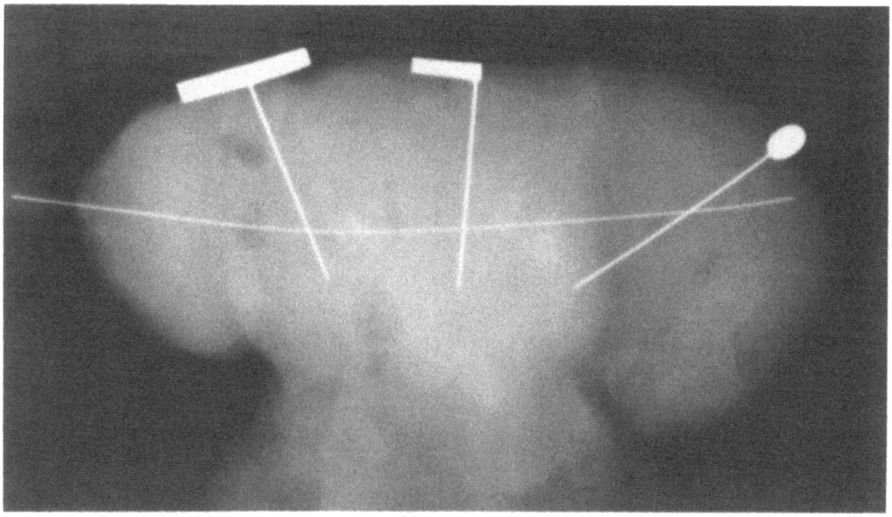

a

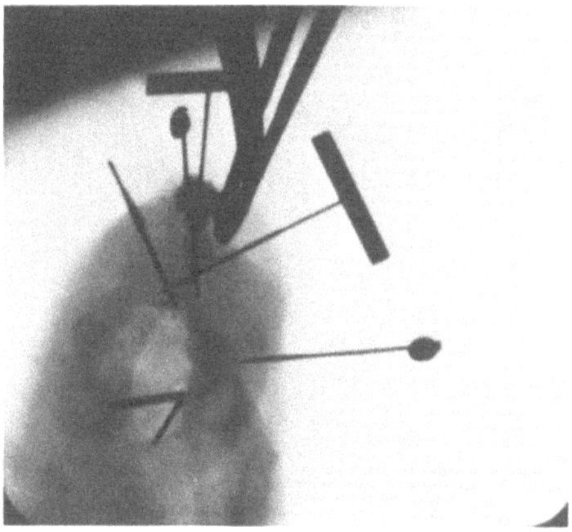

b

Fig. 7a, b. Lateral and transverse intraoperative views of the kidney to demonstrate stones in dorsal or ventral segments

factorily solved by GIL-VERNET (GIL-VERNET and CULLA 1981), who has designed a special film-holding forceps with which the especially-trimmed film can be gripped in a film-holding wallet. The instrument allows intimate contact between film and kidney. Since film placed in this way does not overlap around the renal pedicle and this area of the kidney would thus remain unseen, two types of forceps have been constructed, one designed to close parallel to the long axis, the other to follow the short axis of the kidney (Figs. 8, 9). Although the radiographs thus obtained give good information on the dorsal or ventral segmental site of a stone, a description of the technique and the instruments alone suffices to show that the process is relatively complicated, involving as it does specially not generally available trimmed film and multiple views. If no

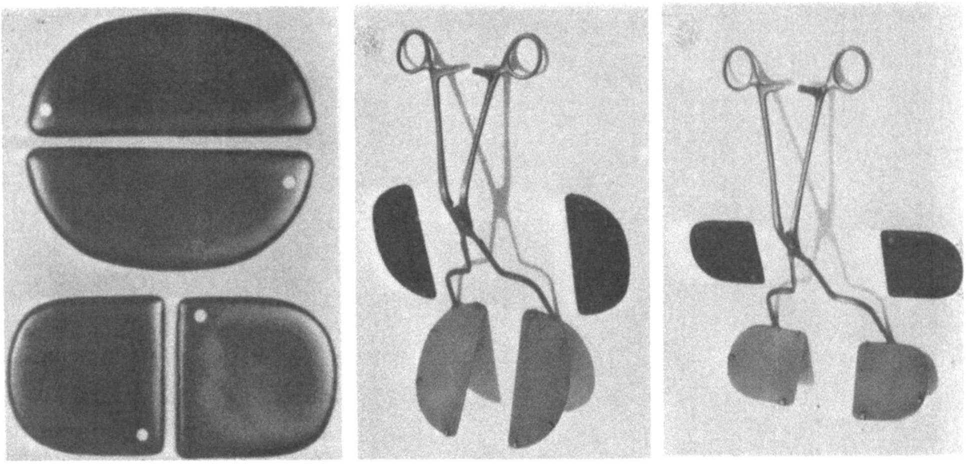

Fig. 8. Film-holding forceps and matching film-wallets (GIL-VERNET and CULLA 1981)

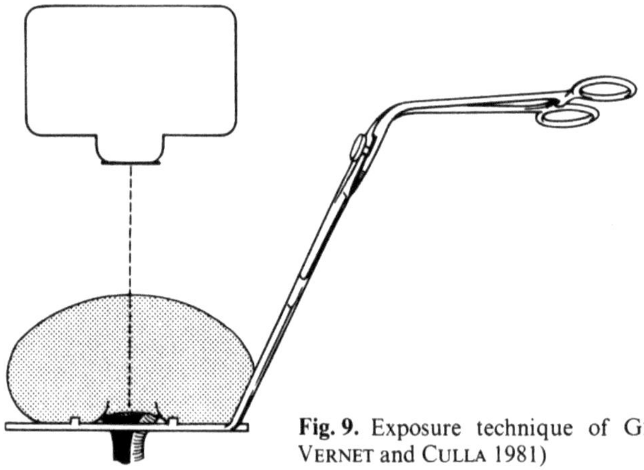

Fig. 9. Exposure technique of GIL-VERNET (GIL-VERNET and CULLA 1981)

other technique is available for localizing stones, objections of this kind may fade into insignificance beside the success rate in terms of freedom from residual stones.

IV. Alternative Techniques

The technique of intraoperative endoscopy should not be thought of as a rival method to intraoperative radiology. Without doubt the results are superior for weakly opaque or radiolucent stones, but since it is not generally possible to inspect the entire collecting system, endoscopy is clearly inferior to radiology at ensuring complete freedom from residual calculi on a whole-kidney basis. The best results come from a rational combination of the two techniques. Whatever approach to the kidney has been employed, endoscopy should aim to extract remaining calculi by that same approach without the need for further incisions. Radiology may indeed be employed to direct endoscopy to the appropriate segment of the collecting system. Only where attempts at extraction under endoscopic vision have failed should radiology be employed to direct further incisions.

On the other hand there are only few restrictions on the extent to which intraoperative ultrasonography can replace radiologic techniques. With the sole exceptions of matrix calculi and loose microlith conglomerates, ultrasound reliably detects stones of any composition (including the radiolucent). The principal practical problem of intraoperative radiology, the three-dimensional detection and localization of stones to dorsal or ventral calyces is without substance for ultrasonography. However, standard ultrasound equipment is not yet able to provide a composite overall picture of the kidney as a record of postoperative stone freedom, and for this purpose radiography remains unavoidable, although a simple lateral view of the kidney is then adequate.

In vivo labelling of calculi with radionuclides (NOBLE et al. 1981) and particularly the labelling of phosphatic calculi with ^{99m}Tc-methylene-diphosphonate is not yet easy to evaluate as a practical clinical tool. In the latter case the use of suitable detectors enables stones of 2–3 mm diameter to be detected.

In the current state of the art the provision of a simple single exposure x-ray set should be regarded as minimum equipment for any operating suite where renal stone surgery is commonly undertaken. First class results are more easily achieved if ultrasound is available in addition, the equipment for which need not be designed specifically for intraoperative use. It is adequate and considerably cheaper to have in the department a general-purpose instrument that can be fitted with a transducer head suitable for intraoperative work.

References

Baskin A, Harvard BM, Janzen AH (1957) Sterile fluoroscopy: Preliminary report of a new technique for localization of renal calculi. J Urol 78:821–826

Baur HM (1972) Intraoperative Röntgenuntersuchung bei Nierensteinoperationen mit dem Röntgengerät „Status-X“. Urologe [Ausg A] 11:190–195

Beck DA (1973) Intraoperative radiography in conservative surgery for renal calculi. J Urol 110:494–497

Boyce WH (1977) The localization of intrarenal calculi during surgery. J Urol 118:152–157

Braren V (1982) Dental film for intraoperative renal stone surgery in children. Urology 20:638

Eisenberger F (1984) The Renodor, an x-ray apparatus for intraoperative localization of kidney stones. In: Wickham JEA (ed) Intrarenal surgery. Churchill, Livingstone Edinburgh, p 271–276

Feldmann RA, Shearer JK, Shield DE, Chase HV (1977) Sensitive method for intraoperative roentgenograms. Urology 9:695–697

Gil-Vernet JM, Culla A (1981) Advances in intraoperative renal radiography: 3-dimensional radiography of the kidney. J Urol 125:614–618

Hanley HG (1967) Flexible renal grid-sling for localizing renal stones during lithotomy. Lancet I:661
Heine G (1980) Doppelaufnahmetechnik und Doppelgitter zur intraoperativen Nierensteinlokalisation. Z Urol Nephrol 73:223–228
Izquierdo F, Rousaud A, Garat JM (1982) Intraoperative Pneumopyelography. Eur Urol 8:148–149
Koshiba K, Ishibashi A, Mashimo S (1980) Use of polaroid film in intraoperative renal radiography: a new technique. J Urol 124:586–587
Leusch G (1970) Ein neues Röntgenverfahren in der Nierensteinchirurgie. Urologe [Ausg A] 9:182–188
Marberger M, Hruby W (1984) Intraoperative radiology: the film. In: Wickham JEA (ed) Intrarenal surgery. Churchill, Livingstone Edinburgh, p 307–315
Marshall FF, Smith NA, Murphy JB, Menon M, Sanders RC (1981) A comparison of ultrasonography and radiography in the localization of renal calculi: Experimental and operative experience. J Urol 126:576–580
Matouschek E (1978) Über eine Methode zur intraoperativen Lokalisation schattengebender Nierensteine in drei Ebenen. Urologe [Ausg A] 17:236–237
Melchior M, Lang G (1981) Three-dimensional intraoperative stone localization. Urol Int 36:390–396
Noble RL, Barker MCJ, Williams RE (1981) The location of urinary calculi using radionuclide imaging. Br J Urol 53:513–515
Roth D, Griffith DP (1983) Operative renal radiography. Urology 21:60–61
Roth RA (1978) Two aids for removal of renal calculi. J Urol 120:666–667
Rubenstein MA, Norris DM, Chun LS (1979) Intraoperative localization of renal calculi using the Polarex 2 C-arm image intensifier. J Urol 121:562–563
Zahm MJ, Bueschen AJ, Lloyd KL, Witten DM (1981) Intraoperative roentgenography in the surgical removal of renal calculi. J Urol 125:284–286
Zink RA, Schmiedt E, Schätzel M (1984) Transrenale and transkorporale Röntgensofortbilddarstellung unter Verwendung von Verstärkerfolien. Urologe [Ausg A] 23:107–108

Percutaneous Manipulation of Renal Calculi

M. MARBERGER

I. Introduction

In 1941, RUPEL and BROWN utilized a nephrostomy tract established by open surgery for endoscopic inspection of the kidney with a cystoscope and extraction of small, obstructing calculi. In the following decades the technique was used sporadically to remove calculi which had been left behind during stone surgery (ENGELKING and ALBRECHT 1969; BRANTLEY et al. 1974; BISSADA et al. 1974; HARRIS 1975), or to remove stones which had formed around permanent nephrostomy tubes (RATHERT et al. 1977; KURTH et al. 1977). Nephrostomy tracts placed at open surgery are, however, usually curved and enter the collecting system at unfavorable positions for reaching calculi, especially if the stones had not been found at the time of surgery. The applicability of this method therefore remained restricted to some anectodal cases. Although GOODWIN et al. had already described a technique of percutaneous nephrostomy providing a straight tract to the kidney in 1955, it was not until two decades later that FERNSTRÖM combined the two methods to a systematic approach to percutaneous removal of kidney stones without the need for open surgery (FERNSTRÖM and JOHANNSON 1976). He reviewed this development in detail in his classical article on "Percutaneous puncture nephrostomy and stone removal" (FERNSTRÖM and ANDERSSON 1977).

II. Anatomical Considerations

Under normal conditions the posterior and lateral margins of both kidneys are immediately adjacent to the lateral abdominal wall, respective psoas major and quadratus lumborum muscles and arcuate ligaments. A transparenchymal puncture of the renal collecting system from a posterolateral approach therefore only transverses the structures of the abdominal wall, Gerota's fascia, the perirenal fat, the fibrous capsule of the kidney and the renal parenchyma (see Fig. 2). With the exception of the pleura in the posterior costo-diaphragmatic recess, which may overlap the upper kidney poles, and the colon, which is in close contact with the medial, anterior aspect of the kidneys, there are no adjacent organs that could be injured. The large vessels of the renal pedicle are almost opposite to the point of entry into the kidney, and if the puncture of the collecting system is noticed and the needle not advanced farther there is little risk of damaging large renal vessels. The only major vessels and nerves coursing posterior to the kidney and lateral of the erector spinae muscle are the 12th intercostal nerve and vessels; unless the puncturing needle is advanced through the abdominal wall slanted upwards and in direct contact with the twelfth rib lesion of these structures are highly unlikely.

The lower line of the pleura usually crosses the twelfth rib at the lateral border of the erector spinae, so that the part of the twelfth rib posterior to this point lies above the line of the pleura. If the puncture is performed at a point below the twelfth rib and approximately 2 finger-breadths lateral to the lateral border of the erector spinae, pleura lesions are avoided. With a supracostal puncture there is of course a high chance of opening the pleura and causing a pneumo- or hydrothorax and even urinary extravasation into the chest.

The relation of the twelth rib to the collecting system shows considerable individual variation, and is influenced by the respiratory movement of the organ and its mobility. WICKHAM and MILLER (1983) investigated the position of the various calyces in relation to the twelfth rib on excretory urograms taken at maximum exspiration with the patient supine: 80% of the lower pole calyces of right kidneys were positioned below the twelfth rib, but only 42% of the middle and 20% of the upper calyces. The left kidney was usually slightly higher, with 78% of the lower pole calyces, 30% of the middle and only 15% of the upper pole calyces in a subcostal position. In females the middle calyces on the right were slightly lower than in males. The figures clearly demonstrate that a lower pole calyx will be the routine port of entry into the collecting system unless specific reasons, like a residual in an upper pole calyx inaccessible by any other approach, justify the high risk of a supracostal puncture.

In the classic type of kidney with a true renal pelvis the anterior and posterior calyces are arranged to the coronal plane of the kidney in an angle of 70° respective 20° (KAYE 1983). On a standard intravenous pyelogram the anterior calyces will therefore appear as the lateral extensions of the collecting system with the typical cup-like structures, whereas the posterior calyces will appear in an orthotopic projection difficult to see due to the overlying pelvis (Fig. 1a). The posterior calyces are clearer to be identified from side-oblique views (Fig. 1b) or by sonography from a side-oblique view. The latter technique also delineates the position of the pleura and colon. Computer tomography, however, is unsurpassed in showing the morphological details of the kidney, stone and perirenal structures (Fig. 2).

The renal arterial vasculature is arranged segmentally, with no collaterals between major vessels. The distribution of the various segments varies greatly (GRAVES 1954), but within the peripheral cortex the feeding interlobular arteries run in a strictly radial direction along the columns of Bertini. When approaching the papilla as peripheral as possible directly from the convexity of the kidney major arteries are rarely encountered and this approach has been used widely for the multiple radial nephrotomy technique. The same approach through the cusp of the papilla is therefore also the entry point of choice for a percutaneous nephrostomy to minimize bleeding. With the blunt dilatation techniques usually employed significant arterial lesions are unlikely to occur,

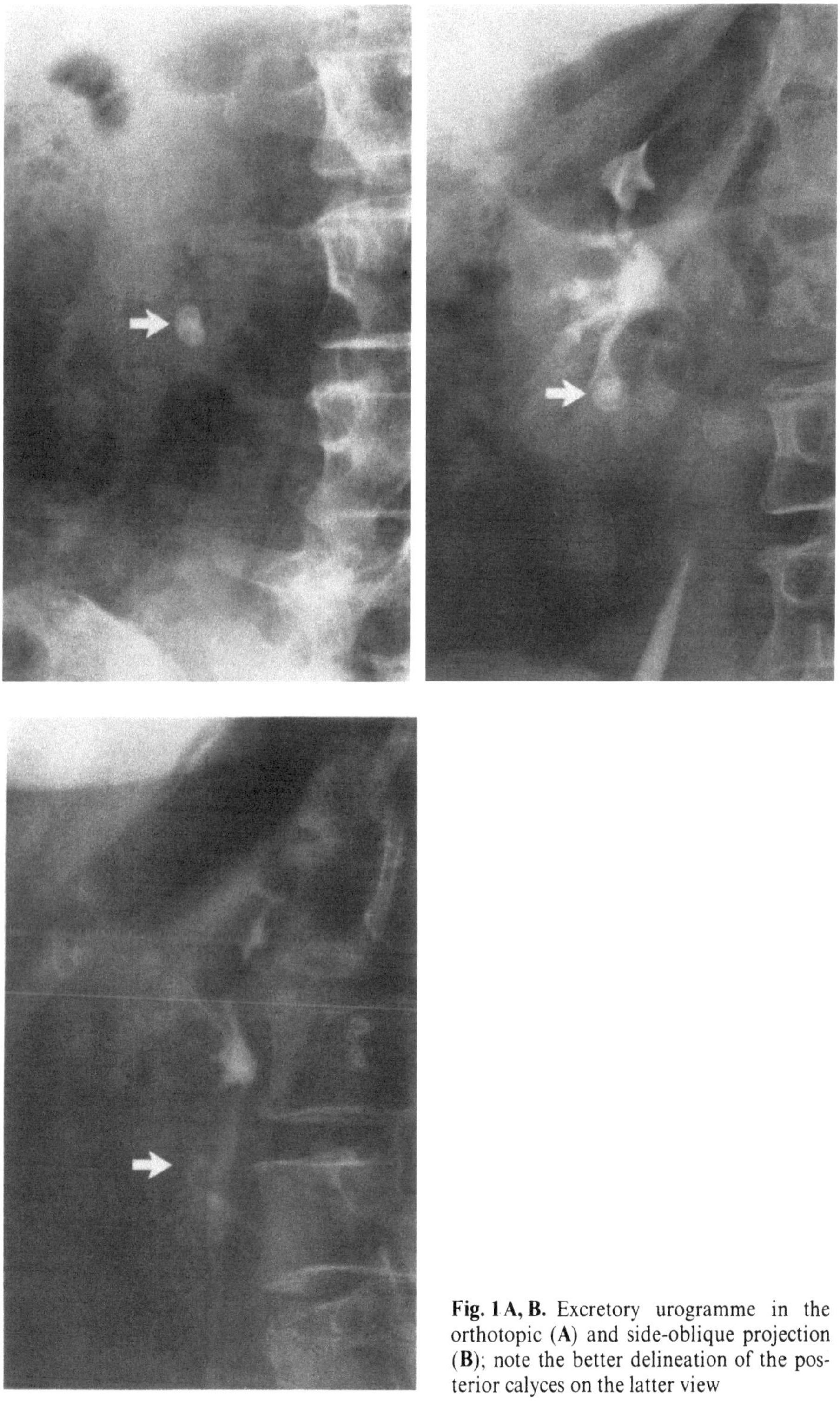

A

B

Fig. 1 A, B. Excretory urogramme in the orthotopic (**A**) and side-oblique projection (**B**); note the better delineation of the posterior calyces on the latter view

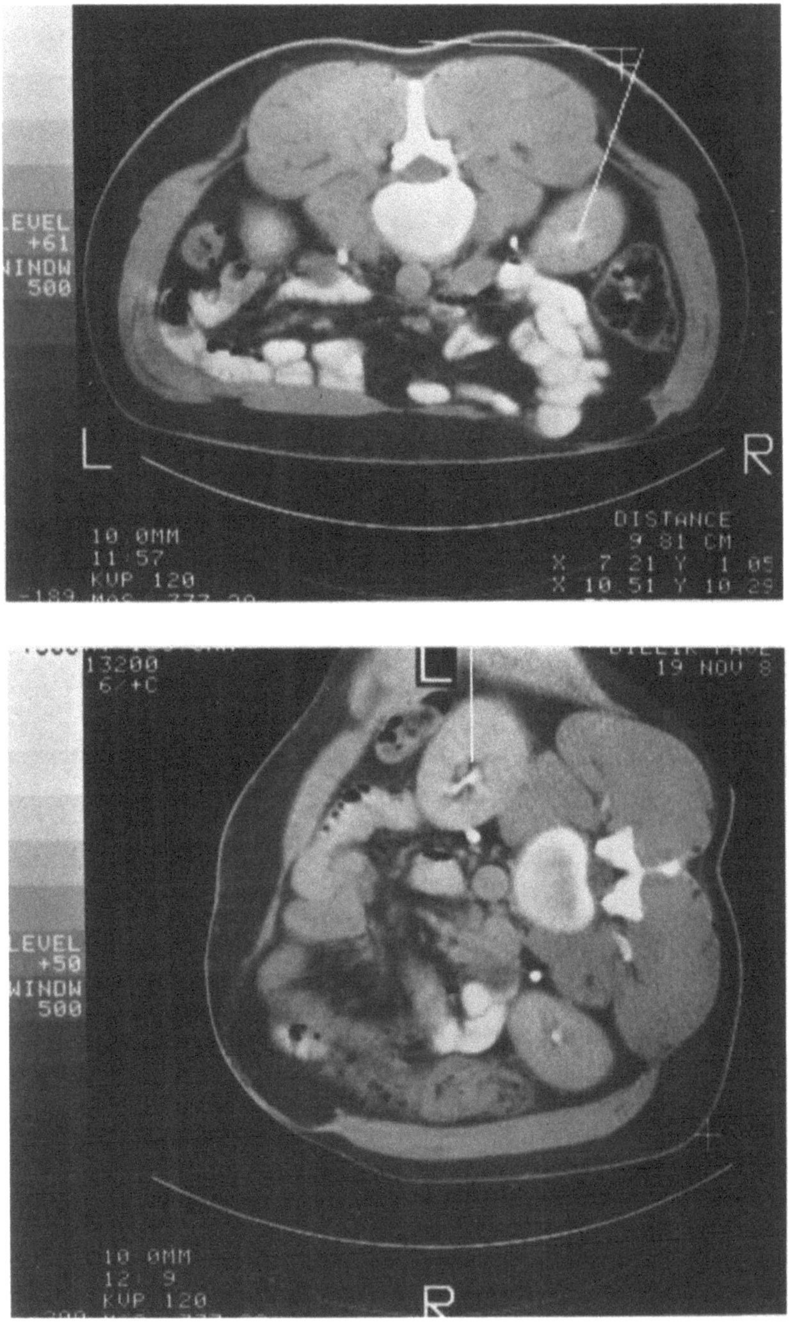

A

B

Fig. 2 A, B. Axial computed tomography of the kidneys with the patient in the prone (**A**) or prone-oblique (**B**) posture; the line of puncture is marked (Courtesy of Dr. W. HRUBY, Rudolfstiftung Vienna)

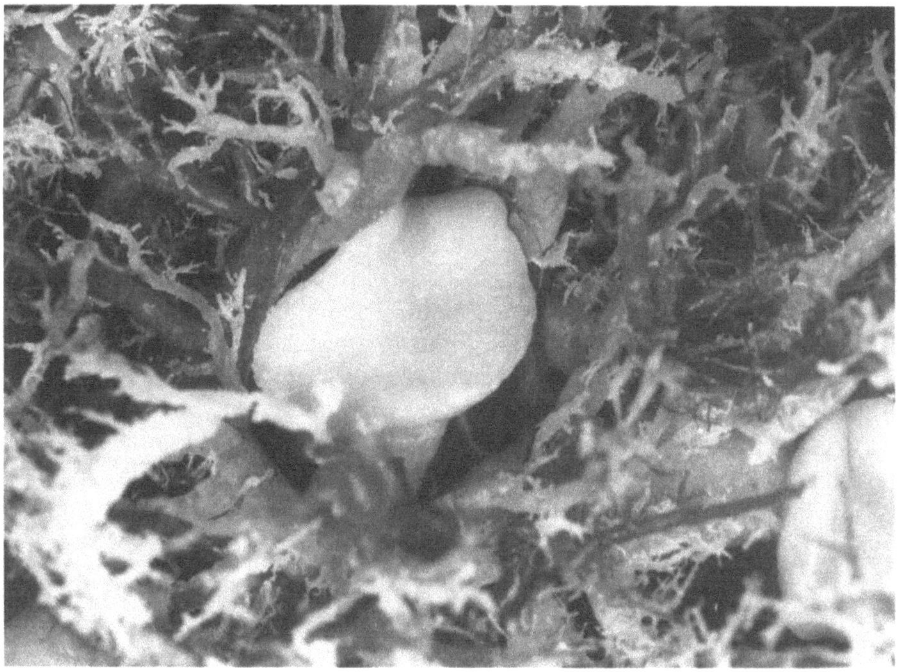

Fig. 3. Corrosion cast of a human kidney showing a calyx and the arterial (darker vessels) and venous vasculature in a view from the peripheral convexity of the kidney, in the direction of a percutaneous puncture. Note the absence of vessels over the calyceal cusp, the radial direction of the arteries and the large veins around the calyceal infundibulum (Courtesy of Dr. I. TSCHABITSCHER, Dept. Anatomy, University of Vienna)

and this puncture direction also avoids the large veins surrounding the calyceal infundibula (Fig. 3).

The success of percutaneous nephrolithotripsy depends entirely on the correct position of the percutaneous nephrostomy. All calculi must be reached through this tract and when rigid endoscopes are used it must be straight. The position of the calculus and the topography of the collecting system therefore ultimately decide on the correct puncture site and must be delineated precisely preoperatively. This is particularly important for peripheral calyceal calculi, as for example a nephrostomy through a posterior lower pole calyx may be absolutely insufficient for reaching a calculus in the adjacent anterior calyx. In general lower pole calyces permit access to the pelvis and most of the lower and upper pole calyces, but to reach a low lying ureteropelvic junction it may be necessary to establish the tract through a middle calyx. With a dilated collecting system the renal pelvis may be punctured directly and this has been advocated to reduce trauma to the parenchyma (BRÜHL 1976), but the collecting system seals poorly around the tube and extravasation frequently occurs (KAYE and GOLDBERG 1982). A transparenchymal approach is therefore mandatory for percutaneous nephrolithotripsy and the tract is the safer the thicker the cortex is at the point of access (STABLES 1982). Intrarenal manipulation is also facilitated by more space for endoscopic maneuvering. The tract should therefore enter the collecting system at a point where a nephrostomy tube or an endoscope can be advanced into the collecting system as far as possible to prevent inadvertent dislocation and loss of the tract. Calyces with a stenosed infundibulum are poorly suited and if they contain a calculus, it is most important for the success of the procedure to pass a guide wire by the stone into the pelvis and an upper pole calyx or the ureter. A transparenchymal access from one calyx into another with active division of the interlying tissue has been employed successfully in selected cases (WICKHAM and MILLER 1983) although this carries some risk of hemorrhage and should be restricted to the hands of the experienced intrarenal surgeon. To summarize, the nephrostomy tract for nephrolithotripsy must be individualized to the specific situation, but it should always be performed via a transparenchymal approach as straight to the stone as possible, preferably through the papilla and infundibulum of a lower pole calyx.

III. Percutaneous Access

With the introduction of percutaneous nephrostomy techniques as routine procedures in every-day urology the literature on this topic has multiplied in an exponential fashion. A complete review of the field exceeds the scope of this presentation and the interested reader is referred to overview articles (BARBARIC 1979; EKELUND et al. 1980; POLLACK and BANNER 1981; STABLES 1982). In most instances, however, the nephrostomy tract is established for draining purposes, i.e. a tube of adequate caliber is inserted somewhere into the collecting system in a position secure enough to achieve this goal. The situation is more complex with nephrolithotripsy: the tube has to be placed precisely in the proximity of the calculus or a part of the collecting system from where the stone can be reached, the majority of kidneys has a delicate, unobstructed collecting system, the tract has to be dilated to admit large caliber instruments and, finally, percutaneous nephrostomy is only the first step of a technically complex procedure requiring an array of special instruments, skills and technical facilities. The details of the approach chosen therefore not only depend on the individual anatomical situation of the patient, but also on the logistic possibilities of the hospital and the experience of the medical staff involved.

1. Patient Preparation

Clotting disorders and renovascular malformations are definite contraindications to percutaneous nephrolithotripsy and must be ruled out preoperatively. This is achieved with a clotting screen including at least a platelet count and determination of the bledding, prothrombin- and partial thromboplastintime (WICKHAM and MILLER 1983), and with screening sonography of the kidney, which may even be performed immediately prior to the procedure. Acotemic patients frequently have a prolonged bleeding time with otherwise normal clotting tests, and preoperative administration of standard red cross cryoprecipitate has been recommended to correct this (JANSON et al. 1980). Hypertension in excess of 200/120 mm Hg increases the risk of hemorrhage and should be controlled prior to percutaneous puncture. Some authors (WICKHAM and MILLER 1983; SEGURA et al. 1982) consider sterile urine mandatory for percutaneous nephrolithotripsy, but frequently urinary infection cannot be abolished in the presence of extensive calculous disease. Provided appropriate antimicrobial agents are administered for at least 48 hours septicemia, renal and perirenal infection have not been a problem after this procedure (MARBERGER et al. 1982; MARBERGER 1983a; CLAYMAN et al. 1983b). Thorough explanation of the procedure, of potential complications and in particular of the possible need for a staged intervention, are mandatory for an informed consent.

Whereas an emergency nephrostomy can frequently be established in obstructed kidneys virtually without anesthesia, good analgesia is essential for a correct access for lithotripsy. This is usually accomplished by infiltration anesthesia with bupivacaine or lidocaine and sedation by small doses of diazepam and pethidine intravenously (MARBERGER et al. 1982; STABLES 1982; KELLETT 1983; HRUBY et al. 1983; CLAYMAN 1983); the patient can then still cooperate sufficiently to suspend breathing on request during puncture (STABLES 1982). Local anesthesia also permits intrarenal manipulation via a mature dilated nephrostomy tract (MARBERGER et al. 1982), in particular when supplemented with butapharnol intravenously until the patient becomes drowsy or his speech becomes blurred (CLAYMAN et al. 1983b). CLAYMAN (1984) even performs complete one-stage nephrolithotripsy with this "assisted" local anesthesia. The movement of large-caliber instruments within the kidney and intermittent distension of the renal capsule is, however, quite painful, and uneasiness of the patient impedes intrarenal manipulation. Regional intercostal (EKELUND et al. 1980) or epidural anesthesia (ALKEN et al. 1983) provide good analgesia, but most authors prefer general anesthesia with endotracheal intubation (MARBERGER 1983; KELLETT 1983; SMITH and LEE 1983) for more aggressive procedures.

Even if only a nephrostomy is established in local anesthesia, the patient should be kept sober for some hours preoperatively to reduce vomitting. For a brisk diuresis fluid is provided intravenously during this phase. The administration of 1 ml/min 20% mannitol intravenously just before commencing with intrarenal manipulation reduces the risk of intratubular reflux and, probably, pyelonephritis (ALKEN 1982). If the nephrostomy is established under fluoroscopic control, the bolus injection of intravenous contrast dye (600 mg iodine/kg) given to opacify the kidney at the time of initiating anesthesia probably fulfills the same purpose (KELLETT 1983).

2. Patient Positioning

The patient may be placed in a prone oblique (STABLES 1982; KELLET 1983) posture, the prone posture (ALKEN 1981; ALKEN et al. 1983; MARBERGER 1983;

HRUBY et al. 1983; SMITH and LEE 1983) or the supine oblique posture (GOODWIN et al. 1955; BABCOCK et al. 1979; GÜNTHER et al. 1979). The latter position, with elevation of the flank to be punctured, is most comfortable for the patient, but the needle must be advanced horizontally and this makes guidance under conventional vertical beam guidance difficult as anterior or posterior deviation of the needle is difficult to assess (STABLES 1982). In addition, sterile endoscopic manipulation is virtually impossible due to the lack of maneuvering space lateral and posterior to the patient; the position is unsuited for nephrolithotripsy.

In the prone oblique position with the patient rotated approximately to 45° obliquity the skin puncture site lies directly over the point of entry into the pelvocalyceal system. When vertical beam fluoroscopy is used for guidance the two points are superimposed, so that the puncture can be performed in a vertical direction directly onto the calyx, parallel to the fluoroscopy beam (see Fig. 2b). Provided the needle is advanced to the correct depth in this direction, puncture is simple. The technique becomes difficult when the needle has to be angled under the costal arch. By comparing the relative movements of the needle tip and the target calyx during respiration, the depth of the needle can frequently be judged by parallax even under single plane fluoroscopy (KELLETT 1983). The use of additional ultrasonic guidance (WALZ et al. 1981; ALKEN et al. 1983; HRUBY et al. 1983) or biplane fluoroscopy (FERNSTRÖM 1983a) obviates the problem.

Nephrolithotripsy is frequently carried out as a staged procedure. With an immature tract this requires identical positioning of the patient at each session to regain the straight tract through the various layers of the abdominal wall. Experience has shown that this is difficult in the prone oblique posture and that barely noticeable variations in obliquity may result in considerable interweaving of the muscular layers along the tract. The prone position is simple to reproduce and in local anesthesia the patient can maintain it with less discomfort than in the prone oblique posture. With general anesthesia correct endotracheal anesthesia is mandatory, as the anesthesist has no possibility to readjust the tube once the patient is prone. Foam rubber rolls are arranged on both sides of the chest to allow for respiratory excursion, and arms and feet must be well padded (SMITH and LEE 1983). A foam rubber cushion in the hypochondrium under the kidney helps to stabilize a mobile organ for puncture (KELLETT 1983; ALKEN et al. 1983). The vertical puncture techniques described above can of course not be employed in the prone position when using vertical beam fluoroscopy, so that puncture is more difficult due to the angled image of the needle. By combining fluoroscopy with ultrasonic guidance (WALZ et al. 1981; ALKEN et al. 1983; HRUBY et al. 1983) or using biplane fluoroscopy (FERNSTRÖM 1983a) this disadvantage can easily be overcome. The routine management of difficult calculi by the percutaneous route increases the number of multi-stage procedures and the prone position is therefore being used more widely (ALKEN et al. 1981; MARBERGER et al. 1982; CLAYMAN et al. 1983).

3. Imaging Guidance

With sonography readily available to many urologists, ultrasound guided puncture has popularized percutaneous nephrostomy of obstructed kidneys (PEDERSEN et al. 1976; STABLES and JOHNSON 1979; HILDEL et al. 1980; BARON et al. 1981; WALZ et al. 1981; OTTO et al. 1982; EICKENBERG et al. 1982; SCHÖLLER et al. 1984). Using B-mode scanning and sterile biopsy transducers (PEDERSEN et al. 1976) or transducers with attachable puncturing devices (WALZ et al. 1981) dilated collecting systems can be delineated sufficiently for puncture, but real-time sonography is employed more frequently (BARON et al. 1981), as it permits simultaneous control of the kidney, calculus and needle.

The most obvious advantage of ultrasonic guidance lies in the fact that opacification of the collecting system is not required. This is difficult to achieve in a poorly functioning kidney, especially if retrograde catheterization fails. The dye also camoflages calculous material. Even with the most sophisticated equipment, however, some details of importance for precise placement of the nephrostomy cannot be delineated in non-dilated collecting systems, such as the calyceal infundibula (ALKEN and GÜNTHER 1983). Fluoroscopic control therefore remains essential for nephrolithotripsy, in particular as it is also needed during the stone manipulation itself. Unless biplane fluoroscopy is available (FERNSTRÖM 1983), sonography is most helpful as an adjunctive imaging technique to conventional vertical beam fluoroscopy. After preliminary screening of the kidney it can be used to decide on the optimal puncture site on the skin and in the collecting system, the necessary angulation of the needle and the depth the needle has to be advanced to (STABLES 1979). With some experience it suffices to mark the point of skin entry and to memorize the angle and depth, and then insert the needle under fluoroscopic guidance (HRUBY et al. 1983).

The choice of the fluoroscopic equipment mainly depends on the availability. Urological tables with overhead tubes are ideal from the aspect of adequate space for sterile maneuvering during lithotripsy, but the radiation exposure of the surgeon is increased at least 100 fold as compared to radiological tables with undertable tubes. Although protective shielding, in particular of eyes and thyroid, scrupulous collimating of the exposed field, and the technical improvements of modern image-intensifying systems with "freeze" monitors significantly reduce radiation hazards (HUTSCHENREITER 1983; SEGURA et al. 1983; BUSH et al. 1984), percutaneous nephrostomies should preferably not be placed on tables with over-head tubes. Together with logistic considerations in the cooperation of urologist and radiologist this factor may be the reason for establishing the nephrostomy and performing nephrolithotripsy as staged procedures, rather than in one session. Lithotripsy must always be performed with the possibility of fluoroscopic control, either on a standard diagnostic table or with the C-arm in the operating theatre, on a radiolucent table. With the latter technique the beam of fluoroscopy may be adapted to the individual situation (SMITH and LEE 1983; CLAYMAN 1983), but there is also significant scatter radiation and the still-image film quality may be insufficient to show residual calculous debris. Kidney puncture is facilitated by inflating the collecting system with saline, contrast dye (CLAYMAN 1983) or methylene blue injected via a

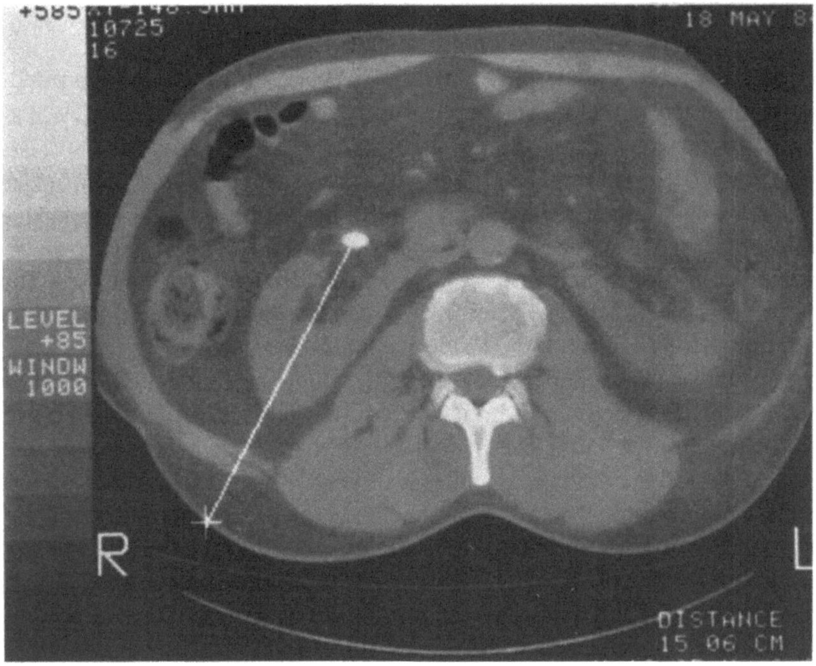

Fig. 4. Horseshoe kidney with calculus in an anterior calyx. Axial computed tomography clearly delineates the posterior calyx to be entered and the position of the stone-bearing calyx to the pelvis (Courtesy of Dr. W. HRUBY, Rudolfstiftung Vienna)

ureteral catheter (KORTH 1983). Guidance under computed tomography is too complicated for routine use, but may be helpful in difficult situations like identifying the relation of a nephrostomy tube to a stone residual in a malformed kidney (HAGA et al. 1977) (Fig. 4).

4. Puncturing the Kidney

Percutaneous nephrostomies may be established directly with trocartype cannulas (GOODWIN et al. 1955; PEDERSON et al. 1966; NEWHOUSE and PFISTER 1981; PFISTER et al. 1983), but these instruments are too traumatizing for use in a non-dilated collecting system and therefore only rarely used for gaining surgical access for endourological procedures. In general variations of the Seldinger technique are employed. According to the instruments used they may be divided into:

a) The Catheter-Over-Needle Method (FERNSTRÖM and ANDERSON 1976; LEVY 1978; WALZ et al. 1981; STABLES et al. 1982; KELLETT 1983; ALKEN et al. 1983): Teflon sheathed needles as used for translumbar aortography are advanced to the collecting system. The needle is then withdrawn and a 0.35 guide wire threaded down the soft sheath into the collecting system.

b) The 3-Part Coaxial Needle Set (GÜNTHER et al. 1979; SADLOWSKY et al. 1979) consisting of an outer blunt cannula, an inner 22-gauge bevelled needle and a stylet: the entire system is advanced through the abdominal wall to the fibrous capsule of the kidney. The collecting system is first punctured with the fine needle until the correct position is reached and the outer cannula is then advanced over it. After withdrawing the inner needle a guide wire can again be inserted.

c) The Double Puncture Technique (STABLES 1982): the pelvocalyceal system is first punctured with a 22-gauge spinal or Chiba needle at a site slightly distant from the optimal puncture site and filled with diluted contrast dye for better delineation and subsequent puncture with a larger needle. The same effect can be achieved by filling the collecting system with dye via a ureteral catheter (CLAYMAN et al. 1982).

d) The Skinny Needle Technique: the collecting system is punctured with a 22-gauge needle, a very fine 0.25 guide wire is threaded through the needle, the needle is removed and a teflon sheathed needle fed over the guide wire under fluoroscopic control.

The point of entry into the pelvocalyceal system depends on the position of the calculus, the anatomy of the collecting system and the position of the 12th rib. In the majority of stone bearing kidneys the lower pole calyx provides good access to the lower pole calyces, the pelvis, and with some limitations, the upper pole calyces. In low kidneys with calculi in the middle calyces these may be punctured directly; this access is also the approach of choice when manipulation at the ureteropelvic junction or in the proximal ureter is to be anticipated.

To reduce the risk of tube kinking in the supine position the tract should enter the skin from the dorso-lateral aspect of the flank at an angle of approximately 45° to the sagittal plane (STABLES 1982). The latissimus dorsi and serratus posterior inferior muscles forming this part of the abdominal wall are relatively thin and easy to be transversed, and the 12th intercostal nerve and vessels are protected by the 12th rib. Using one or several of the imaging techniques described above the ideal point of skin entry is determined and marked and the correct angle of puncture and depth at which the collecting system is reached noted. After notching the skin the puncture needle is advanced to the fibrous capsule of the kidney. If a coaxial 3-part needle set is used, the parenchyma is first pierced with the inner needle and the outer needle is only advanced over it after urine dripping from the needle signalizes a correct needle position. With the other techniques the larger bore needles are advanced through the parenchyma under frequent fluoroscopic control to document adherance to the projected path.

In a kidney with a dilated collecting system the experienced urologist will notice a slight give as the collecting system is entered, but in a non-dilated system urine dripping from the needle is the usual sign of success. An appropriate guide wire (usually 0.35) with a soft J-tip is now fed down the needle and into the collecting system; in case of resistance or an obviously inappropriate position it is withdrawn and the position of the needle controlled with diluted contrast dye. To reduce respiratory movement of the kidney the patient is asked to breath rather quietly; puncture in maximum inspiration or after the request to stop breathing may result in an angled tract difficult to negotiate with rigid instruments. With high lying kidneys this may nevertheless be the only possibility of entering the collecting system via a subcostal approach.

The guide wire directs the successive dilatation instruments or tubes and prevents loss of the tract if problems occur during this phase. It is therefore imperative that it is advanced into the collecting system as far as possible, preferably directly, passing the calculus, into an upper pole calyx (ALKEN et al. 1983; HRUBY et al. 1983) or down the ureter (SEGURA et al. 1983).

The limited availability of fluoroscopy facilities for urologists, but also the increasing experience with ureterorenoscopy and retrograde endourology has sparked interest in retrograde nephrostomy techniques (HUNTER et al. 1983; LAWSON et al. 1983). With these methods a catheter is directed into a calyx suitable for percutaneous access in the retrograde direction via the ureter. The catheter serves as sheath to guide a semirigid needle stylet to this point, from where it is then advanced through the parenchyma and abdominal wall in an outward direction to be retrieved outside the skin. The nephrostomy is established over the puncture wire. Purpose built sets are commercially available, and HUNTER et al. reported only 3 failures in a clinical trial in 30 patients (HUNTER et al. 1985). The main difficulty of the technique arises from correct placement of the wire in the correct calyx. In spite of incorporating special tip-deflecting catheters or torque wires (LAWSON et al. 1983; HUNTER et al. 1983; MILLER et al. 1983a) this may be difficult for lower pole calyces, and penetration into adjacent organs, in particular the pleura, liver and colon, has been reported (HUNTER et al. 1983). MILLER et al. (1983a) suggested that the complication rate could be further reduced by retrieving the stylet already at the level of the fibrous capsule with the help of lumboscopy.

5. Tract Dilatation

In the early days of endourology percutaneous stone manipulation was almost exclusively performed via a mature tract which had been established in steps by introducing nephrostomy tubes of gradually increasing diameter. The constant effort to reduce treatment periods, but also to reduce tube complications between the time of tract formation and endoscopic surgery, has continuously shortened this period. Most authors today routinely perform the entire procedure in a single session (KELLETT and WICKHAM 1983; ALKEN et al. 1983). This requires the use of special instruments for rapid tract dilatation.

Derived from fascial dilators as used in angiography semirigid teflon dilators were first utilized for this purpose (ALKEN et al. 1981b; KELLETT 1983). Dilators of increasing diameter are advanced into the collecting system one after the other, under radiological control, and over the guide wire. Instruments from F 5 to F 34 are commercially available. Alternatively, polyethylene coaxial dilators may be used (SMITH and LEE 1983). After inserting a F 8 polyethylene dilator over the guide wire the succeeding dilators 2 F larger than the previous one are passed in turn over the initial F 8 dilator. After dilatation the final endoscopic instrument is advanced into the kidney over the guide-wire with both approaches. This carries a high risk of kinking of the guide wire and loss of the tract. The development of teflon sheaths which are slid into the collecting system directly over the largest dilator significantly improved the efficiency of these systems (RUSNAK et al. 1982). The dilators are then removed through the sheath which stays in place during the manipulation and compresses the parenchyma along the tract, thus reducing intraoperative hemorrhage. In this manner any endoscopic instrument may be introduced through the sheath without traumatizing the kidney. The irrigation fluid drains freely around the instrument so that an increase of intrarenal pressure during endoscopic surgery is avoided. If the surgeon considers the continuous leakage of fluid and drenching of the field annoying, the system can be sealed with a snap-on cap on the sheath (RUTNER 1983) and an overflow cannula.

Properly used, semirigid instruments are safe and economical, as they can be re-used. With very dense tissues, however, in particular after multiple previous operations, they tend to buckle at the levels of the fascia and fibrous capsule of the kidney. This can result in dislocation of the guide wire and a false passage. Metal dilators help avoid this hazard. ALKEN (1981) developed a telescope-dilator system in which aerial dilators increasing in increments of F 2 are advanced one over the other, along a central metal rod. Nephrostomy tubes or the sheaths of nephroscopes may be inserted directly over the appropriate dilators which can then be retrieved through the lumen of the instrument with the help of a retriever knob at the distal end of the central rod (Fig. 5). In the

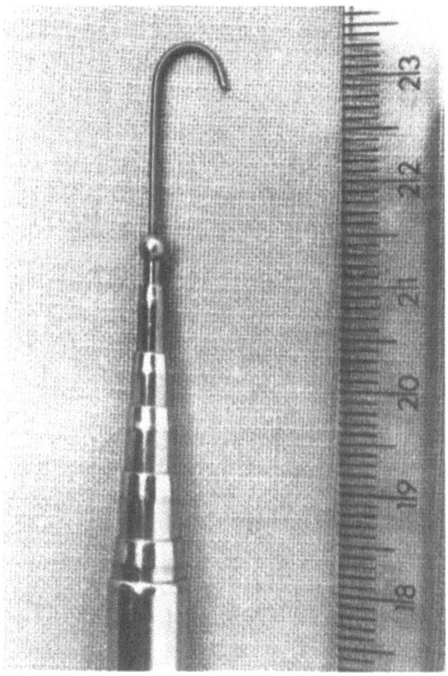

Fig. 5. Telescope dilator and semirigid Lunderquist guide-wire

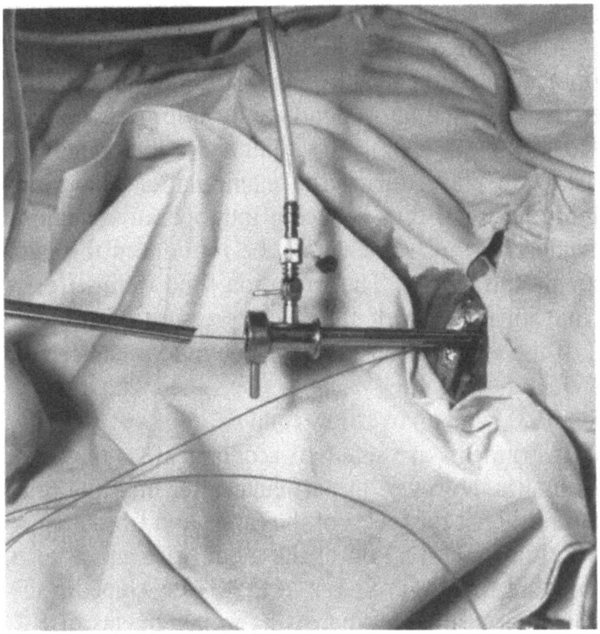

Fig. 6. Nephroscopy: the F 24 sheath was introduced over the telescope dilator, which was then withdrawn. The Lunderquist guide-wire is still in place and is threaded through the nephroscope to facilitate initial intrarenal orientation. Note "safety" guide-wire outside the sheath

original version presented by ALKEN (1981) this rod had no axial perforation, so that it could not be directed over a guide wire, but this modification added substantially to the safety of the system (MARBERGER et al. 1983a). Passage of the fascial layer and scar tissue can further be facilitated by cutting these structures with a rigid instrument with cruciate adjustable blades (KORTH 1984).

Balloon catheters originally developed for transluminal angioplasty tolerate pressures in excess of 10 atmospheres and can be employed for rapid tract dilatation (KELLETT 1982). With the balloon deflated the catheter is positioned over a guide wire, so that the balloon covered part is located along the tract to be dilated. With obese patients repeated in- and deflation of the balloon and repositioning of the catheter may be required. The balloon is rapidly filled with diluted contrast dye to inflate it along the entire tract. After several seconds it is collapsed again, the catheter removed and the endoscopic instrument advanced into the tract over the guide wire. CLAYMAN et al. (1983c) solved the problem of buckling of the working wire and false passage when introducing the instrument by using a 10 mm Olbert angioplasty balloon catheter which is backloaded with a teflon working sheath or the nephroscope sheath. The balloon only needs to be inflated for several seconds; after deflation the backloaded instrument is slipped into the collection system directly over the balloon.

No system is without draw-backs and complications; experienced endourologists use a variety of dilatation instruments. Semirigid dilatators are safest for dilating the tract from the caliber of the puncture needle to ca. F 16. Larger flexible dilators buckle at fascial layers and may be extremely difficult to be advanced through extensive scar tissue. Metal dilators are highly efficient and safe once the central rod is properly positioned in the collecting system and dilatation is performed under fluoroscopic control, but it may be difficult to insert the rod over the guide wire if the original tract was not straight. Balloon catheters are very costly and can usually not be re-used. With significant perirenal scarring they may not inflate completely when insufficient inflation pressures are used, and they may require repositioning during the dilatation phase. The author therefore relies on a combined approach with dilatation of the tract to ca. F 16 with fascial dilators and subsequently to F 24 with the metal telescope dilators.

In addition to the improvement of dilatation instruments the complication rate of this phase of the procedure has been significantly reduced by using Lunderquist guide wires as working guides, and an additional safety guide wire in case the first is dislocated (Fig. 6). The Lunderquist guide wire is made of rigid polished steel with a soft floppy end (see Fig. 5) and guides the dilators unfailingly into the collecting system once positioned properly (Marberger 1983; Smith and Lee 1983; Kellett et al. 1983).

6. Nephrostomy Tubes

The requirements a nephrostomy tube suitable for percutaneous stone manipulation has to meet exceed those of an instrument designed for simple drainage purposes. Its lumen must open at the blunt-tipped end and be large enough not only to permit drainage of bloody urine and even clots, but also passage of guide-wires and even a F 6 angiography catheter. They should be rigid enough to be advanced down the tract over a guide wire with little tendency to kink, buckle or collapse. These prerequisites rule out all pig-tail catheters and angiography catheters, and basically limit the choice to straight tubes. A variety of purpose-built tubes of this type are today commercially available. Some feature radiopaque markings to facilitate fluoroscopic control. Spontaneous tube displacement is a major problem in pre- and postoperative drainage, and various retention disks to secure the tubes to the skin, malecot tipped and balloon tipped catheters and even a tube with a balloon for fixation in the perirenal fat (Hohlbrugger and Janetschek 1984) were designed to prevent this. In the author's experience all are not completely satisfying. The malecot tips tend to provoke hemorrhage and do not reliably eliminate dislocation. The balloon tipped catheters drain poorly and may even obstruct upper pole calyces in kidneys with an intrarenal collecting system. The author routinely uses straight, blunt-tipped polyethylene tubes with an end- and one side hole and a caliber of at least F 12 which are secured to the skin with a suture and tape. Recently tubes made of polyurethane have become available that have the same construction and rigidity, yet better tissue tolerance, radiopaque markers and a detachable funnel-shaped end so that they can be inserted through a nephroscope sheath (Fig. 7).

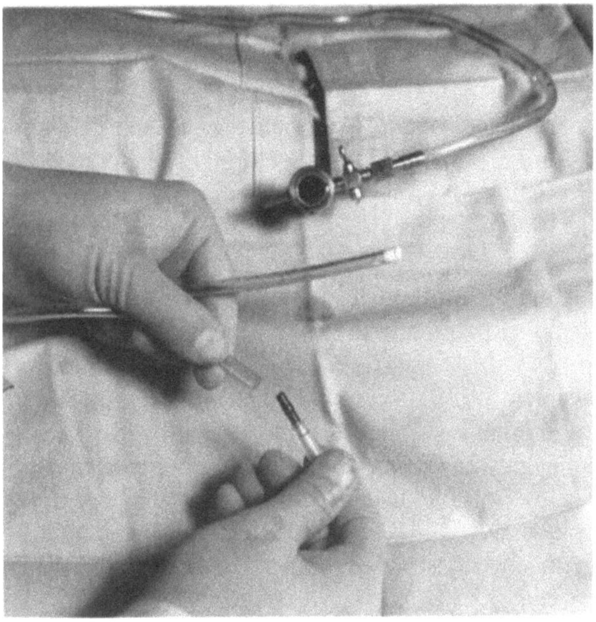

Fig. 7. Polyurethane nephrostomy tube with end-and-side hole tip, radiopaque markings and detachable funnel to pass tube through the nephroscope sheath (Rüsch)

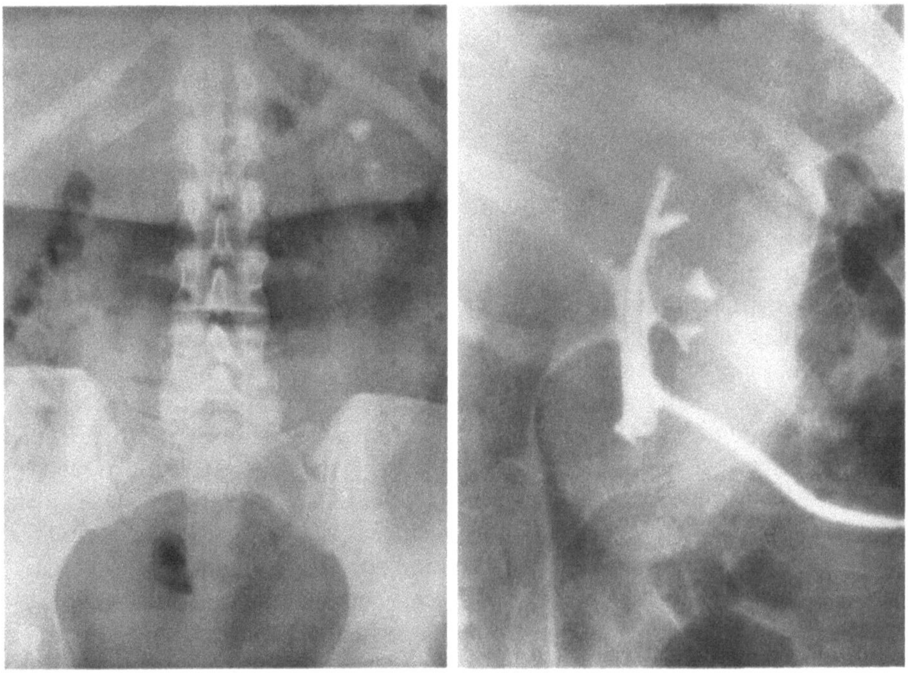

a b

Fig. 8. Correct position of nephrostomy tube for percutaneous stone manipulation: it enters the system through a lower pole calyx and permits access to all calculi; there is adequate length of the tube within the collecting system to prevent dislocation from respiratory movement

Even when properly secured to the skin, the tubes are dislocated rather easily from the kidney because of the respiratory movement, in particular in obese patients with very mobile kidneys. This is best prevented by advancing the tube as far into the collecting system as possible, at least 5–6 cm. Tubes advanced down the ureter are safest, but large caliber catheters obstruct urinary drainage and promote extravasation. The standard position of the tube in the author's approach is therefore entry of the tube into a lower pole calyx and passage through the pelvis into an upper pole calyx, in immediate proximity of the calculus to be removed (Fig. 8).

Postoperatively many authors recommend a large caliber tube > F 24 to tamponade the tract and reduce venous bleeding; standard Foley balloon catheters with slight traction applied to them have likewise been used, and recently the Kaye tamponade catheter resembling a modified angioplasty catheter has become available for this purpose. Provided the nephrostomy tract is dilated bluntly, hemorrhage is practically always of venous origin and will stop spontaneously. Large caliber tubes left in the tract for a longer postoperative period tend to provoke fresh bleeding and to prevent collapsing of the tract so that morbidity is increased. The author therefore routinely inserts a 14 F tube which is left in place for only 24 hours, unless a residual stone or extravasation require further manipulations or longer drainage. In case of significant venous hemorrhage, which usually corresponds with the opacification of major renal veins at injection of contrast dye through the tube, the tube is simply stoppered for some time until the tract tamponades itself. Only rarely has it been necessary to insert large caliber tubes or a special short-tipped balloon catheter with a detachable end that can be placed through the nephroscope sheath (Fig. 9).

IV. Nephroscopy

With the development of percutaneous needle puncture techniques nephrostomies could be placed within the close vicinity of renal calculi. It was therefore only a natural next step to attempt their removal via the percutaneous tract. The pioneers of these methods (FERNSTRÖM and JOHANSSON 1976; FERNSTRÖM and ANDERSSON 1977) only relied on fluoroscopy for intrarenal guidance during stone manipulation. In spite of the use of biplane fluoroscopy, steerable instruments and modified Mazzariello-Caprini forceps interposing soft tissue frequently resulted in failures, so that most authors reported anecdotal cases only (ENGELKING and ALBRECHT 1969; BRANTLEY and SHIRLEY 1974; KARAMCHETI and O'DONELL 1977; WEISS et al. 1977; HELLSTRÖM and PALESTRANT 1981; CLAYMAN et al. 1983a).

Already RUPEL and BROWN (1941) had pointed out the solution: percutaneous nephroscopy. Using a cystoscope advanced down a surgical nephrostomy tract they successfully identified and extracted an obstructing renal stone. Endoscopes originally designed for the lower urinary tract proved to greatly facilitate percutaneous stone manipulation, and together with the wider availability of percutaneous nephrostomy formed the basis for establishing per-

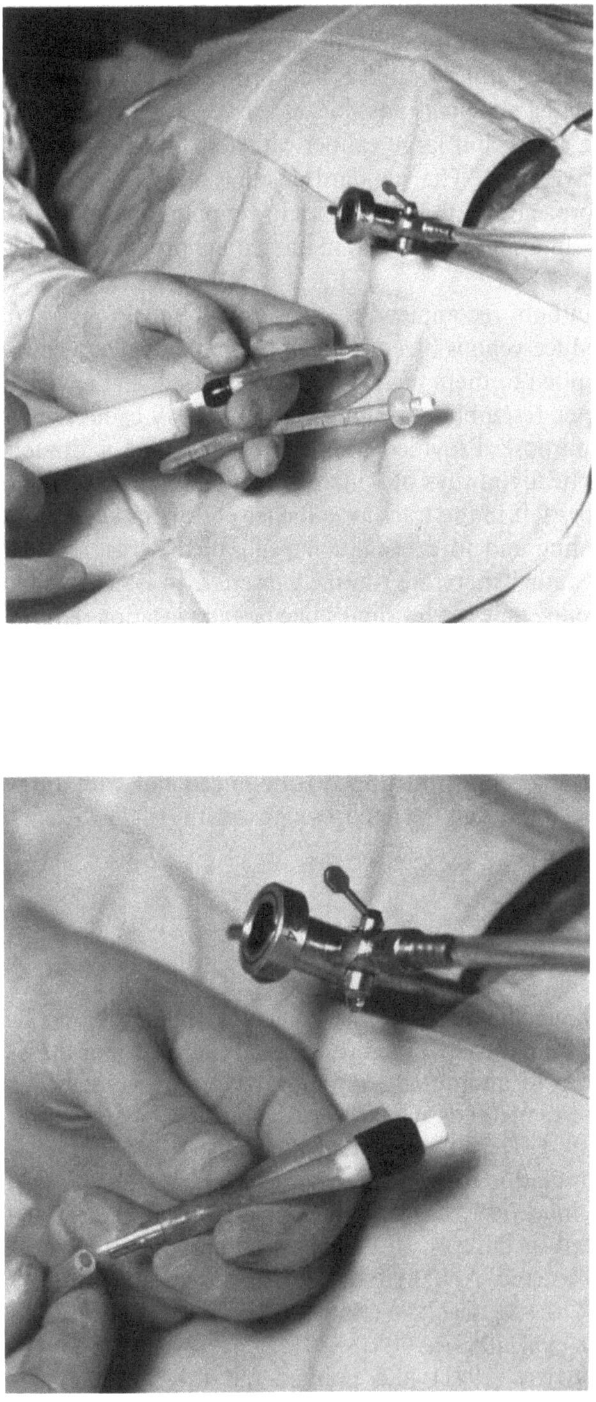

Fig. 9. Modified polyurethane nephrostomy tube (see Fig. 7) with balloon and detachable end to introduce it through the nephroscope sheath

cutaneous stone manipulation as a standardized treatment modality (BRANTLEY and SHIRLEY 1974; BISSADA et al. 1974; KURTH et al. 1977; SMITH et al. 1978; WICKHAM et al. 1981; ALKEN et al. 1981). In general 30° F 20 to F 24 pan-endoscopes or F 20 urethrotomes were used (CLAYMAN 1983; MILLER and WICKHAM 1983), which permitted antegrade vision without protruding instrument beaks. Irrigation was provided by gravity perfusion with saline either intermittently through the in- and outflow channels of the instrument or with an outflow down the ureter or along the instrument by using a nephrostomy sheath. The high optical quality of the rigid-rod-lens systems for the first time permitted true endoscopic inspection of the kidney and provided the basis for the first large patient series treated percutaneously. The main disadvantage of the instruments, however, was their lack of an operating port which permits a direct approach to a calculus with a straight, rigid instrument. Calculi had to be removed with baskets or flexible forceps which proved to be difficult to be manipulated inside the kidney or too small for larger stones. The ultrasonic lithotrite originally developed for bladder calculi was also used in the kidney (KURTH et al. 1977; ALKEN et al. 1981; ALKEN 1982), but was too awkward.

1. Rigid Nephroscopes

The break-through came with the development of purpose-built nephroscopes. In 1981 the author designed a 24 F universal nephroscope for percutaneous surgery (MARBERGER et al. 1981; MARBERGER et al. 1982). It incorporated a sheath and shaft system with a 15° endoscope and a straight, 11 F working channel. The eyepiece of the endoscope was right-angled from the working port to permit sterile manipulation. An integrated continuous flow irrigation system provided a continuous exchange of irrigation fluid at high flow rates; as the diameter of the outflow channel exceeded that of the inflow channel, an increase of intrarenal pressure was avoided (Fig. 10). The inflow channel, working port

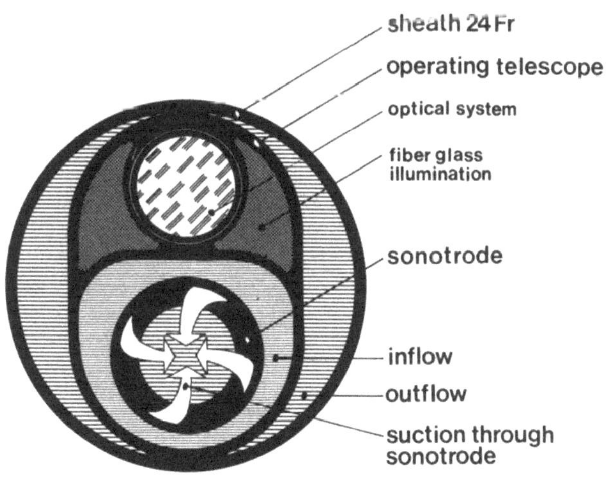

Fig. 10. Cross-section of F 24 nephroscope (Wolf) demonstrating continuous irrigation system. The outflow port is larger than the inflow port, so that an increase of intrarenal pressure is avoided even when suction through the sonotrode is not used (Reproduced with permission from MARBERGER, M.: Urol Clin N Am 10: 729, 1983)

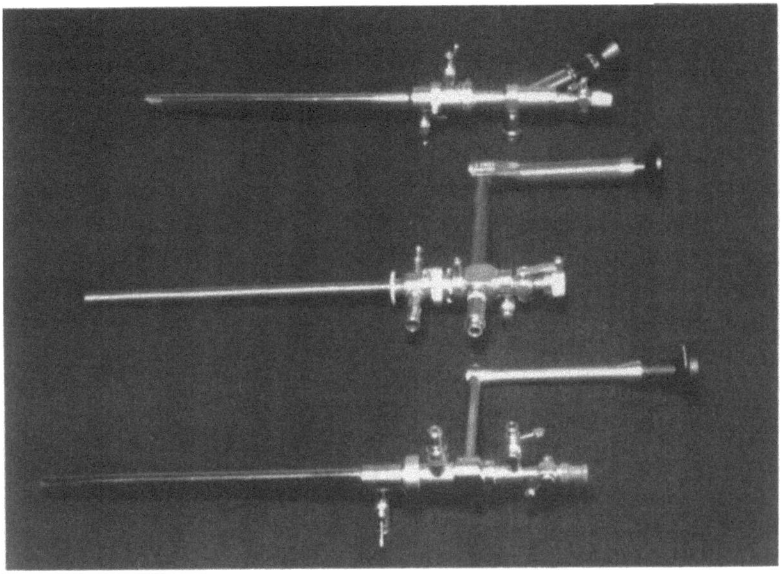

Fig. 11. Rigid nephroscopes for percutaneous stone manipulation (From top to bottom: Olympus, Storz, Wolf)

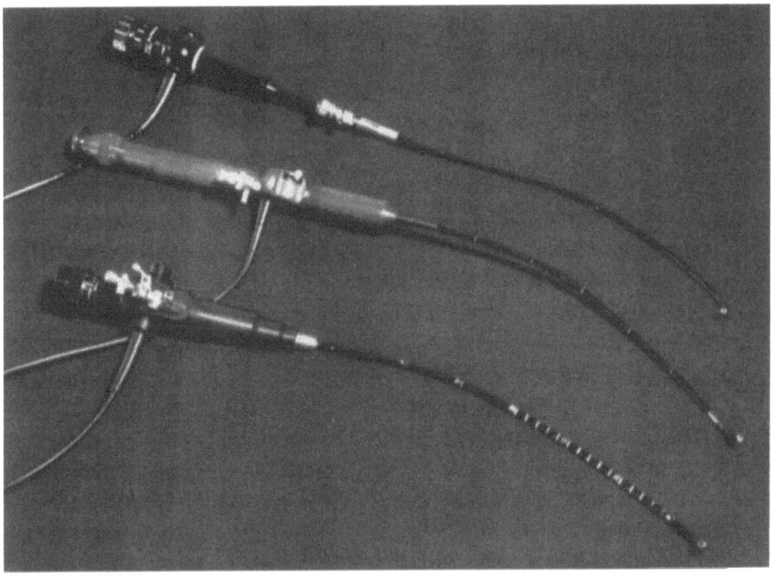

Fig. 12. Flexible nephroscopes for percutaneous stone manipulation (Olympus, Storz, Wolf)

and endoscope were integrated to one unit, so that the instrument could also be used without its sheath, for example within a nephrostomy sheath. Modifications of the irrigation system improved the flow rate to 650 ml/min with a free working port and to 420 ml/min with an F 10 instrument inserted (gravity perfusion at 60 cm). The design principles of this nephroscope are today in general employed in all commercially available nephroscopes (Fig. 11; MARBERGER et al. 1983; MILLER and WICKHAM 1983; KORTH 1983; CLAYMAN 1983).

In obese patients and high kidneys the right-angle eye-piece of the instrument may interfere with the patient's buttocks, and it has also been claimed to have a "back-heavy" lateral torque effect. Instruments with an acute-angle eye-piece have recently been designed to avoid this disadvantage (MILLER and WICKHAM 1983). They are easier to manipulate in difficult situations, yet many urologists find it unaccustomed not to work in the direction of vision. With straight forward 0°-vision instruments introduced into the working port are only marginally visible and therefore difficult to control, so that a downward view of 10 to 25° appears preferable. Wide angle "fish-eye" lenses (100°+) theoretically improve intrarenal orientation, but the systems presently available suffer from significant optical distortion in the margins of the optical field; although more complicated, the use of an additional insert telescope with a 70° or 110° angle through the working port provides a wider field of vision at better quality (MARBERGER et al. 1983).

2. Flexible Nephroscopes

In 1975, HARRIS and MCLAUGHLIN reported on the first use of a fibre-optic bronchoscope for extracting residuals after stone surgery through a nephrostomy. Since then flexible nephroscopy has received continuous interest (MIKI et al. 1978; WILBUR et al. 1981; BURCHARDT 1982; CLAYMAN et al. 1982; MCANINCH and KAHN 1983; CLAYMAN 1983a, MARBERGER 1983; CLAYMAN et al. 1984). The obvious advantage of this approach lies in the possibility of guiding a rather thin instrument under optical control through tortuous tracts and to remote areas of the kidney that cannot be reached with a rigid instrument.

Originally flexible endoscopes designed for other organs were used, in particular choledochoscopes, but recently purpose-built flexible nephroscopes have become available (Fig. 12). Varying from a length of 50 to 70 cm and an outer diameter of F 15 to 18, the tips can be flexed upwards 100–180° and downwards 30–130°. The deflector length varies from 25 to 35 mm (CLAYMAN 1983a). All instruments provide an instrumentation port 2–2.6 mm in diameter; most incorporate a locking feature to stabilize the flexed tip in a certain position and are fully immersible for sterilization. They can be locked watertight into the sheaths of rigid nephroscopes either with a metal connector or a rubber-shod connector. The length of flexible endoscope protruding from the working side of the nephroscope can be adapted to the individual situation (MARBERGER 1983; KORTH 1983). Irrigation is accomplished via the working port. The use of a nephroscope sheath or a nephrostomy sheath permits continuous flow irrigation; an F 18 instrument with 2 irrigation taps even provides simultaneous in- and outflow through the flexible instrument itself (MARBERGER 1983). A wide array of flexible baskets, triradiate graspers, diathermy, cutting, coagulation and F 3.5 to F 5 electrohydraulic probes are available as surgical accessories.

In the hands of experts flexible nephroscopes have proven highly versatile and effective for all types of intrarenal surgery (CLAYMAN et al. 1984). All instruments presently available, however, have significant drawbacks in comparison to rod-lens nephroscopes. Even with the best fibre bundles the optical qualities are significantly poorer both in respect to resolution and illumination. Urologists are spoiled by the brilliance of modern rigid endoscopes, and the grit-like haze on the image caused by the arrangement of the fibre bundles is initially most annoying. With the entire port available for irrigation adequate flow rates for good visibility can usually be attained, especially when a higher level of gravity irrigation is chosen. The insertion of an instrument into the port, for example a basket to extract a calculus, virtually abolishes irrigation in all instruments with channels smaller in diameter than F 6. Even with a larger port and a high level of the irrigation container the flow rate is insufficient to clear even the slightest hemorrhage. Flexible nephroscopes can therefore only be used in mature tracts. The narrow working ports limit the size of the instruments available for stone manipulation; the branches of F 5 flexible alligator forceps only permit the engagement of calculi up to 5 mm (CLAYMAN 1983). Finally insertion of instruments into the working port also reduces the flexibility of the tip by at least 20°. Frequently a calculus in a remote calyx can be seen with the flexible instrument, but the instrument has to be deflected to insert an appropriate grasping instrument. It may then prove to be impossible to reenter the calyx due to the reduced maneuverability of the tip.

In general at least 90% of all percutaneous stone manipulations are performed with rigid nephroscopes today, and flexible instruments are only employed for specific situations, such as entering an anterior medial calyx or the proximal ureter (WICKHAM and MILLER 1983; MARBERGER 1983). In the remaining 10% of the procedures they may, however, ultimately, decide between failure and success. In spite of their technical complexity, high cost and fragility they should therefore be available at endourological centers, especially as with continuous practice their efficiency increases sharply.

V. Mechanical Stone Extraction

Percutaneous extraction of an intact renal calculus via the nephrostomy tract is the most satisfactory method of percutaneous stone manipulation. There is no risk of residual fragments, the technique is simple and does not require sophisticated stone disintegration techniques and is rapidly performed with minimal morbidity. There can be no doubt that it is the treatment modality of choice wherever applicable. The only limiting factor is a disproportion between the size of the calculus and the diameter of the tract respective sheath it has to be removed through.

Whereas some authors are reluctant to dilate nephrostomy tracts to over F 26 (MARBERGER et al. 1982; MARBERGER 1983; WICKHAM and MILLER 1983; ALKEN et al. 1983; SEGURA et al. 1983), others routinely dilate up to F 34 (CLAYMAN et al. 1983; SMITH and LEE 1983). The risk of damaging the kidney certainly increases with the diameter of the tract, but blunt dilatation seems to prevent severe functional and morphological deterioration. A F 24 nephrostomy left no significant impact on the morphology and over-all function of canine kidneys (WEBB and FITZPATRICK 1984). KELLETT et al. (1983) observed a 10% decrease in the DMSA scan in only one of 14 kidneys after percutaneous nephrolithotripsy and it had been subjected to three subsequent punctures; MARBERGER et al. (1985) noticed no deterioration of split ^{131}I-hippuran renograms and renal morphology in 82 patients at late follow-up studies after nephrolithotripsy through a F 24 tract. Functional studies after dilatation to F 34 are not available, but the immediate complication rate does not appear to be higher. It therefore appears justified to attempt to extract any calculus that will pass through a F 34 tract, i.e. up to a diameter of ca. 1.2 cm. The alignment of the stone along its longest axis with jagged ends preferably covered by the grasping forceps naturally is also most important for successful extraction.

The size and type of the grasping instrument used likewise limits the size of the calculus that can be managed by extraction. Grooved Randall or Mazzariello-Caprini forceps worked under fluoroscopic control permit manipulation of large stones, but because of the lack of endoscopic control they carry a high risk of renal damage and should therefore not be used routinely (CLAYMAN et al. 1983). Baskets are difficult to use in non-tubular systems as the stones tend to elude engagement; special floppy, flush-ending 4-wire baskets are more effective but usually also fail with stones larger than 1 cm in diameter. The length of the branches of alligator forceps in mm corresponds to the maximum diameter of a calculus that can be grasped with the instrument (CLAYMAN 1984). The working ports of flexible nephroscopes only admit F 5 flexible alligator forceps, so that only stones up to a diameter of 5 mm can be removed with them. Larger panendoscopes permit the use of larger flexible forceps but they are still too small for most symptomatic stones. Flexible 3-prong graspers have a wide-opening angle and are therefore difficult to be worked through flexible nephroscopes; they also tend to get hooked in the renal parenchyma and cause bleeding. Rigid forceps inserted through rod-lens nephroscopes are far more effective.

A variety of instruments of the alligator 2-prong, triradiate or 3-prong type are available. When used through the nephroscope the stone is usually rapidly identified and engaged, but in general too large to be extracted through the working port. By extracting it together with the nephroscope through the sheath calculi up to 8 mm in diameter can be extracted in this manner. 3-prong rigid forceps with spring type handles are ideal for this approach because the prongs open completely within 1.5 cm from the tip of the nephroscope and forceps and nephroscope can be extracted with one hand while the sheath is stabilized with the other. Alligator forceps are used for smaller stones or calculi in narrow confinements, where 3-prong graspers need too much space to open. They are also employed to remove matrix or clots, if these materials can not be aspirated.

2-prong forceps opening with parallel jaws are particularly helpful for extracting calculi wedged into the ureteropelvic junction as they need not be opened very much more than the maximum diameter of the calculus. By using the nephroscope in combination with a nephrostomy sheath even larger stones are amenable to extraction. Calculi up to ca. 1.1 cm in cross diameter pass through the largest sheath, which protects the renal tissue, reduces hemorrhage and facilitates repeated reinsertion of the nephroscope.

In view of the risk of residual fragments after stone disintegration it is tempting to also extract stones slightly too large to pass through a sheath by grasping them with strong forceps and extracting them together with the sheath. The safety guide-wire is then used for regaining percutaneous access (WICKHAM and MILLER 1983; SMITH and LEE 1983; CLAYMAN 1984). Although feasible, the calculus frequently slips out of the forceps at the level of the fibrous renal capsule or the lumbodorsal fascia, where it is lost along the tract. Although there is no evidence at the time that it acts as a nidus for a perirenal abscess, the appearance of this "residual" stone on follow-up films is annoying to patient and doctor. Most of the lost stones can be retrieved by entering the tract again under optical control along the safety guide-wire and attempting to grasp the stone again with forceps or by a cut-down on the stone, but the author has been reluctant to extract stones in this manner.

The development of a special optical tri-radiate grasper by WICKHAM and MILLER (1984) has significantly reduced the risk of loosing the stone during extraction: special tri-radiate graspers with powerful jaws that provide a vice-like grip securely engage the stone so that calculi up to a diameter of 1.5 cm can be extracted intact together with the instrument and sheath. Extraction is performed under fluoroscopic control and by gently turning the instrument to adapt to the tissues as resistance is encountered; incision of the lumbodorsal fascia with a knife at the time of tract dilatation facilitates the procedure. The powerful jaws of the grasper may crush soft stones, so that these are better disintegrated if they cannot be removed through the sheath. The mechanical trauma to the tissue surrounding the tract is naturally larger as is reflected by more significant hemorrhage after the extraction. Provided the upper-limit of 1.5 cm stone diameter is respected the method nevertheless seems to be safe and highly effective. Larger calculi can also be forced through the tract, but this tends to split the renal tissue and may result in significant vascular damage (SMITH and LEE 1983).

VI. Intrarenal Stone Disintegration

1. Mechanical Disintegration

Disruption of urinary calculi by mechanical crushing with an instrument requires considerable force with the risk of trauma to the surrounding structures, so that it is practically limited to the treatment of bladder calculi. The size requirements a double-jaw-type lithotrite has to meet in order to provide adequate strength and efficiency prohibits its use through a nephrostomy tract. The "punch" lithoclast significantly reduced the size-requirements of these instruments, as the calculus is broken up mainly by shearing forces (MAUERMAYER and HARTUNG 1976). This provides space for an irrigation system and an integrated sheath, within which the lithotrite is worked and the calculous debris removed without injury to the surrounding tract. Although developed for bladder calculi, the Mauermayer-Punch Lithoclast has been employed through percutaneous nephrostomy tracts (SMITH et al. 1982). KORTH (1983) promotes a modified version for intrarenal surgery that can be used through a standard nephroscope sheath. Regardless of the type used, the instrument acts by counteracting movement of the lithoclast cylinder against the sheath over a distance at least the length of the lithoclast window, i.e. at least 2 cm, plus the length of the reinforced lithoclast tip distal to the window. This requires a spacious collecting system, which in the author's experience is only rarely available in renal calculi. To reduce mechanical movement the stone window has to be minimized, but this also reduces the size of calculi that can be disrupted with this technique, as they have to fit into the window at least with a segment. Finally, with the lithotrite advanced vision is severly impaired to a barrel-type view. With a good continuous flow system the collecting system may fold up within sheath and lithotrite window without this being seen. A punch type lesion of the pelvis may result, which because of the large defect is considerably more serious than a simple perforation. Although most manufacturers producing nephroscopes also provide purpose built punch-lithoclasts, they are only sporadically used for percutaneous manipulation.

2. Ultrasonic Lithotripsy

Attempts to overcome the structural adhesive properties of urinary calculi by exposing them to ultrasound of high frequency failed (MULVANEY 1953; COATS 1956). By changing the concept and using ultrasound only to propell a steel probe to high frequency sinus vibrations, urinary calculi may be disintegrated by a drill-like action. Longitudinal and transverse vibrations result in a jack-hammer type impact of the probe on the stone, which disintegrates to sand at the contact site. With ultrasound of 20–27 kHz all urinary calculi may in vitro be disintegrated with instruments of this type (LUTZEYER et al. 1970; GASTEYER 1971), provided the probe remains in good contact with the stone and the stone debris is removed continuously. LUTZEYER et al. (1970) and GASTEYER (1971) solved this problem by using a hollow sonotrode and connecting its central lumen to a vacuum pump which aspirates the stone dust continuously with the irrigation fluid and cools the probe. Their prototypes later became commercially available as lithotrites for vesical calculi and have been in clinical use for this purpose for over a decade (TERHORST et al. 1972; MARBERGER 1979; HAUTMANN et al. 1983). In 1977, KURTH et al. and RATHERT et al. (1977) used an instrument of this type to disintegrate renal calculi via the tract of a preexisting U-tube nephrostomy. ALKEN et al. (1981, 1982a) subsequently extended the approach to the treatment of kidney stones via a percutaneous nephrostomy.

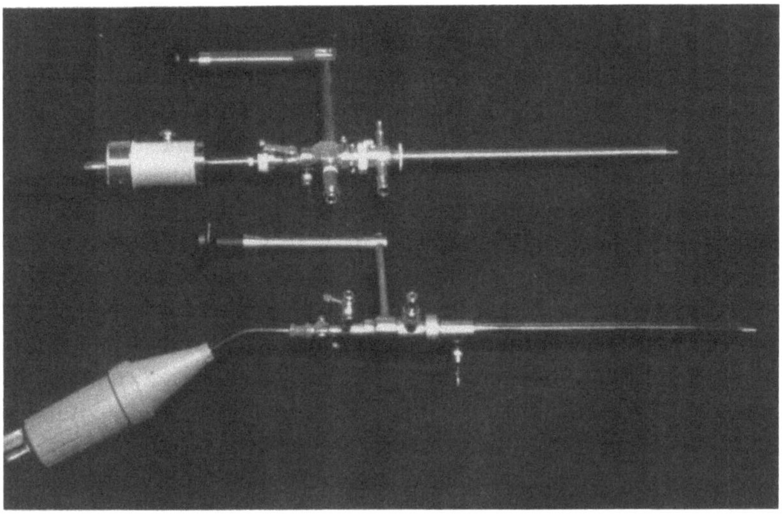

Fig. 13. Nephroscopes with sonotrode for ultrasonic lithotripsy introduced through the working port (Storz, Wolf)

However, vesical lithotrites proved to be too awkward and cumbersome for intrarenal lithotripsy, and purpose-built ultrasonic lithotrites for renal calculi were therefore developed (MARBERGER et al. 1981; MARBERGER et al. 1982; ALKEN et al. 1983).

The instruments presently available consist of an ultrasound transducer with an integrated sonotrode and an external generator (Fig. 13). Powered at about 100 Watt the piezoceramic elements in the ultrasonic transducer produce ultrasound at a frequency of 23 to 27 kHz, depending on the manufacturer. With an accoustical horn bolted to the accoustical end-parts the integrated steel probe protruding from the transducer is propelled to longitudinal and transverse vibrations, which are utilized to disintegrate the calculus. For this the probe must tip the calculus at the site of disintegration. It is therefore advanced through the working port of a nephroscope and manipulated under optical control like a drill. The efficiency of the probe increases the better the contact between stone and sonotrode. The probe is hollow and connected to a vacuum pump to remove the irrigation fluid and stone dust. This maintains vision and cools the probe. Whereas one model (Wolf) can be connected to any type of aspiration apparatus, the other (Storz) has an integrated roller pump system for aspiration, which is operated with the same foot-switch as the lithotrite. The generator permits 3 power setting, which influence the vibration amplitude and thus the efficiency of the probe. When measured under the microscope at setting 1 the maximum amplitude of the Wolf sonotrode was 20 μ for transverse and 20 μ for longitudinal vibrations (MARBERGER et al. 1985). At setting 2 this increased to 20 μ rsp 30 μ and at setting 3 to 30 μ rsp 50 μ. The author in general uses medium setting.

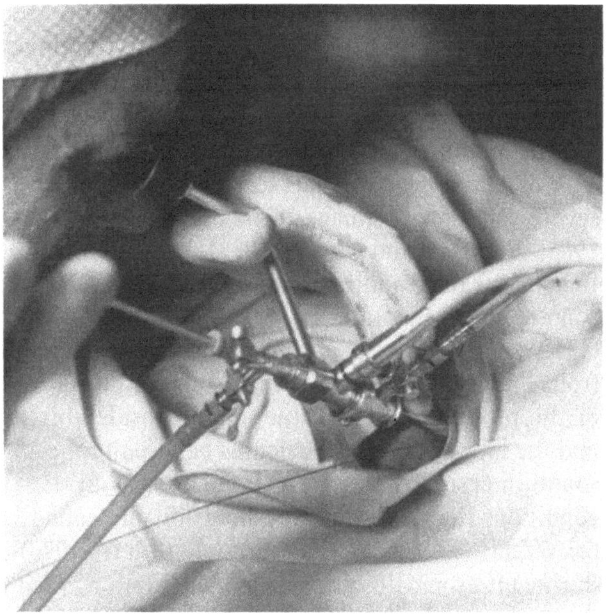

Fig. 14. Ultrasonic lithotripsy: the sonotrode is worked like a drill with the right hand and the left hand stabilizes the instrument and controls irrigation inflow; note the "safety" guide-wire

Once the calculus is identified through the nephroscope, the probe is advanced to it and worked like a drill (Fig. 14). Usually the stone surface rapidly disintegrates and the calculus breaks up into larger fragments. Aspiration through the probe clears the kidney of stone dust and smaller fragments and approximates larger remnants. These are then removed step-by-step, preferably under fluoroscopic control to avoid loosing bits. If the stone proves to be rather resistant, this procedure is shortened by extracting larger fragments with forceps. During the entire manipulation it is most important to avoid a flow of irrigation fluid away from the probe to prevent spillage of calculous material throughout the kidney. This is best achieved by continuous aspiration during lithotripsy and precise control of an effective high outflow with low inflow during phases of mechanical extraction. The effect of ultrasonic lithotripsy on soft tissues is well investigated. Theoretically damage could result from heat development, from ultrasound induced cavitation processes, mutagenic ultrasound effects and mechanical trauma from the oscillating probe.

Heat development at the tip of the probe correlates in a linear fashion to the time of energy exposure and the ratio of density differences at accoustical interphases (LEHMANN et al. 1978). Without irrigation cooling the probe reaches temperatures >40 °C within seconds, so that it should never be operated in this manner. Already the dissipating capacity of a cylinder of 10 ml water at 20 °C slows the temperature increase to 3 °C after 30 seconds, and with continuous irrigation with saline at 20 °C and a flow of 30 ml/min the temperature increase is reduced to only 1.4 °C even after 5 minutes of continuous energy exposure (MARBERGER 1983b). MARBERGER et al. (1985) repeated this experiment under identical conditions in vivo in leporine bladders and found a mean increase of the bladder wall temperature at the site of probe contact of 4 °C. This temperature was reached after approx. 3 minutes of continuous energy exposure, but did not increase further during the following 2 minutes. As intrarenal endoscopy requires a flow rate of at least 100 ml/min for adequate vision, thermic damage is therefore avoided reliably under clinical conditions.

Cavitation processes at accoustical interphases are known to be reasons for severe soft tissue damage of focused ultrasonic energy (COWDEN and ABELL 1963; WICKHAM and MILLER 1983). Measurements of the sound intensity levels in under-water conditions representative of the clinical situation using Wolf sonotrodes at medium power level showed a maximum sound intensity of 0.35 W/cm² at the tip of the probe. The levels rapidly decayed with distance from the probe to 0.037 W/cm² 5 mm and 0.006 W/cm² 10 mm straight ahead of the probe's tip. The values were considerably lower in oblique directions, and the interposition of a calculus between probe and microphones reduced the sound intensity by ca. 50% (MARBERGER et al. 1985). As even under optimum conditions the cavitation threshold for ultrasound at this frequency is at least 0.7 W/cm² (LEHMANN et al. 1978; LEHFELDT 1973), cavitation does not occur during ultrasonic lithotripsy. Stone disruption is achieved purely by mechanical forces due to the oscillation of the probe. There has been speculation that ultrasound may cause DNA breakdown by mechanisms other than cavitation (LEHMANN et al. 1978), but extensive investigations in this respect have not provided any evidence for this in diagnostic ultrasound in this intensity range (LIEBESKIND et al. 1978; PIZARELLO et al. 1978). Human leukocyte cultures exposed to ultrasound in the frequency and intensity range as used for lithotripsy showed no significant change of the sister chromatid exchange rate (STACKL et al. 1984), and analysis of the DNA of rat kidneys by gel diffusion subjected to a similar procedure showed no abnormalities (MILLER et al. 1983 b).

The sequelae of the mechanical trauma from the oscillating probe are minimal (GASTEYER 1971; TERHORST et al. 1972; GOODFRIEND 1973; HOWARDS et al. 1974). TERHORST et al. (1975) found even direct contact of the probe with leporine bladders and continuous ultrasound exposure over 5 minutes to cause only mild edema, which only slightly exceeded the edema caused by the same probe connected to the vacuum pump only. Lesions of deeper bladder wall layers were only noted when the vibration exceeded 25 µ, but experimental details of their model were not provided. MARBERGER et al. (1985) therefore repeated the experiments under precise monitoring of the vibration amplitude. In spite of amplitudes of the transverse vibration of up to 30 and the longitudinal vibration of up to 50 µ perforations were never observed. This was confirmed for the canine pelvis and ureter by WEBB and FITZPATRICK (1984). MILLER et al. (1983) studied the structural effects of ultrasound lithotripsy on rat kidneys by light and electron microscopy and likewise found no abnormalities. Metal flakes are frequently chipped from the probes due to contact between the probe and the nephroscope during disintegration. MARBERGER et al. (1985) found that the flakes were completely washed out of leporine bladders within 24 hours when injected into the cavity of leporine bladders. When rubbed into the mucosa they completely disappeared within one week, but when trapped within the bladder wall at the cystostomy site they remained unchanged within the musculature during the follow-up period of 10 weeks. Tissue reaction around the foreign-bodies, was, however, minimal, and always less pronounced than for example from polyglycolic suture material. The minimal soft tissue damage inflicted by ultrasonic lithotripsy is in the meantime also well documented by large clinical series (MARBERGER et al. 1983, 1984; SEGURA et al. 1983; ALKEN et al. 1983; HAUTMANN et al. 1983).

In vitro and theoretically also in vivo all urinary calculi can be disintegrated with ultrasound. The time of energy exposure required for this mainly depends on the surface structure, hardness, density, porosity and, to a lesser extent, the chemical composition of the stone; good contact between the stone and probe accelerates fragmentation. In clinical practice very smooth and hard calculi, mainly uric acid stones and occasionally calcium oxalate stones, may prove to be quite resistant and to require very long disintegration times. Based on in vitro studies a baffle-plate loosely fitted to the tip of the sonotrode increases the drilling properties multifold (TERHORST et al. 1972, 1975). Clinical experience has not confirmed this (MARBERGER 1979; MARBERGER 1983a) and the experimental studies of TERHORST et al. (1975) even suggest slightly more mechanical trauma by the jagged crown of the baffle-plate. In the author's experience of now over 1000 patients subjected to ultrasonic lithotripsy the calculi proved to be too hard in only 3 patients; electrohydraulic lithotripsy likewise failed in these very smooth and round calcium oxalate stones of particularly high density. Large stones, stones with a very smooth surface and very dense stones may, however, occasionally require very long disintegration times of up to several hours. This time can be reduced by extracting larger fragments or supplementing ultrasonic lithotripsy with electrohydraulic fragmentation.

Like with any technique of intrarenal stone disruption residual calculi are an inherent problem of this method. Although residual rates of up to 54% have been reported (MILLER et al. 1983b), this problem can be reduced considerably by a careful step-by-step fragmentation technique, with peripheral smaller fragments being removed first before the bulk of the stone is further disintegrated (MARBERGER et al. 1983) (Fig. 15). A carefully monitored continuous flow-irrigation system reduces the spillage of fragments, and a ureteral catheter prevents fragments from entering the ureter. Residuals in remote calyces can be located with a 110° insert endoscope and removed with a retro-steerable forceps (MARBERGER et al. 1982) or the flexible nephroscope. The availability of fluoroscopic control during all phases of intrarenal manipulation is mandatory. In general a residual stone rate of 6 to 12% is achieved (ALKEN et al. 1983; MARBERGER 1983a; SEGURA et al. 1983). The residual rate naturally also depends on the type of stone being treated: in a series of 272 patients treated by the authors with ultrasonic lithotripsy the residual rate was 9% for simpler, smaller stones, 12% for large stones completely moulding the pelvis or several calyces, and 38% for staghorn stones. In this series 11% of the patients were subjected to a second procedure in general anesthesia to remove fragments. The residual rate could certainly have been reduced further by additional percutaneous manipulation, but usually the residual material was just calculous "dust" of a particle size that could be expected to be passed spontaneously, in particular when compared to the particles produced by extracorporeal shock-wave lithotripsy. WICKHAM and

A
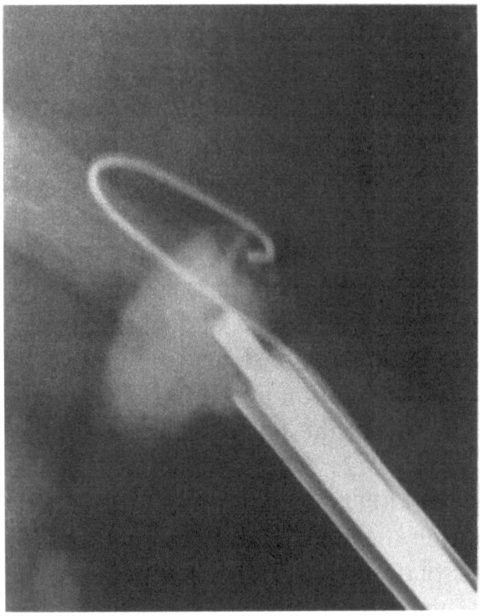
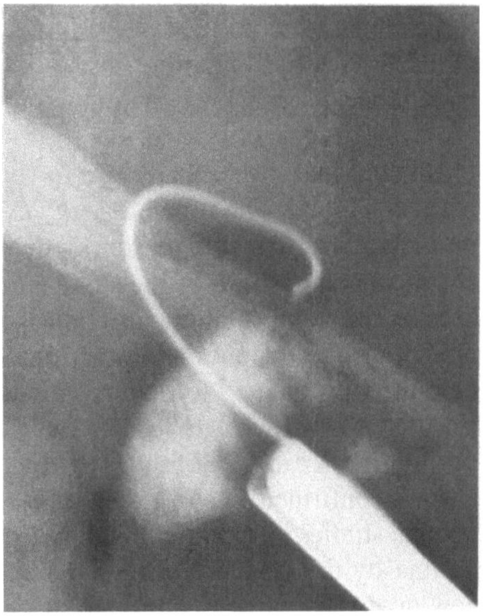
B

C
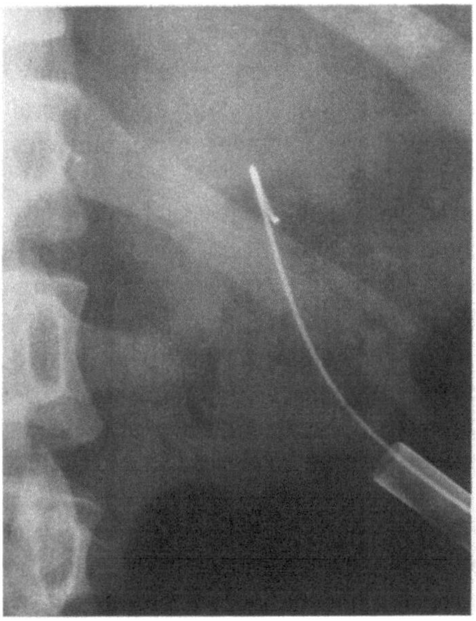

Fig. 15 A – C. Ultrasonic lithotripsy: the calculus is disintegrated step-by-step, beginning at an edge (**A**) and removing smaller fragments first before reducing the main segment further (**B**), until the kidney is stone free (**C**)

MILLER have questioned this (1983) and reported on 2 early recurrent stones after ultrasonic lithotripsy in 42 patients. This has not been the experience of other authors (ALKEN et al. 1983; MARBERGER 1983; SEGURA et al. 1983).

The authors conducted a precise follow-up study in 82 patients who had been treated 4 to 1 years previously by ultrasonic lithotripsy (MARBERGER et al. 1985). 62 patients also underwent axial computed tomography. In 9/82 patients residuals had been documented at discharge. In 2 of them larger fragments were dislocated into calyces where they could not be reached during the procedure, and subsequently dropped into the pelvis again where they were removed from percutaneously 4 rsp. 7 months after the initial procedure. 2 patients passed all residuals spontaneously, usually with a renal colic. In 5 asymptomatic patients the residuals remained unchanged, and computed tomography showed that in fact they were located in the parenchyma in one respective peripelvic fat in another patient. In the same series 2 patients who were documented stone-free at discharge, developed a recurrent stone after 12 resp. 14 months, which again had to be removed percutaneously. In 23 of 83 patients in the series stones had already been removed by open surgery from the same kidney prior to percutaneous surgery. A review of this group revealed that 6 patients had formed the recurrencies within 24 months after open surgery. Although of course the follow-up period is too short for a final statement, there is at the present time no evidence for an increased stone growth-rate after ultrasonic lithotripsy.

The main draw-back of ultrasonic lithotripsy lies in the inability to transport the disintegrating energy around curves. By combining the technique with multiple nephrostomies, the use of the flexible nephroscope and in selected cases electrohydraulic lithotripsy, practically all clinical situations requiring stone disruption can, however, be handled. Early technical problems with sterilization (MARBERGER 1979), overpowering and probe failure (WICKHAM and MILLER 1983) and probe clogging (MARBERGER et al. 1983) have largely been overcome by technical modifications.

As air-borne sound levels of up to 103 db at 20 kHz and 127 db at 25 kHz had been measured near the ultrasound probes (MILLER et al. 1983b), there has been considerable concern on a possible hearing damage to the surgeon's ear closest to the probe. Although sound levels of this magnitude do not cause noticeable temporary or permanent hearing losses after one hour of continuous exposure (ACTON and HILL 1977; GRIGOR'EVA 1966; HERMAN and POWELL 1981), the producers have improved noise insulation. Audiofrequency studies of 5 new Wolf probes (Nr. 2167.10) revealed air-borne sound levels in the 3-octave band centered on a frequency of 16 kHz from 72 to 92 db and at 20 kHz from 95 to 107 db. Whereas these levels at 20 kHz do not even cause subjective complaints, tinnitus, headaches, and fatigue has been reported when workers were exposed to sound levels over 78 db at 16 kHz for an entire working day (ACTON and CARSON 1967). Exposure limits have not been defined on an international legal basis, but for industrial settings the exposure limits for the third octave band centered at 16 kHz are 75 db (United Kingdom), 80 db (Canada), 85 db (US Air Force), 90 db (FRG, USSR) (HERMAN and POWELL 1981; VDI-Richtlinien 1970). Although these recommendations are given for industrial workers exposed to the sound levels for an entire working day and this rarely occurs under clinical conditions, protection of the ear closest to the probe with an ear-muff appears advisable. This provides an attenuation factor of 10–15 db, so that even subjective discomfort is eliminated.

3. Electrohydraulic Lithotripsy

In 1950 the Russian engineer JUTKIN (GOLDBERG 1960) discovered the destructive effect of electrohydraulic shock-waves on solid bodies within a liquid medium. GOLDBERG and ROSE (GOLDBERG 1960) applied the principle to the treatment of bladder calculi, and designed an electrohydraulic lithotrite for disintegration of bladder calculi. Slightly modified, this apparatus named URAT I became commercially available in Western Europe in the late sixties.

Basically the stone is exposed to repeated bursts of hydraulic shock-waves, which are produced by high voltage under-water discharges at the tip of a coaxial cable with an axial inner and tubular outer electrode. This results in a short but steep pressure impulse with a large amplitude which spreads spherically in water at a speed of 1500 m/sec. The pressure curve rapidly decays with the distance from the point of discharge so that the calculus must be approximated with the lithotrite probe. The pressure front of the impulse is partially reflected by the calculus, resulting in a rebound phase and subsequently in additional high strain forces and cavitation phenomena within the calculus. The stress resistance of the stone exceeds its strain resistance a 100 fold; although both stress and strain disintegrate the calculus, the stress waves are more effective.

The URAT I's pulse generator incorporates a high voltage rectifier and permits pulse voltages to a maximum of 3 kV with an impulse current of a minimum of 500 ampere and a pulse duration of 1 – 5 msec, with a repetition rate of 30 to 100 cycles per second (EATON et al. 1972). The energy thus supplied suffices to disintegrate all urinary calculi, the time required for complete disintegration depending mainly on the chemical composition, surface, size and porosity of the stone as well as the proximity between probe and stone. Uric acid and oxalate stones are usually more resistant than calcium phosphate calculi (MARBERGER 1979), but the technique is far more efficient than any other physical method of stone disintegration.

Unfortunately any tissue within 5 mm of the point of discharge is likewise hit by the full impact of the shock-wave. In soft tissues like the bladder wall or renal pelvis this may result in disruption of the tissue integrity, sloughing, and edema of the adjacent structures, an effect very similar to the blast effect of an explosion (KIERFELD et al. 1969; TERHORST et al. 1975; PELANDER et al. 1980; NASR 1982). Heat obviously also plays a major role (ROUVALIS 1970; PUROHIT et al. 1980), but the damaging effect is further increased by calculous fragments which are blasted off the stone and impacted shrapnell-like on underlying surfaces (TIDD et al. 1976; WEBB and FITZPATRICK 1984). These hazards are easier to avoid by an improved triggering mechanism of the discharges and better modulation, providing extremely steep impulse curves of extremely short duration. Newer lithotrites provide pulses at 3 power levels, the frequency of which can be modified in an ungraded range of 1 ("Single-shot") to up to 70 per second, and the duration of which can be adjusted between 1 and 5 seconds (RANEY 1975a; BÜLOW et al. 1981; CLAYMAN 1984). This permits the use of higher energy up to a maximum discharge of 8 kV (BÜLOW et al. 1981).

In spite of the technical refinements optical control of electrohydraulic lithotripsy is imperative at all times. The tip of the electrode must be within

1 mm of the calculus, but at least 5 mm away from all soft tissues and the observation endoscope, which may otherwise also be shattered. This is easily accomplished in the bladder, and the technique has therefore today become the standard method of vesical lithotripsy in Europe (REUTER 1970; ROUVALIS 1970; ANGELOFF 1972; ALFTHAN and MURTOMAN 1972; ALBRECHT et al. 1972; MARBERGER 1979; BÜLOW et al. 1981). The space requirements for safe lithotripsy within the confined dimensions of the renal collecting system are more difficult to meet. RANEY and HANDLER (1975) were the first to employ electrohydraulic lithotripsy in the kidney to disintegrate stones either at open surgery or via a nephrostomy tract which had been placed by open surgery. They reported no complications, and this has in the meantime been confirmed by other authors who used the technique through a percutaneous nephrostomy (ALKEN et al. 1981; CLAYMAN 1984; WICKHAM and MILLER 1984; KORTH 1984). BUSH et al. (1982) even reported successful electrohydraulic disintegration of renal calculi with electrodes advanced to the renal pelvis via the ureter. The main attraction of the technique certainly lies in its high efficiency. Stones are disintegrated far more rapidly than with ultrasonic lithotripsy. Electrodes F 3.5, F 5 and F 9 in diameter are available today. As they are flexible, the thinner electrodes can be used through a flexible nephroscope and therefore be utilized to disintegrate stones in remote calyces not amenable to a rigid nephroscope (CLAYMAN 1984).

Although WICKHAM and MILLER (1984) and KORTH (1984) consider electrohydraulic lithotripsy their technique of choice for intrarenal stone disintegration, and have not reported serious complications, the potential risks are well established from experimental studies. PUROHIT et al. (1980) noticed perforations of the canine ureter in 33–40% after intraureteral discharge and WEBB and FITZPATRICK (1984a) reported similar results for the canine renal pelvis. This corresponds to experimental data from vesical lithotripsy (KIERFELD et al. 1969; TERHORST et al. 1975; TIDD et al. 1976). The safety requirements of intrarenal electrohydraulic lithotripsy are therefore essential: the entire procedure must be performed under vision with the probe within 1 mm of the calculus and at least 5 mm away from the tip of the nephroscope and all soft tissues. The electrohydraulic unit should be set at a low discharge voltage (ca. 75 to 85 V) and primarily at single-shot discharge. Voltage and discharge frequency is increased as needed (CLAYMAN 1984). The objective is to fragment a larger stone to 4–5 smaller segments, which are then extracted, rather than to multiple, difficult to remove minute fragments.

The insulation of the electrode rapidly wears down with use and the probe may then be disintegrated itself. To prevent blasting foreign bodies into the kidney it must therefore be discarded when the insulation is worn off at the tip. As F 5 electrodes have a life-span of an average 20–30 discharges only, the F 9 electrode is preferably employed for stones amenable for the straight nephroscope. A 1/6 to 1/7 normal saline solution has been recommended as the optimum irrigant for electrohydraulic lithotripsy (CLAYMAN 1984), but in the author's experience the efficiency of the lithotrite is not severely reduced when used with standard saline. Smaller, smooth stones are very difficult to shatter, as they bounce away from the probe and the optimum range of the shock-wave.

To prevent this the surgeon may tend to press the calculus against the mucosa with the electrode at the time of discharge, but this must be avoided within the kidney. WICKHAM and MILLER (1984) stated that with electrohydraulic lithotripsy less small fragments are impacted on the mucosa than with ultrasonic lithotripsy. Other authors have not made the same observation (MARBERGER 1983; ALKEN et al. 1983), and WEBB and FITZPATRICK (1984a) noticed multiple fragments impacted in the mucosa after electrohydraulic lithotripsy in the canine kidney which showed little tendency to be passed. In contrast the fragments after ultrasonic lithotripsy were obviously mainly impacted in clots, and washed out within a week.

The author at the present time prefers ultrasonic lithotripsy as the routine technique for intrarenal stone disintegration, because of less significant side effects and risks to soft tissues. Some selected cases, in particular very large calculi (Fig. 16), very hard and smooth stones and larger stones positioned at the entry of a wide upper pole calyx are better managed primarily with electrohydraulic lithotresis. In the latter case the need for good contact between sonotrode and calculus frequently results in dislodgement of the stone into the upper pole calyx, where it may then occasionally not be reached with a rigid instrument. The flexible F 5 electrode is helpful in disintegrating peripheral calyceal stones, but most are easier to be removed with simpler techniques. Ideal is the availability of both techniques, i.e. the calculus is first fragmented into large pieces with electrohydraulic discharges and then reduced farther and removed with the ultrasonic lithotrite. The aspirator of the latter instrument facilitates removal of calculous debris.

4. Microexplosion Lithotripsy

In 1977, WATANABE et al. suggested the use of an explosion to disintegrate calculi, as it has a simple mechanism and efficient power to mass ratio with easy carriage to target organs.

An explosive suitable for microexplosion techniques has to be sensitive enough to ignite even in small quantities, yet not too sensitive for ordinary manipulation. After in vitro studies they chose lead azide which detonates at 350° and generates 0.37 calories per mg, i.e. has a detonation power similar to usual industrial explosives (WATANABE et al. 1979). In extensive in vitro studies with artificial calculi of physical properties similar to those of urinary calculi they determined that a calculus 10 mm in diameter required 2 mg explosive, and a calculus of 20 mm 5 mg (KANEKO et al. 1979). Experiments with isolated segments of canine bladders showed the danger range of soft tissue injury to be within 7.5 mm from the site of the explosion, provided it was detonated under water (WATANABE et al. 1980). Soft tissue damage occurred from the expansive reaction of the stone fragments within this area; distant to 7.5 mm and at a discharge 2 mg, the shock-wave passed through soft tissues without damage. This was confirmed in in vivo experiments with pig bladders (WATANABE et al. 1983).

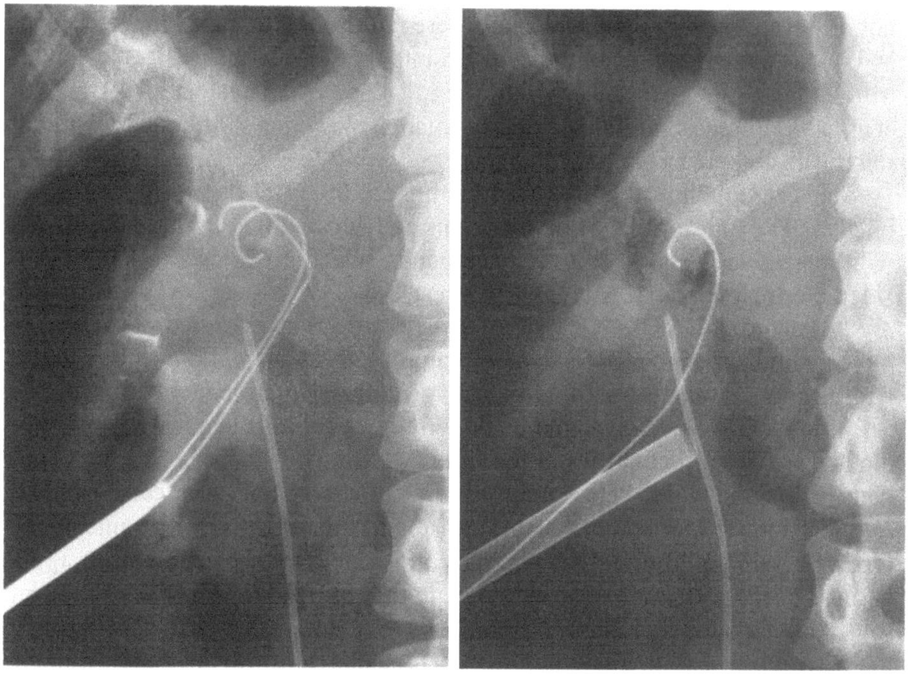

A B

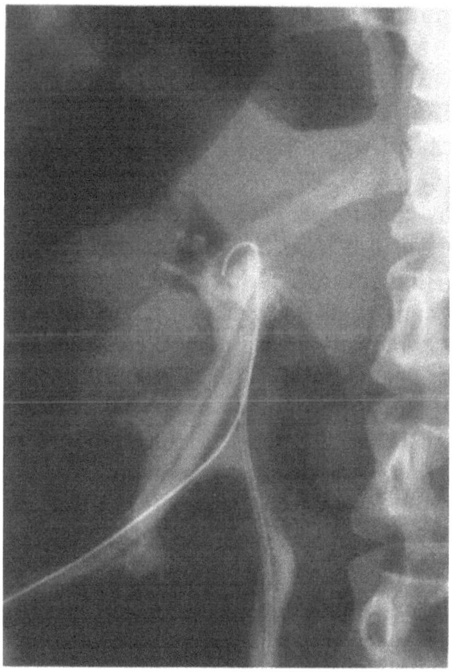

C

Fig. 16 A – C. Electrohydraulic lithotripsy of a large cystine stone in a solitary kidney: In one session percutaneous nephrostomy directly onto the stone, tract dilatation (**A**; minimal dye residuals in upper pole calyces; note ureteral catheter and "safety" guide wire), and electrohydraulic disintegration and mechanical removal of the fragments. The stone was extremely hard and quite resistant to ultrasonic lithotripsy. After 120 minutes the kidney was stone free (**B**) and there was no extravasation (**C**)

After construction of a special cystolithotriptor they employed the technique for disintegrating vesical calculi in three patients. Complications were not observed, but multiple explosions were required to disrupt the large stones and in one patient holes had to be drilled into the stone with an ultrasonic lithotrite to deposit the explosive within the calculus (WATANABE et al. 1983). XUI et al. (1981) used a similar method of microexplosion-cystolithotripsy without significant complications in 20 patients.

The technique must, however, at the present time still be considered experimental. At explosion the stone fragments and surrounding tissues are sprayed with ionized lead and lead azide compounds, which are known to have a considerable toxic effect (RANEY 1983; MILLER and WICKHAM 1983b). Although WATANABE et al. (1983) observed no increase of lead levels in red blood cells in their animal experiments or signs of carcinogenesis in mutation rate studies with E. coli and Salmonella typhimurium cultures contaminated with lead, the activation of toxic lead compounds certainly prohibits clinical use of this method in Western countries at the time. MILLER (1984) observed a very limited therapeutic width between an insufficient charge and an excessive explosive reaction. Urinary stones break up irregularly. Often larger fragments are formed needing additional microexplosions, which are then difficult to apply because of the reduced size of the stone. In the confined renal collecting system soft-tissue damage including perforations from stone fragments shot through the pelvocalyceal wall is impossible to be avoided with the presently available technique (MILLER 1984). With improved explosives and the adaption of shockwave focusing systems as used for military explosions, the technique may one day become useful (MILLER 1984).

5. Stone Disintegration by Laser Irradiation

Disruption of calculi can be achieved by continuous wave or pulsed laser irradiation. With the former approach the calculus is reduced by thermic effects only, i.e. it is melted or even burned at the site of irradiation. Coupling the energy to the urinary calculus is difficult, in particular when working under water, and requires the risk of damaging the costly instrument (PENSEL et al. 1981). Although it has been employed for disintegrating urinary calculi in vivo in dog bladders and even to treat vesical calculi in patients (TANAHASHI et al. 1979; TANAHASHI et al. 1981; PENSEL et al. 1981), the poor correlation between efficiency and thermic side effects render this method rather impractical.

By using pulsed lasers, i.e. lasers emitting energy at higher levels, but in pulses of extremely short duration in the nanosecond range, the calculus is reduced by thermic strain forces without being melted (MULVANEY and BECK 1968; PENSEL et al. 1981). The energy can be stepped up further by Q-switching so that the light energy is optimally converted to mechanical energy and the calculus disintegrated by mechanical rather than thermic strain forces (TANAHASHI et al. 1979; PENSEL et al. 1981). Even more efficient the laser can be used indirectly with an opto-mechanical coupler (FAIR 1978). By irradiating a thin aluminium sheet with a 20 nsec pulsed laser microexplosions are induced on the metal substrate, which exert a shock-wave on the calculus capable of rapid disintegration of every urinary calculus. Thermic side-effects are completely avoided and disintegration becomes independent of the surface structure and color of the stone. PENSEL et al. (1981) compared the various methods in vitro, and came to the conclusion that only the latter method promisses clinical practicability. Although CO_2 lasers are more effective in vitro (MULVANEY and BECK 1968; TANAHASHI et al. 1979; TAHIRA et al. 1979), the use of Neodynium-Yag lasers appear more rewarding, as their light can be directed through rod-lens or flexible telescopes with flexible quartz fibres. Appropriate endoscopes are already available for endoscopic surgery in the bladder and urethra. Laser disintegration is at the present time purely experimental and considerable technological refinements are required before it will have clinical applicability, in particular in view of the high price of the equipment.

VII. Percutaneous Chemolysis

In vitro all urinary calculi can be dissolved by appropriate chemolytic agents and for over half a century chemolysis has been pursued with ingenuity and perseverance. BÜSCHER (1961) reviewed the extensive literature on this topic in detail. Since then the dissolution of uric acid calculi by oral alkalinization has been the only real triumph in the field; uric acid calculi are today non-surgical stones and their management is covered in VAHLENSIECK (1985). With some exceptions in cystine (LOTZ and BARTTER 1965; SHAW and SUTOR 1972) and sterile struvite (GRIFFITH et al. 1979) calculi chemolytic agents cannot be concentrated within the collecting system at a sufficient concentration when administered by the oral route.

The problems of direct irrigation of the calculus for chemolysis using retrograde ureteric catheters or operatively introduced nephrostomy tubes is best reflected by the extensive experience of TIMMERMANN and KALLISTRATOS (1966). Using acetic acid (EDTA), they completely dissolved calculi in 66% of 260 patients, and partially in 34%. This success rate, however, was clouded by the inconvenience and expense of many weeks of hospitalization of the patient, who was frequently immobilized by a large caliber ureteric catheter, and a significant rate of complications from infection, local irritation and metabolic imbalances. In view of these drawbacks topical chemolysis did not seem to offer decisive advantages over standard stone surgery and therefore remained limited to the dissolution of retained fragments after stone surgery (BLAIVAS et al. 1975; NEMOY and STAMEY 1976; JACOBS and GITTES 1976) or for recurrent calculi in severe stone formers like in patients with spinal-cord injury (FAM et al. 1976). With the advent of endourology and extracorporeal shock-wave lithotripsy the disadvantages of topical irrigation became even more obvious, but there remain specific situations where the approach still seems appropriate.

Successful chemolysis depends on knowledge of the chemical composition of the stone to choose the correct solvent, an adequate concentration of the agent at the site of action, and the absence of metabolic, toxic and infectious complications. Important contributions have been developed in the last years to achieve this aim: Computed tomography permits a rather reliable analysis of the stone composition by radiological means (Mitcheson et al. 1981). Percutaneous nephrostomy techniques provide a short direct access to virtually any part of the collecting system, so that one or several tubes can be brought into close vicinity of the calculus. This not only helps maintain a high concentration of the chemolytic agent around the stone, but also prevents problems from obstruction and infection; poorly draining, uncomfortable ureteral catheters are completely avoided (Spataro et al. 1978; Drettler et al. 1979; Smith et al. 1979; Weirich et al. 1982; Sheldon and Smith 1982; Pfister et al. 1983). The percutaneous access can also be used to obtain stone samples for a precise analysis if chemolysis seems to fail. In spite of these advances, dissolution still requires long hospitalization periods: for percutaneous chemolysis of uric acid stones Pataro et al. (1978) needed 14–21 days and Hedgecock et al. (1982) a mean 21 days; Pfister et al. reported treatment periods of 2–30 days for dissolution of struvite stones and 6–42 days for cystine stones; Weirich et al. (1981, 1982) required 12 days for the dissolution of struvite stones and 21 days for cystine stones.

In view of the minimal morbidity of endourological stone treatment and extracorporeal shock-wave lithotripsy percutaneous chemolysis must therefore be limited to selected cases where the other techniques fail or permit only incomplete stone clearance. These are almost exclusively patients with recurrent struvite stones forming on the basis of chronic urinary tract infection and impaired urinary drainage, cystinuric patients and patients with poorly functioning, obstructed kidneys and uric acid stones. Extracorporeal shock-wave lithotripsy is hazardous in the presence of infection and obstruction, cystine stones are poorly disintegrated (Schmeller et al. 1984) and uric acid stones are difficult to visualize for proper focusing. Many of these stones can successfully be removed by percutaneous lithotripsy, but minute struvite residuals in remote calyces are frequently the nidus for rapid recurrencies and complete stone clearance may also be impossible in branched cystine or uric acid stones. In these patients the risks of recurrent surgical intervention may outweigh the disadvantages of a prolongued treatment by irrigation chemolysis.

Phosphatic stones are managed with acidifying solutions such as hemiacridine (Renacidine; Mulvaney 1959) or Suby's solution G (Suby and Albright 1943; Suby et al. 1952); both have a pH of 4.0. A 10% renacidine solution is today used most commonly. After reports of letal septicemia (Kohler 1962; Fostved and Barnes 1963), hypermagnesemia from magnesium absorption (Cato and Tulloch 1974) and severe tissue damage (Kohler 1962; Boyce 1979) after renacidine irrigation the agent was temporarily withdrawn from use in the upper urinary tract in the United States. The key to these complications proved to be impaired drainage of the irrigant rather than urinary infection, which may be difficult to be eradicated in struvite stones. Provided intrapelvic pressures are maintained below 30 cm water, urinary tract infection is treated by appropriate antimicrobial agents and irrigation is discontinued at signs of discomfort, hematuria, persistent fever or metabolic disorders serious complications can reliably be avoided (Nemoy and Stamey 1976; Fam et al. 1976; Jacobs and Gittes 1976; Blaivas et al. 1975).

This is best achieved by placing two large caliber nephrostomy tubes at each side of the calculus and by using one for irrigation and the other for drainage. 24 hours after nephrostomy placement irrigation is begun with normal saline at 30 ml/hour and slowly increased to 120 ml/hour, or a rate tolerated without pain or intrarenal pressures over 30 cm water; this is guaranteed by a 3-way safety valve incorporated in the irrigation system (PFISTER et al. 1983). Infection must be treated vigorously prior to renacidine irrigation; with a sterile urine prophylactic antibiotics are administered. Once the urine is sterile and saline irrigation tolerated without pain irrigation is commenced with a 10% hemiacridine solution at 120 ml/hour or less, so that intrarenal pressures do not exceed 30 cm water (PFISTER et al. 1983). Patient cooperation is important. He is instructed in the mechanisms of the irrigation system and monitoring of the safety valve, and told to immediately interrupt irrigation with significant discomfort. Slight fever, flank pain or hematuria are frequent and may require temporary interruption or reduction of irrigation. With septicemia, signs of deteriorating renal function or the presence of resistent urinary infection chemolysis has to be discontinued permanently. PFISTER et al. (1983) also recommend discontinuation of treatment if there is no decrease in stone size within 7 days or failure of 50% dissolution within two weeks. In 28 kidneys subjected to hemiacridine irrigation they observed complete dissolution of the calculi in 19 and partial chemolysis in 6 kidneys; dissolution failed in 3 kidneys.

Cystine is far more soluble in alkaline than in acid urine and maintenance of dilute alkaline urine is the foundation of both treatment and prevention. Topical irrigation with sodium bicarbonate usually fails to dissolve the stone, but tromethamine-E (THAM-E) with a pH of 10.2 is very efficient (CRISSEY and GITTES 1979; SHELDON and SMITH 1982; PFISTER et al. 1983). More frequently thiol-containing agents such as acetylcysteine (MULVANEY et al. 1975; KALLISTRATOS 1978; SMITH et al. 1979; WEIRICH et al. 1981; PFISTER et al. 1983), thiopronin (HAYASE et al. 1980) or d-penicillamine (STARK and SAVIR 1980) are used, which convert the cystine dimer to more soluble compounds on the basis of a thiol-disulfide exchange (KALLISTRATOS 1975, 1977; SCHMELLER et al. 1984). Additional systemic treatment improves the effect. PFISTER et al. (1983) successfully dissolved cystine stones in 7 of 11 kidneys, using the same protocol as outlined above. Treatment was well tolerated and no significant complications were observed. Mixed stones with components of struvite, apatite or calcium oxalate in an amount sufficient to interfere with chemolysis were apparently the main reason for failure (SHAW and SUTOR 1972) and additional irrigation with hemiacridine or EDTA may be necessary (PFISTER et al. 1983).

Uric acid stones rarely require aggressive treatment. If they do not respond to oral alkalinization they dissolve readily upon topical irrigation with sodium bicarbonate or THAM-E (PFISTER et al. 1983; SPATARO et al. 1978).

The main disadvantage of percutaneous stone dissolution, the long treatment period, can be reduced significantly by combining the technique with percutaneous lithotripsy or ESWL. The bulk of the calculus, which is usually easily accessible for rigid nephroscopes, is removed by ultrasonic or electrohydraulic lithotresis and the difficulty to reach peripheral residuals are dissolved by chemolysis (Fig. 17). As a precise stone analysis is available, the optimum ir-

A

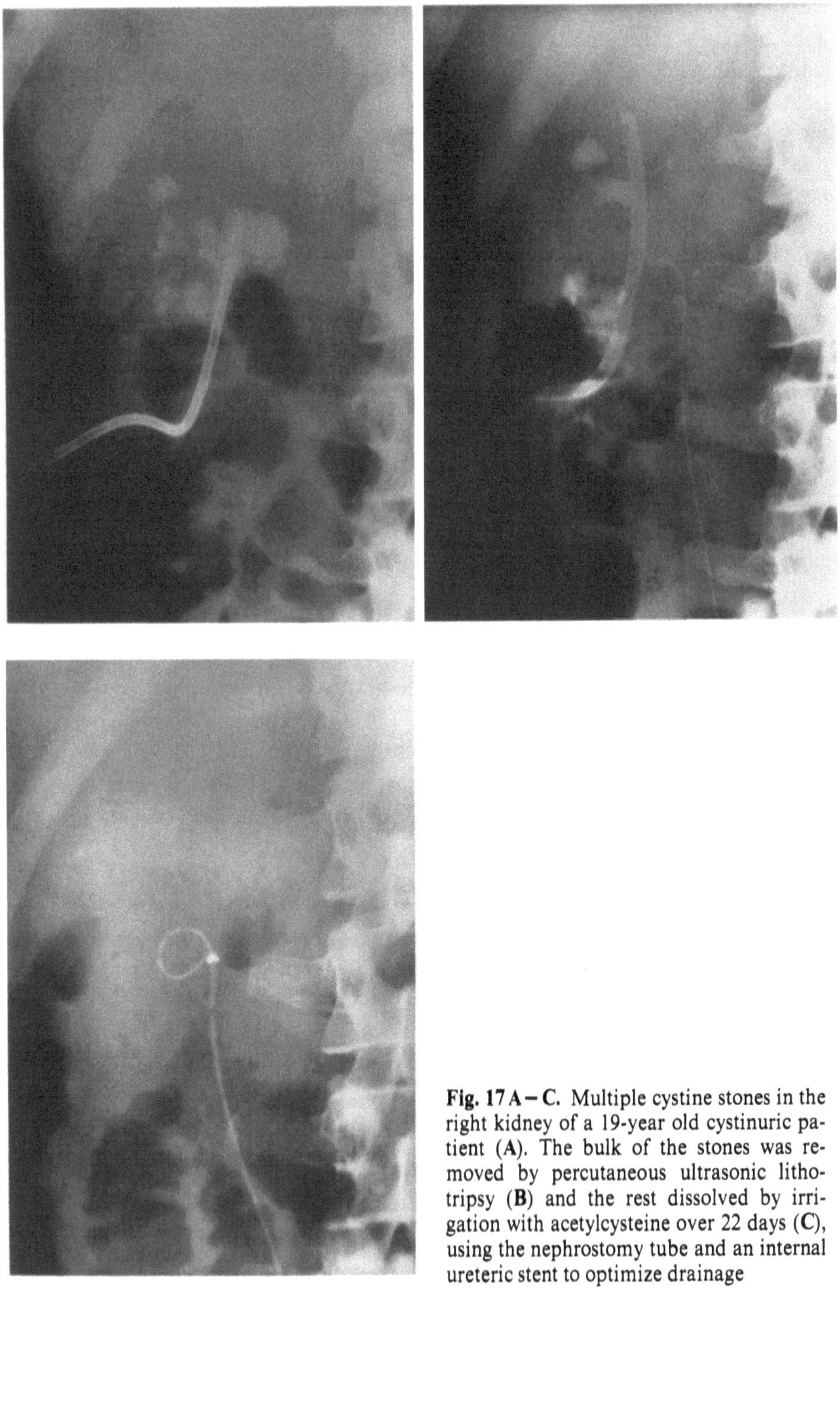

B

C

Fig. 17 A – C. Multiple cystine stones in the right kidney of a 19-year old cystinuric patient (**A**). The bulk of the stones was removed by percutaneous ultrasonic lithotripsy (**B**) and the rest dissolved by irrigation with acetylcysteine over 22 days (**C**), using the nephrostomy tube and an internal ureteric stent to optimize drainage

rigant can be chosen without having to wait for a radiographic response after a trial treatment period.

VIII. Results and Complications

The success rate of percutaneous lithotripsy depends on patient selection, the experience of the surgeon and the available equipment. Both percutaneous nephrostomy and endoscopic manipulation require considerable training and all statistics reflect a learning curve. The author experienced a failure rate of 15% in his first 16 patients subjected to percutaneous lithotripsy (MARBERGER et al. 1982), and it dropped to 6% in the first 1000 patients inspite of including difficult stones. Once the learning problems are overcome and provided a full armamentarium of equipment including a flexible nephroscope is available, the results mainly depend on the type and localization of the calculus being treated. With pelvic calculi in a rather dilated collecting system the success rate approaches 100%, whereas for calyceal stones in an anterior middle calyx with a delicate collecting system and a very mobile kidney failures are frequent. Complicated stones may require multiple interventions, usually to remove fragments from calyces or the ureter but in general, the success rates in large series today exceed 95% (ALKEN et al. 1983; KAHN 1983; SEGURA et al. 1984; CLAYMAN et al. 1984). Once the initial learning problems are overcome, postoperative morbidity is minimal. Although experience at more centers and over longer follow-up periods is necessary to define the ultimate complication rates of these procedures, they are obviously significantly lower than for equally effective open surgery (Table 1). Procedure related mortality is extremely rare and usually as-

Table 1. Complications of percutaneous nephrolithotripsy in 1000 kidneys (Rudolfstiftung Vienna); complications requiring open surgery are given in parenthesis

	Pelviceal calculi[a] (n=725)	Calyceal calculi[a] (n=178)	Branched calculi (n=97)
Mortality	1	–	–
Secondary nephrectomy	–	–	–
Insufficient tract	15 (9)	4 (2)	1 (1)
Hemorrhage	7 (3)	1	2
Residual stones[b]	25 (2)	15	32 (2)
Stone too hard for disintegration	3 (2)	–	–
Myocardial infarction	–	–	–
Exacerbation of renal tuberculosis	–	1	–

[a] with pelviceal and calyceal calculi the more difficult stone was used for group assignment
[b] Noticed on plain film at discharge; usually just "dust". Both stones that had to be removed surgically were dislocated into the ureter and a ureteral catheter had not been used

sociated with cardio-vascular or respiratory disease, and probably unavoidable in this magnitude in any series of patients of this size regardless of the treatment.

The impact on renal function is in general insignificant (see page 203) and there are no limitations to use the technique in solitary kidneys, poorly functioning kidneys or kidneys that have been subjected to previous surgery. The author treated patients aged 7 to 87 years; FITZPATRICK (1984) successfully removed a renal calculus percutaneously from a 9 year old child. Postoperative hospitalization depends on the type of stone, the condition of the patient and the local medico-social system. In 80 consecutive patients treated at this institution it averaged 4.2 days inspite of staging percutaneous nephrostomy and lithotripsy in the majority of patients. Other authors give similar figures (ALKEN et al. 1983; SEGURA et al. 1984; WICKHAM et al. 1983; CLAYMAN et al. 1984) and with good out-patient supervision the period can probably be reduced further. Almost all patients are painfree and asymptomatic at the time of hospital discharge, and fit for office or light housework.

Aside from problems with an incorrect nephrostomy tract (see page 85) and stone residuals (see page 209 and page 214) hemorrhage is the most important intraoperative complication. Provided the contraindications of percutaneous manipulation, namely clotting disorders, reno-vascular malformations and severe hypertension, are respected, it rarely presents a grave problem. If bleeding obscures vision during intrarenal surgery it is imperative that the procedure is stopped to prevent damage from uncontrolled manipulation. Hemorrhage is almost always of venous origin and rapidly stops spontaneously. Large caliber nephrostomy tubes (ALKEN et al. 1983) or balloon catheters (CLAYMAN et al. 1983b) have been reported to tamponade the bleeding tract, but in the author's experience freshly dilated tracts collapse rapidly and a thin F 14 tube suffices. If the bleeding continues inspite of forced diuresis, the tube is simply stoppered for some time for self-tamponade of the tract (see page 197). With continuing hemorrhage an arterial lesion is to be suspected and an arteriogramme has to be obtained. Arterial lesions are best managed by superselective embolization (GÜNTHER et al. 1977). Provided the patients' circulatory situation is stable, open exploration should be avoided at all means, as intraoperative inspection of the kidney rarely permits delineation of the bleeding vessel and the procedure frequently ends with a nephrectomy. The author explored 4 kidneys because of hemorrhage so far: 1 patient bled from an intercostal artery and in one hemorrhage had stopped by the time the kidney was exposed and the bleeding point could not be defined any more; both patients could have been managed conservatively.

Inadvertent injury to the pleural cavity, the colon, the liver and the gall bladder have been reported (WICKHAM and MILLER 1983; HUNTER et al. 1983; CLAYMAN et al. 1984); injuries to the duodenum, the pancreas and the large abdominal vessels theoretically appear possible. The pleura is almost exclusively opened at puncture over the 12 rib and this frequently results in pneumo- and hydrothorax, requiring drainage by a chest tube (WICKHAM and MILLER 1983; FERNSTRÖM 1983b). Injury of the colon may be noticed at the time of puncture by the escape of gas from the needle; after redrawing the needle the lesion seals spontaneously without further problems. Occasionally the colon is intubated with a tube, and this is noticed only at an attempted nephrostomogramme; antibiotic coverage and gradual withdrawal of the tube over some days seems to be the only therapeutic measure needed (ALKEN et al. 1983). Postoperative bowel distention is, however, observed frequently after percutaneous lithotripsy and this may be an indirect sign of minor bowel lesions. In the author's experience it always resolves with conventional measures.

With significant perforations of the collecting system intrarenal manipulations should be interrupted, although even large amounts of saline are mobilized without a problem from the retroperitoneum. If electrolyte-free solutions as used for transurethral surgery are employed as irrigant, a "TUR-syndrome" may develop. Characterized by severe hyponatremia, hypoosmolarity and water intoxication it has been one of rare reasons for a fatal complication of percutaneous renal surgery (SCHULTZ et al. 1983); saline must be used exclusively. Frequently massive extravasation is noticed unexpectedly at the final nephrostomogramme. The leaks seal within hours, provided the kidney is drained with a properly positioned nephrostomy tube.

In the author's experience urinary infection has not been a problem. Preoperative infection is treated appropriately and all patients are covered with an antimicrobial agent for the time of nephrostomy drainage. Occasionally a patient experiences chills or a sharp rise of temperature in the immediate postoperative period, but this is almost always due to incorrect drainage and responds immediately to repositioning of the tube. With fever the kidney is screened by sonography at short intervals. Abnormal extrarenal fluid collections are drained percutaneously and do not refill, provided the kidney itself is drained correctly (Fig. 18). Late urinomas or perirenal abscesses were not observed.

With an unobstructed ureter the nephrostomy tract usually closes within 24 hours after removal of the tube, otherwise the ureter is stented with a double-J stent. SEGURA et al. recommend this routinely (1982), but in the author's experience it is usually unnecessary if a thin tube is left in place postoperatively for only 24 hours.

SEGURA et al. (1984) reported a 0.6% rate of late hemorrhage from pseudoaneurysms or arterio-venous malformations. Although MARBERGER et al. (1984) noted no a.v. malformations in a late follow-up study of 82 patients, this complication certainly must be considered the most important potential hazard of the procedure. It seems to be directly related to the dilatation and manipulation trauma (see page 204; SMITH and LEE 1983) and is best prevented by blunt dilatation and gentle manipulation only, which avoids tearing or cutting of renal tissue. MARBERGER et al. (1984) found no evidence for significant late complications from hypertension or urinary tract infection. At computed tomography 79% of the kidneys appeared absolutely normal after lithotripsy, and this figure rose to 85% if kidneys which had been subjected to previous surgery were excluded. Only 1 of 62 kidneys showed a cortical scar 1.2×1.5 cm in diameter as a sign of cortical infarction, but the function of the kidney was not impaired. The former nephrostomy tract could only be recognised in 46% of the patients, usually by a delicate scar through the abdominal

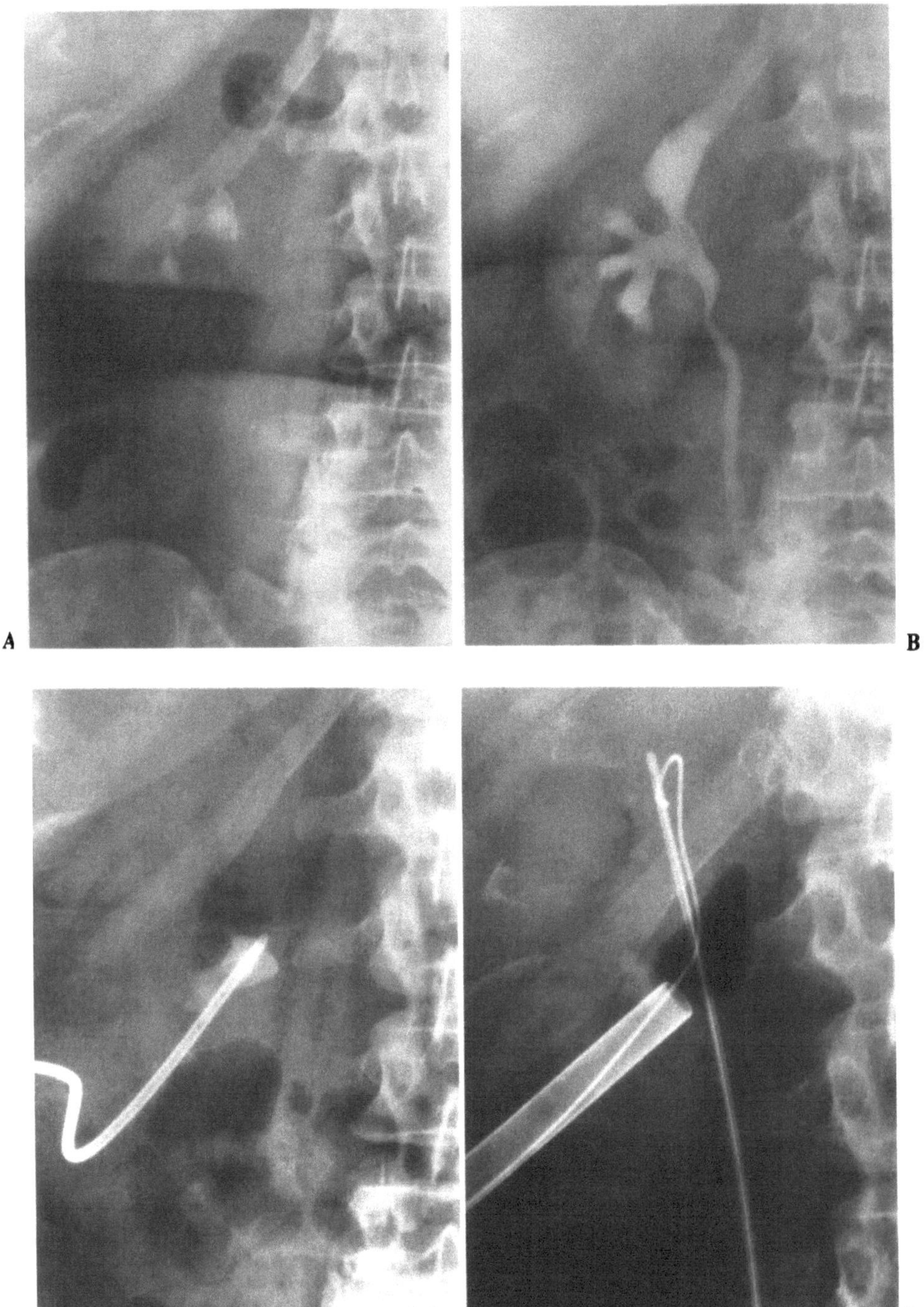

Fig. 18A–G. Plain film (**A**) and excretory urogramme (**B**) of large apatite stone in the right kidney: Percutaneous nephrostomy (**C**) and ultrasonic lithotripsy (**D**; during disintegration) in one session. 24 hours later the patient developed fever; dislocation of the tube outside the kidney and an extrarenal fluid collection was demonstrated (**E**). A double-J-ureteric stent was in-

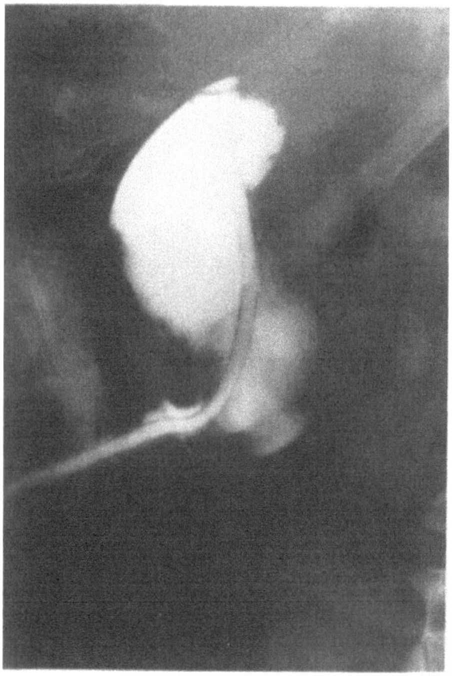

E

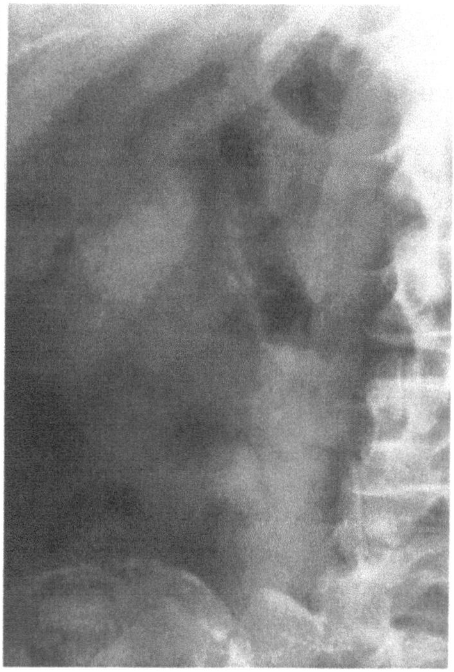

F

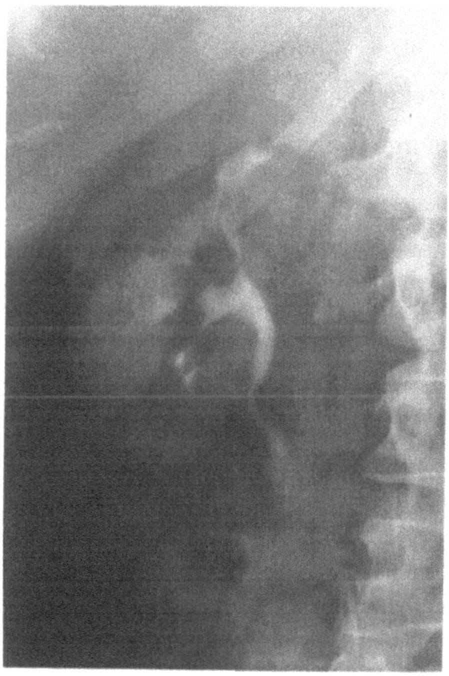

G

serted and the nephrostomy tube left in place until it stopped draining and sonography showed no fluid collections. Further recovery was uneventful, and an excretory urogramme (**F, G**) after removal of the stent two weeks later demonstrated complete stone removal and a normal kidney

Table 2. Surgical procedures performed to remove upper urinary tract calculi at the Rudolfstiftung Vienna 1/1/1984–31/12/1984 (ESWL not available)

Percutaneous nephrolithotripsy	391	85%
Ureterorenoscopy	59	
Ureterorenoscopy and percutaneous lithotripsy	56	
Zeiss loop extraction	65	
Open ureterolithotomy	44	15%
Pelviolithotomy	9	
Extended pelviolithotomy and multiple nephrolithotomies	31	
Partiall nephrectomy	3	
Nephrectomy	14	
Total reno-ureteral units treated	672	

wall; only 1 patient showed more significant alterations of the psoas muscle from resorption of a larger hematoma.

IX. The Choice of Treatment

The majority of renal calculi can be managed endoscopically. At the Rudolfstiftung Vienna 85% of all kidney stones requiring a therapeutic intervention are treated in this manner at the present time (Table 2). Most of the patients still subjected to open surgery either require reconstructive procedures to improve urinary drainage or ablative operations to remove completely destructed, usually pyonephrotic organs. A limited number of patients with uretero-pelvic stenosis can be managed with percutaneous pyelolysis (Wickham and Miller 1983; Whitfield et al. 1983), although late results of this procedure are not yet available. There remains a small group of patients, who could be treated percutaneously, but in whom the percutaneous approach is considered to be more complicated and disadvantageous for the patient than open surgery. This group comprises patients with branched staghorn stones or multiple peripheral calculi in different calyces. Some authors routinely manage stones of this type percutaneously, too (Kahn 1983; Clayman et al. 1983). In the author's experience, however, complete stones clearance from these kidneys usually requires multiple nephrostomies and staged interventions, adding up to many hours of endoscopic manipulation and weeks of treatment. Just like with any surgical intervention the choice of treatment also has to consider the volubility of the procedure. Prolongued endoscopic treatment may be justified to remove recurrent calculi of this type, which are difficult to remove by open surgery, but a simple, large staghorn calculus in a kidney which has not been operated on before may be managed more advantageously by open surgery. These considerations equally apply to the decision for percutaneous stone dissolution.

The concept of mainly basing the treatment of renal calculi on percutaneous manipulation as outlined above has to be revised. With the development of extracorporeal shock-wave lithotripsy (ESWL) an even less invasive procedure became available, that completely avoids direct manipulation on the patient (CHAUSSY et al. 1982; see chapter on "Extracorporeal Shockwave Lithotripsy (ESWL) in the Treatment of Kidney and Ureter Stones"). In view of its high efficiency and low complication rate there can be no doubt that it will be the treatment of choice for the majority of renal calculi in the future. The main disadvantage of the procedure, the need of spontaneous passage of the calculous material via the ureter, represents the main limitation in the applicability of the technique, and failure to pass the material has been the main source of complications. With the availability of percutaneous nephrostomy techniques and uretero-renoscopy these situations are easily managed. As nephrostomy tubes do not interfere with ESWL, they can already be placed prior to stone disintegration to facilitate the discharge of the stone debris. The amount of energy needed for stone disintegration with ESWL, i.e. the number of discharges rsp. sessions, depends on the volume of the calculus, and large stones may require multiple sessions. Treatment is facilitated considerably by combining ESWL with percutaneous lithotripsy: the bulk of the stone, which is usually well accessible for a rigid-rod nephroscope, is removed by ultrasonic or electrohydraulic lithotripsy, and the difficult to reach calyceal remnants are treated by ESWL. In this manner over 95% renal stones can be managed without open surgery (FUCHS et al. 1984). Again the multiple procedures and long treatment periods required with this therapeutic approach must be weighed against the disadvantages of open surgery (ALKEN 1984). ESWL does not render percutaneous endoscopic procedures unnecessary. There is unanimous consent among authors using ESWL that the latter techniques are essential adjunctives to ESWL and needed in 14 to 18% of the patients treated by ESWL (SCHÜLLER et al. 1984; SCHMELLER et al. 1984; WILBERT et al. 1984; NAGEL et al. 1984; FUCHS et al. 1984; ALBRECHT et al. 1984).

References

Acton WI, Carson MB (1967) Auditory and subjective effects of airborne noise from industrial sources. Br J Ind Med 24:297

Acton WI, Hil CR (1977) Hazards of industrial ultrasound. Protection 114:12

Albrecht D, Nagel R, Kölln CP (1972) Electrohydraulic waves (Urat 1) for the treatment of vesical calculi. Int Urol Nephrol 4:45

Albrecht KF, Lazica M, Gleiner J, Moncada J (1984) Experiences gained with ESWL of kidney and ureter stones. 2nd W Congr Perc Ren Surg, Mainz, June 14–15, Abstract No. 52

Alfthan O, Murtoma M (1972) Experiences with the clinical and experimental use of URAT-1 lithotriptor. Scand J Urol Nephrol 6:23

Alken P (1981) Teleskopbougierset zur Perkutanen Nephrostomie. Akt Urol 12:216

Alken P (1982) Percutaneous ultrasonic destruction of renal calculi. Urol Clin North Am 9:145

Alken P (1982) Intrarenaler Reflux beim Hund. Klin Padiatr 194:49

Alken P, Hutschenreiter G, Günther R, Marberger M (1981) Percutaneous stone manipulation. J Urol 125:463

Alken P, Hutschenreiter G, Günther R (1982) Percutaneous kidney stone removal. Eur Urol 8:304

Alken P, Günther R, Thüroff J (1983) Percutaneous nephrolithotomy – A routine procedure? Br J Urol [Suppl] 1

Almgard LE, Fernström I (1973) Percutaneous Nephropyelostomy. Acta Radiol [Diagn] (Stockh) 15:288

Angeloff A (1972) Hydroelectrolithotripsy. J Urol 108:867

Babcock JR, Shkolnik A, Cook WW (1979) Ultrasound-guided percutaneous nephrostomy in the pediatric patient. J Urol 121:327

Barbaric ZL (1979) Interventional uroradiology. Radiol Clin North Am 17:413

Baron RL, Lee JKT, McClennan BL (1981) Percutaneous nephrostomy using real-time sonographic guidance. Am J Roentgenol 136:1018

Bartley O, Chidekel N, Radberg C (1965) Percutaneous drainage of renal pelvis for uremia due to obstructed urinary flow. Acta Chir Scand 129:443

Bigongiari LR (1981) The Seldinger approach to percutaneous nephrostomy and ureteral stent placement. Urol Radiol 2:141

Bissada NK, Meacham KR, Redman JF (1974) Nephrostoscopy with removal of renal pelvic calculi. J Urol 112:414

Blaivas JG, Pais WM, Spellman RM (1975) Chemolysis of residual stone fragments after extensive surgery for staghorn calculi. Urology 6:680

Boyce WH (1977) Comment in: The Yearbook of Urology. Med Publishers, Chicago

Brantley RG, Shirley SW (1974) U-tube nephrostomy for postoperative retained stones. J Urol 111:7

Brock WA, Nachtsheim DA, Parsons CC (1980) Hemiacridin irrigation of renal pelvic calculi in patients with ileal conduit urinary diversion. J Urol 123:345

Brühl P (1976) Indikation und Technik der radioskopischen perkutanen Nierenbeckenfistel. Urologe [Ausg A] 15:260

Bülow H, Frohmüller HGW (1981) Electrohydraulic lithotripsy with aspiration of the fragments under vision – 304 consecutive cases. J Urol 126:454

Büscher HK (1961) Therapie der Nieren und Harnleitersteinen. In: Andersson L, Gittes RF, Goodwin WE, Lutzeyer W, Zing E (eds) Die Steinerkrankungen. La lithiase urinare. (Handbuch der Urologie/Encyclopedia of Urology, vol X), Springer, Berlin Heidelberg New York, p 283

Burchardt P (1982) The flexible Panendoscope. J Urol 127:479

Bush IV, Guinan P, Laungers J (1982) Ureterorenoscopy. Urol Clin North Am 9/13

Carson CC, Moore AV, Weinerth JC, Ford KK, Dunnick NR (1984) Percutaneous dissolution of renal calculi using ultrasonic litholapaxy. South Med J 77:196

Castaneda-Zuniga WR, Clayman RV, Smith AD, Rusnak B, Herreda M, Amplatz K (1982) Nephrostolithotomy. Percutaneous techniques for urinary calculus removal. Am J Roentgenol 139:721

Castaneda-Zuniga WR, Miller RP, Amplatz K (1982) Percutaneous removal of kidney stones. Urol Clin North Am 9:113

Cato AR, Tulloch AGS (1974) Hypermagnesemia in a uremic patient during renal pelvis irrigation with renacidin. J Urol 111:313

Chaussy C, Schmiedt E, Jocham D, Brendel W, Forssmann B, Walther V (1982) First clinical experience with extracorporeally induced destruction of kidney stones by shock waves. J Urol 127:417

Clayman RV (1983a) Percutaneous nephroscopy. A non-operative approach to the diagnosis and treatment of renal disease. Br J Urol [Suppl] 11

Clayman RV (1983b) Percutaneous removal of renal calculi: use of the backloaded balloon catheter for rapid dilatation and instrumentation of the nephrostomy tract. Br J Urol [Suppl] 19

Clayman RV (1984) Techniques in percutaneous removal of renal calculi. Urology 23: special issue, 11

Clayman RV, Surya V, Castaneda-Zuniga WR, Miller RP, Lange PH (1983a) Percutaneous nephrostolithotomy with Mazzariello-Caprini Forceps. J Urol 8:26

Clayman RV, Miller RP, Surya V, Castaneda-Zuniga WR, Smith AO, Amplatz K, Lange PH (1983b) Nephrostolithotomy: Percutaneous removal of renal and ureteric calculi. Br J Urol [Suppl] 6
Clayman RV, Castaneda-Zuniga WR, Hunter D, Miller RP, Lange PH, Amplatz K (1983c) Rapid balloon dilatation for stone removal radiology. Radiology 147:884
Clayman RV, Surya V, Miller RP, Castaneda WR, Smith AD, Hunter DH (1984a) Percutaneous nephrolithotomy: extraction of renal and ureteral calculi from 100 patients. J Urol 131:868
Clayman RV, Hunter D, Surya V, Castaneda-Zuniga WR, Amplatz K, Lange PH (1984b) Percutaneous intrarenal electrosurgery. J Urol 131:864
Coats EC (1956) The application of ultrasonic energy to urinary and biliary calculi. J Urol 75:865
Coleman CH, Witherington R (1979) A review of 117 partial nephrectomies. J Urol 112:11
Cowden JW, Abell MR (1983) Some effects of ultrasound radiation on normal tissues. Exp Mol Pathol 2:367
Crissey MM, Gittes RF (1979) Dissolution of cystine ureteral calculus by irrigation with tromethamine. J Urol 121:811
Das S (1981) Transurethral ureteroscopy and stone manipulation under direct vision. J Urol 125:112
Drettler St, Pfister RC, Newhouse JH (1979) Renal stone dissolution via percutaneous nephrostomy. New Engl J Med 300:341
Eaton JM Jr, Malin JM, Glenn JF (1972) Electrohydraulic lithotripsy. J Urol 108:865
Ekelund L, Karp W, Klefsgård Ö (1980) Percutaneous nephrostomy – indicational and technical considerations. Urol Radiol 1:227
Engelking R, Albrecht KR (1969) Die sekundäre transrenale Entfernung von Nierenbeckenkonkrementen über eine Nephrostomie. Urologe [Ausg A] 28:198
Fair OF (1978) In vivo destruction of urinary calculi by laser induced stress waves. Med Instrum 12:100
Fam B, Rossier AB, Yalla S, Berg S (1976) the role of hemiacridin in the management of renal stones in the spinal cord injury patient. J Urol 116:697
Fernström I (1983) Complications of percutaneous nephrostomy. Br J Urol [Suppl] 23
Fernström I (1983b) Percutaneous extraction of renal calculi: Technique and results. Br J Urol [Suppl] 25
Fernström I, Andersson I (1977) Percutaneous puncture nephrostomy. In: Andersson L, Gittes RF, Goodwin WE, Lutzeyer W, Zingg E (eds) Encyclopedia of Urology. Vol V/1, Suppl Springer, Berlin Heidelberg New York
Fernström I, Johannson B (1976) Percutaneous pyelolithotomy. A new extraction technique. Scand J Urol Nephrol 10:257
Fernström I, Johansson B (1982) Percutaneous extraction of renal calculi. Front Eur Radiol 1:1
Fitzpatrick JM (1984) Personal communication
Fostvedt GA, Barnes RW (1963) Complication during lavage therapy for renal calculi. J Urol 89:329
Fuchs G, Miller K, Bub P, Eisenberger F (1984) Extracorporeal shock-wave lithotripsy (ESWL): Clinical experience and results. 2nd W Congr Perc Ren Surg, Mainz, June 14–15, Abstr No. 53
Furlow WL, Bucchiere JJ (1976) The surgical fate of ureteral calculi. Review of Mayo clinic experience. J Urol 116:559
Gasteyer KH (1971) Eine neue Methode der Blasensteinzertrümmerung: Die Ultraschallithotripsie. Urologe [Ausg A] 10:30
Goldberg BB (1969) Electrohydraulic lithotripsy. In: Proc Kiev. Conference of Russian urologists, p 31, Moscow
Goodfriend R (1973) Disintegration of ureteral calculi by ultrasound. Urology 1:260
Goodwin WE, Casey WC, Woolf W (1955) Percutaneous trocar (needle) nephrostomy in hydronephrosis. JAMA 157:891
Graves FT (1954) The anatomy of the intrarenal arteries and its application to segmental resection of the kidney. Br J Surg 42:132
Gridor'eva WM (1966) Ultrasound and the question of occupational hazards. Maschinstrochiya 8:32. Ultrasonics [Abstract] 4:214

Günther R, Alken P (1982) Percutaneous nephropyelostomy and endo-urological manipulations. Frontiers in European Radiology. Vol. 1. In: Baental, Boyssen E, Fuchs WA, Heuck FHW (eds) Springer, Berlin Heidelberg New York
Günther R, Schubert U, Georgi M, Marberger M (1977) Technik der therapeutischen Katheterembolisierung der Niere mit Histoacryl (Butyl-2-Cyanoacrylat). Akt Urol 8:299
Günther R, Alken P, Altwein JE (1979) Percutaneous nephropyelostomy using a fine-needle puncture set. Radiology 132:228
Griffiths DR, Moskowitz RA, Carlton CE Jr (1979) Adjunctive chemotherapy of infection-induced staghorn calculi. J Urol 121:711
Haaga JR, Zelch MC, Alfidi RJ (1977) CT-guided antegrade pyelography and percutaneous nephrostomy. Am J Roentgenol 128:621
Harris RD, McLaughlin AP, Warrell JH (1975) Percutaneous nephroscopy using a fiberoptic bronchoscope. Removal of renal calculus. Urology 6:376
Hayase Y, Fukatsu H, Segawa A (1980) The dissolution of cystine stones by irrigated tiopronin solution. J Urol 124:775
Hedgcock MV, Eisenberger RL, Williams RA (1982) Antegrade catheter technique to dissolve uric acid ureteral calculi. Urology 19:467
Hellsten S, Frank B, Hildell J (1980) Percutaneous pyelolithotomy: case report and technique. Eur Urol 6:50
Herman BA, Powell D (1981) Airborne Ultrasound: measurements and possible adverse effects. U.S. Dept. Health and Herman Services Publication (FDA) 81:8163
Hildell J, Aspelin R, Sigfusson B (1980) Percutaneous nephrostomy. Acta Radiol [Diagn] (Stockh) 21:485
Hohlbrugger G, Janetschek G (1984) A new self-retaining nephrostomy catheter. 2nd World Congr. Percutaneous Surg, Proceedings, Abstr 8
Howards SS, Merill E, Harris S, Cohn J (1974) Ultrasonic lithotripsy: Laboratory evaluations. Invest Urol 11:273
Hruby W, Marberger M (1984) Percutaneous nephrostomy for lithotripsy of difficult renal calculi. World J Urol, accepted for publication
Huffman JC, Bagley OH, Lyon ES (1982) Treatment of distal ureteral calculi using rigid ureteroscope. Urology 20:574
Hunter PH, Hawkins IF, Nanni G, Senor D, Finlayson B, Hawkins-Hunter (1983) Retrograde transcutaneous nephrostomy: a new technique. Urology 22:583
Hunter PH, Finlayson B, Drylie DM, Leal J, Hawkins IF (1985) Retrograde nephrostomy and percutaneous nephrolithotomy in 30 patients. J Urol 133:369
Hutschenreiter G, Müller SC, Ewen K (1984) Strahlenexposition am urologischen Röntgenarbeitsplatz. Akt Urol 15:25
Jacobs StG, Gittes RF (1976) Dissolution of residual renal calculi with hemiacridin. J Urol 115:2
Janson PA, Jubelirer S, Weinstein MJ (1980) Treatment of the bleeding tendency in uremia with cryoprecipitate. N Engl J Med 303:1318
Jonsson M, Lindberg B, Risholm L (1972) Percutaneous nephropyelostomy in cases of ureteral obstruction. Scand J Urol Nephrol 6:51
Kahn RI (1983) Complications of percutaneous renal and ureteral manipulations. Endourology – AUA Videoconference. AUA – Office of Education – Videothec
Kallistratos G (1975) Litholyte agents with bacterostatic properties in consecutive treatment of kidney stones. Eur Urol 1:261
Kallistratos G (1978) Synthese neuer potentieller L-Cystein lösender Verbindungen. In: Vahlensieck W, Gasser G (Hrsg) Pathogenese und Klinik der Harnsteine V, p 324, Steinkopff, Darmstadt
Kaneko H, Watanabe H, Takahashi T, Watanabe K, Akiyama K, Kondo K, Furue H, Oinuma S (1979) Studies on the application of microexplosion to medicine and biology. IV. strength of wet and dry urinary calculi. Jp J Urol 70:61
Karamcheti A, O'Donnell WF (1977) Percutaneous nephrolithotomy. An innovative extraction technique. J Urol 118:671
Kaye K (1983) Renal anatomy for endourological stone removal. J Urol 30:647
Kaye KW, Goldberg ME (1982) Applied anatomy of the kidney and ureter. Urol Clin North Am 9:3

Kellett MJ (1983) Percutaneous access to the kidney: radiology and ultrasound. In: Wickham JEA, Miller RA (eds) Percutaneous Renal Surgery. *Churchill Livingstone,* Edinburgh London Melbourne New York

Kellett MJ, Miller RA, Wickham JEA (1983) The role of the radiologist in percutaneous renal surgery. Br J Urol [Suppl] 27

Keyser LD, Scherer PC, Claffey WW (1948) Studies in the dissolution of urinary calculi: experimental and clinical studies. J Urol 59:826

Kierfeld G, Mellin R, Damm H (1969) Blasensteinzertrümmerung durch hydraulische Schlagwellenwirkung im Tierexperiment. Urologe [Ausg A] 9:99

Korth K (1983) A new percutaneous pyeloscope with permanent irrigation. Br J Urol [Suppl] 31

Korth K (1984) Perkutane Nierensteinchirurgie: Springer, Berlin Heidelberg New York Tokyo

Krawitt LN (1978) Percutaneous renal calculus extraction. J Urol 120:647

Kurth KH, Hohenfellner R, Altwein JE (1977) Ultrasound litholapaxy of a staghorn calculus. J Urol 117:242

Lawson RK, Murphy JB, Taylor AJ, Jacobs SC (1983) Retrograde method for percutaneous access to the kidney. Urology 22:580

Leadbetter WF (1950) Instrumental visualization of the renal pelvis at operation as an aid to diagnosis; presentation of a new instrument. J Urol 63:1006

Lehfeldt W (1973) Ultraschall. Vogel, Würzburg

Lehmann JF, Warren CG, Guy AW (1978) Ultrasound: its applications in medicine and biology. In: Fry FJ (ed) vol 2, Elsevier, Amsterdam, p 561

Levy JM, Potter WM, Stegman CJ (1979) A new catheter system for permanent percutaneous nephrostomy. J Urol 122:442

Liebeskind D, Bases R, Elequin F, Neuborts Leifer R, Goldberg R, Koenigsberg M (1978) Diagnostic ultrasound: effects and growth patterns of animal cells. Radiology 131:177

Lotz M, Bartter FC (1965) Stone dissolution with d-penicillamine in cystinuria. Br Med J 2:1408

Lutzeyer W, Pohlmann R, Terhorst B, Cichos M (1970) Die Zerstörung von Harnsteinen durch Ultraschall. Experimentelle Untersuchungen. Urol Int 25:47

Marberger M (1979) Ultrasonic destruction of bladder stones. In: Resnick MI, Sanders RC (eds) Ultrasound in Urology. Williams & Wilkins, Baltimore

Marberger M (1983a) Disintegration of renal and ureteral calculi with ultrasound. Urol Clin North Am 10:729

Marberger M (1983b) Ultrasonic lithotripsy of renal calculi: A 3-year experience. Br J Urol [Suppl] 41

Marberger M, Stackl W (1983) New developments in endoscopic surgery for ureteric calculi. Br J Urol [Suppl] 34

Marberger M, Hruby W, Stackl W (1981) Percutaneous litholapaxy of renal calculi with ultrasound. Scientific exhibit 76. Convention of AUA Abstract p 5–35, Boston, U.S.A

Marberger M, Stackl W, Hruby W (1982) Percutaneous litholapxy of renal calculi with ultrasound. Eur Urol 8:236

Marberger M, Stackl W, Hruby W, Kroiss A (1985) Late sequelae of ultrasonic lithotripsy of renal calculi. J Urol 133:170

Marberger M, Stackl W, Hruby W, Wurster H, Schnedl W (1985) Ultrasonic lithotripsy and soft tissue. W J Urol 3:27

Mauermayer W, Hartung G (1976) Der Stein-Punch, ein neues Prinzip zur Sicht-Lithotripsie. Urologe [Ausg A] 15:164

McAninch JW, Kahn RI (1983) Nephroscopy. AUA Update Series, Lesson 10, vol II:1

Menanze SG, Pollack HM, Banner MP (1982) The use of grasping forceps in the upper urinary tract: Technique and radiologic implications. Radiology 144:171

Miki M, Inabe Y, Machida T (1987) Operative nephroscopy with fiberoptic scope: Preliminary Report. J Urol 119:166

Miller RA (1983) Nephroscopy: Endoscopic instruments and their accessories. In: Wickham JEA, Miller RA (eds) Percutaneous renal surgery. Churchill, Livingstone

Miller RA (1984) Experimental studies on microexplosion presentation. 2nd World Congr Percut Surg, Mainz, June 14

Miller RA, Wickham JEA (1983) Percutaneous nephroscopy. Br J Urol [Suppl] 55

Miller RA, Wickham JEA, Kellett MJ (1983a) Transuretero pyelostomy: A new technique for percutaneous renal access. Br J Urol [Suppl] 60
Miller RA, Wickham JEA, Kellett MJ (1983b) Percutaneous destruction of renal calculi: Clinical and laboratory experience. Br J Urol [Suppl] 51
Mitcheson HD, Zamenhof RG, Bankoff MS, Prien EL (1983) Determination of the chemical composition of urinary calculi by computerized tomography. J Urol 130:814
Mulvaney WP (1953) Attempted disintegration of calculi by ultrasonic vibrations. J Urol 70:704
Mulvaney WP (1960) Renacidin in urinary calcifications. J Urol 84:206
Mulvaney W, Beck CW (1968) The laser beam in urology. J Urol 99:112
Mulvaney WP, Quitter T, Mortera A (1975) Experiences with acetyl-cysteine in cystinuric patients. J Urol 114:107
Nagel B, Berendsen GU, Böhle A, Roggenbruck R (1984) Extracorporeal shock wave therapy for kidney and ureteric stones. 2nd W Congr Perc Ren Surg, Mainz, June 14–15, Abstract No 54
Narayan P, Smith AD (1982) Percutaneous nephrostomy as an adjunct in the management of ureteral calculi. Urol Clin North Am 9:121
Nasr ME (1982) Studies on the fracture mechanism in urinary concretions by lithotriptor devices. Master Thesis, University of Florida
Nemoy JN, Stamey ThA (1976) Use of hemiacridin in management of infection stones. J Urol 116:693
Newhouse JH, Pfister RC (1981) Therapy for renal calculi via percutaneous nephrostomy: dissolution and extraction. Urol Radiol 2:165
Otto R, Hauri D, Meier J, Wellauer J (1982) Perkutane ultraschallgeleitete Nephrostomie unter permanenter Sicht. Fort Röntgenstr 137:665
Ouchi T, Takashi H (1967) Zertrümmerung von Harnsteinen durch Ultraschall. Proc 14th Congress of the Int Soc Urol, Munich
Pedersen JF, Cowan PF, Kristensen JK (1976) Ultrasonically guided percutaneous nephrostomy. Radiology 119:429
Pelander WM, Kaufman JM (1980) Experience with the electrohydraulic disintegrator. J Urol 117:159
Pensel J, Frank F, Rothenberger KH, Hofstetter A, Unsöld E (1981) Destruction of urinary calculi by neodymium-yag laser irradiation. 4th Congr Int Soc Laser Surg, Tokyo, p 10-4
Pfister RC, Dretler SP, Yoder IC (1983) Percutaneous catheter dissolution of renal stones. Br J Urol [Suppl] 69
Pfister RC, Johnson RD, Pollack HM, Banner MP, Yoder IC (1983) Removal of pyeloureteric foreign bodies using a percutaneous approach. Br J Urol [Suppl] 75
Pfister RC, Yoder IC, Newhouse JH (1983) A trocar-cannula unit for percutaneous procedures. Br J Urol [Suppl] 64
Pizarello DJ, Vivino A, Madden B, Wolsky A, Keegan AF, Becker M (1978) Effect of pulsed low-power ultrasound on growing tissues. Exp Cell Biol 46:179
Pollack HM, Banner MP (1981) Percutaneous nephrostomy and related pyeloureteral manipulative techniques. Urol Radiol 2:147
Purohit GS, Pham D, Raney AM (1980) Electrohydraulic ureterolithotripsy: An experimental study. Invest Urol 17:462
Raney AM (1975a) Electrohydraulic lithotripsy: Experimental study and case reports with the stone disintegrator. J Urol 113:345
Raney AM (1978) Electrohydraulic ureterolithotripsy. Urology 12:284
Raney AM (1983) Comment. J Urol 129:28
Raney AM, Handler J (1975) Electrohydraulic nephrolithotripsy. Urology 6:439, 1
Reddy P, Smith AD (1982) Circle tube nephrostomy and nephroureterostomy. Urol Clin North Am 9:69
Reuter HC, Kern E (1973) Electronic lithotripsy of ureteral calculi. J Urol 110:181
Reuter HJ (1970) Electronic lithotripsy: transurethral treatment of bladder stones in 50 cases. J Urol 104:834
Rouvalis P (1970) Electronic lithotripsy for vesical calculus with "Urat-1". Br J Urol 42:486
Rupel E, Brown R (1941) Nephroscopy with removal of stone following nephrostomy for obstructive calculous anuria. J Urol 46:177
Rusnak B, Castaneda-Zuniga WR, Smith AD (1982) An improved dilator system for percutaneous nephrostomy. Radiology 144:74

Sadlowski RW, Finney RP, Branch WT (1979) New technique for percutaneous nephrostomy under ultrasound guidance. J Urol 121:559
Saxton HM (1981) Percutaneous nephrostomy-technique. Urol Radiol 2:131
Schmeller NT, Kersting H, Schüller J, Chaussy C, Schmiedt E (1984) Combination of chemolysis and shock-wave lithotripsy in treatment of cystine renal calculi. J Urol 131:434
Schüller J, Schmeller NT, Kersting H, Walther V (1984) Ultrasound-guided percutaneous one-step nephrostomy. Br J Urol 56:342
Schüller J, Chaussy Ch, Brandl H, Liedl B (1984) Expansion of ESWL by auxiliary methods. 2nd W Congr Perc Ren Surg, Mainz, July 14–15. Abstract No 60
Schultz RE, Hanno PM, Wein AJ, Levin RM, Pollack HM, Van Arsdelen KN (1983) Percutaneous ultrasonic lithotripsy: choice of irrigant. J Urol 130:858
Segura JW, Patterson DE, Le Roy AJ, McGaugh PF, Barrett DM (1982) Percutaneous removal of kidney stones. Mayo Clin Proc 57:615
Segura JW, Patterson DE, Leroy AJ, May GR, Smith LH (1983) Percutaneous lithotripsy. J Urol 130:1051
Segura JW, Patterson DE, Le Roy AJ, May GR (1984) Results of percutaneous removal of ureteral and renal stones. 2nd W Cong Perc Ren Surg, Mainz, June 14. Abstract No 2
Shaw DG, Sutor DJ (1972) Cystine stone dissolution. Br J Radiol 45:664
Sheldon CA, Smith AD (1982) Chemolysis of calculi. Urol Clin North Am 9:121
Smith AD, Lee WJ (1983) Endourological management of upper ureteric stones. Br J Urol [Suppl] 82
Smith AD, Lee WJ (1983) Percutaneous stone extraction. Br J Urol [Suppl] 84
Smith AD, Lee WJ (1983) Technique and complications of nephrostomy tract dilatation and tube insertion. Br J Urol [Suppl] 86
Smith AD, Lange PH, Miller RP, Reinke DB (1979) Dissolution of cystine calculi by irrigation with acetylcysteine through percutaneous nephrostomy. Urology 13:422
Smith AD, Reinke DB, Miller RP, Lange PH (1979) Percutaneous nephrostomy in the management of ureteral and renal calculi. Radiology 133:49
Smith AD, Clayman RV, Castaneda-Zuniga UR (1982) Use of Mauermayer stone punch via percutaneous nephrostomy. J Urol 128:1285
Spataro RF, Linke CA, Barbaric ZL (1978) The use of percutaneous nephrostomy and urinary alkalinization in the dissolution of obstructing uric acid stones. Radiology 129:629
Stables DP (1982) Percutaneous nephrostomy: techniques, indications and results. Urol Clin North Am 9:15
Stables DP, Johnson ML (1979) Percutaneous nephrostomy: the role of ultrasound. Clin Diagn Ultrasound 2:73
Stables DP, Ginsberg NJ, Johnson M (1978) Percutaneous nephrostomy: A series and review of the literature. Am J Roentgenol 130:75
Stark H, Savir A (1980) Dissolution of cystine calculi by pelviocalyceal irrigation with D-penicillamine. J Urol 124:895
Strijk SP, Boetes C, Froeling P (1982) Dissolution of bilateral renal calculi via percutaneous nephrostomy. Acta Radiol [Diagn] (Stockh) 23:599
Suby HI, Albright F (1943) Dissolution of phosphatic urinary calculi by retrograde introduction of citrate with magnesium. N Engl J Med 228:81
Suby HI, Suby RM, Albright FW (1952) Dissolution of urinary calculi. J Urol 68:96
Tahira K, Fukatsu T, Miyakawa T, Tanahashi Y (1979) Laser perforation of extracted urinary calculi and a simple model of perforation process. Acta Engl Def Acad 17:203
Takayasu H, Aso Y, Takagi AT, Go T (1971) Clinical applications of fiber optic pyeloureteroscope. Urol Int 26:97
Tanahashi Y, Orikasa S, Chiba R, Tahira K, Fukatsu T, Miyakawa T (1979) Disintegration of urinary calculi by laser beam. Tokyo J Exp Med 128:189
Tanahashi Y, Orikasa S, Numata I, Miyakawa T, Tanira K, Satoh K, Yammoto H (1980) The use of laser beam in urology: Disintegration of extracted urinary calculi using optical waveguides. Jpn J Urol 71:28
Tanahashi Y, Numata I, Kambe K, Harada K, Chiba Y, Toyota S, Orikasa S (1981) Transurethral disintegration of urinary calculi by the use of laser beam. 4th Congr. Int Soc Laser Surg Tokyo, p 10–30
Terhorst B, Lutzeyer W, Cichos M, Pohlmann R (1972) Die Zerstörung von Harnsteinen durch Ultraschall. Urol Int 27:458

Terhorst B, Cichos M, Versin F, Buss H (1975) Der Einfluß von elektro-hydraulischer Schallwelle und Ultraschall auf das Uroepithel. Urologe [Ausg A] 14:41
Tidd MJ, Wright HC, Oliver Y, Wallace DM, Proteous M (1976) Hazards to bladder and intestinal tissues from underwater electrical discharges. Urol Res 4:49
Timmermann A, Kallistratos G (1966) Modern aspects of chemical dissolution of human renal calculi by irrigation. J Urol 95:469
Trattner HR (1948) Instrumental visualisation of the renal pelvis and its communications: Proposal of a new method. J Urol 60:817
Tseng CH, Talwalkar YB, Tank ES, Hatch T, Alexander SR (1982) Dissolution of cystine calculi by pelviocalyceal irrigation with tromethamine-E. J Urol 128:1281
Vahlensieck W (1985) Diagnosis of urinary calculi. In: Schneider H-J (Ed) Urolithiasis: Etiology, Diagnosis. Springer, Berlin Heidelberg New York Tokyo (Handbook of urology, Vol. 17/II, p 335–424)
VDI-Richtlinien (1970): Beurteilung von Arbeitslärm am Arbeitsplatz hinsichtlich Gehörschäden. VDI-Richtlinien, VDI 2058, Blatt 2, Oktober 1976
Voltonen EJ (1968) Histologic method of measuring influence of U/S on living tissue under experimental conditions. Acta Rheum Scand 14:35
Walz PH, Riedmiller H, Alken P, Hutschenreiter G (1981) Technik und Fehlermöglichkeiten der perkutanen Nephrostomie unter sonographischer Kontrolle. Akt Urol 12:232
Watanabe H, Oinuma S (1977) Studies on the application of microexplosion to medicine and biology. I. Development of special explosive for the experiments. Jpn J Urol 68:243
Watanabe K, Watanabe H, Takahashi H, Akiyama K, Kaneko H, Kondo K, Uchida M, Oinuma S, Shiino K, Tanaka I (1980) Studies on the application of microexplosion to medicine and biology. V. Development of experimental apparatus for microexplosion and histological change in dog bladder wall by blast in air. Jpn J Urol 71:15
Watanabe H, Watanabe K, Shiino K, Oinuma S (1983) Microexplosion cystolithotripsy. J Urol 129:23
Watson GM, Miller RA, Coluin BT, Wickham JEA (1983) The ancrod coaculum for extraction of residual stone fragments after percutaneous nephrolithotomy. Br J Urol [Suppl] 89
Webb DR, Fitzpatrick JM (1984a) Percutaneous nephrolithotomy: Structural and functional effects. Abstract 3, proceedings, 2nd World Congress on percutaneous renal surgery, Mainz, June 14–15
Webb DR, Fitzpatrick JM (1984b) Ureterolithotripsy: An experimental model. Abstract 40, proceedings, 2nd World Congress on percutaneous renal surgery, Mainz, June 14–15
Weirich W, Ackermann D, Alken P, Riemiller H (1979) Die Auflösung von Cystin-Steinen mit N-Acetylcystein nach perkutaner Nephrostomie. Akt Urol 12:224
Weirich W, Haas H, Alken P (1982) Perkutane Chemolyse von Struvitsteinen bei Nierenbecken- und Kelchhalsobstruktion. Akt Urol 13:256
Weiss EQ, Levya A, Hernandez A (1976) Treatment of lithiasis by forced injection of liquid and ureteral catheter by translumbar route. Int Surg 61:419
Whitfield HN, Mills V, Miller RA, Wickham JEA (1983) Percutaneous pyelolysis: An alternative to pyeloplasty. Br J Urol [Suppl] 93
Wickham JEA, Kellett MJ (1981) Percutaneous nephrolithotomy. Br Med J 283:1571
Wickham JEA, Miller RA (1983a) Percutaneous renal surgery. Churchill Livingstone, Edinburgh London Melbourne New York
Wickham JEA, Kellett MJ, Miller RA (1983b) Elective percutaneous nephrolithotomy in 50 patients: Analysis of technique, results and complications. J Urol 129:904
Wickham JEA, Miller RA, Kellett MJ (1983c) Percutaneous nephrolithotomy results and cost effectiveness. Br J Urol [Suppl] 103
Wickham JEA, Miller RA, Kellett MJ (1984) Percutaneous disintegration of renal calculi. Proc, 2nd World Congr Perc Surgery, Mainz, June 14–15. Abstract No 15
Wilbert DM, Müller StC, Alken P, Hohenfellner R (1984) Extracorporeal shock-wave lithotripsy (ESWL) – Mainz experience. 2nd W Congr Perc Ren Surg, Mainz, July 14–15. Abstract No 55
Wilburg HJ (1981) The flexible choledochoscope. A welcome addition to the urological armamentarium. J Urol 126:380
Xui M, Chang J, Xui Z, Cheng W, Bao Z, Shi Z, Wang J (1981) Microexplosion of bladder stone. Chin J Med 61:341

The Instrumentation and Surgery of Ureteric Calculi

P. ALKEN

I. Introduction

It emerges from pooled epidemiological data that 30 to 50% of episodes of stone disease are due to ureteric calculi.

However, this figure reflects only hospital admissions and stone analyses, the true incidence no doubt being higher. Since 80% of ureteric calculi pass spontaneously patients may be reluctant to seek hospital admission. Also, some stones pass asymptomatically. The often minute quantities of material or apathy on the part of the physician prevent small stones coming to analysis. There is considerable disagreement on the recommended treatment, which ranges from surgical intervention in ⅔ of cases through instrumental manipulation for 90% to conservative treatment for almost 80% of patients (BANDHAUER 1970).

New treatments such as percutaneous nephrolithotomy, ureterorenoscopy and shockwave lithotripsy will no doubt generate their own sets differing figures.

II. History

Patients with recurrent stone disease frequently report previous spontaneous passage of stones of varying caliber, indirect data from which to predict whether or not the present stone is likely to pass of its own accord. Past operations are also significant. Partial obstruction due to strictures at the site of previous surgery will reduce the likelyhood of spontaneous passage. The same will be true where there is radiological evidence of the stone being impacted at the same ureteric level for several weeks: surrounding inflammation and reactive mucosal proliferation will tend to arrest the stone. A history of febrile episodes and associated symptoms may lead to a more active therapeutic approach.

III. Significance of Symptoms

Neither the periodicity, the duration nor the frequency of attacks of colic provide a firm basis for deciding on treatment, nor does the occurrence of vomitting or partial ileus. In general the intensity of such symptoms bears no relationship to the size of a stone or to its ability to pass of its own accord.

IV. Investigations

A plain X-ray of the kidneys, ureters and bladder should always be the first investigation and will reveal the presence, site and size of radio-opaque stones within the ureter. As a rule ultrasound merely reveals obstructive changes in the proximal tract, since stones themselves can only be demonstrated immediately distal to the renal pelvis. Because of their anatomical position the distal ureters are difficult to see on ultrasound, although some calculi at the immediate vesicoureteric junction can sometimes be seen if the bladder is full.

If, as is frequently the case, the proximal system is obstructed and dilated, contrast excretion is often delayed on intravenous urography, the proximal ureter sometimes not opacifying until 24 hours after injection. The column of contrast then points like a finger to the level of obstruction (Figs. 1, 2). Delayed films are particularly important if no stone was seen on the plain film, either because the stone is radiolucent or because an opaque stone was masked by a vertebral transverse process or the bones of the iliosacral region (Figs. 1 and 2). If the stone is not causing significant obstruction, the ureter will opacify up to the level of the stone virtually without delay and contrast will be seen streaming past into the distal ureter.

Stones immediately above the bladder are often difficult to distinguish from pelvic phleboliths. Their relationship to local ureteric obstruction may be demonstrated on the urogram by a post-micturition film.

Forniceal rupture is the classical but rare (reported in 1% of cases) complication of intravenous urography in the presence of stone obstruction. The contrast medium provokes an osmotic diuresis with a subsequent rise in pressure in the proximal collecting system, followed by radiological evidence of extravasation where the calyces insert into the renal parenchyma. This complication is equally rare in our own experience and occurred only where urography was performed during an attack of colic. The use of low osmolarity contrast medium reduces osmotic diuresis and avoids the complication of forniceal rupture. Little time is usually lost furthermore by delaying urography until a colic-free interval.

All cases of forniceal rupture require antibiotic treatment, but the need for additional measures will depend on the size of the calculus. If the latter appears likely to pass spontaneously, conservative treatment can usually be justified. In the presence of larger stones temporary decompression of the renal pelvis may be undertaken by ureteric catheter or percutaneous nephrostomy. The stone may then be dealt with on a separate occasion.

Attempts to use isotopic renal function studies at the time of diagnosis as a criterion for active or conservative treatment have not yielded any firm results (ANDREN-SANDBERG et al. 1980; HOLM-NIELSEN et al. 1981; LUNDSTAM et al. 1983).

Fig. 1. Patient A.M.: Plain film with faintly radiopaque left ureteral stone (*arrow*). Stone is masked by the vertebral transverse process

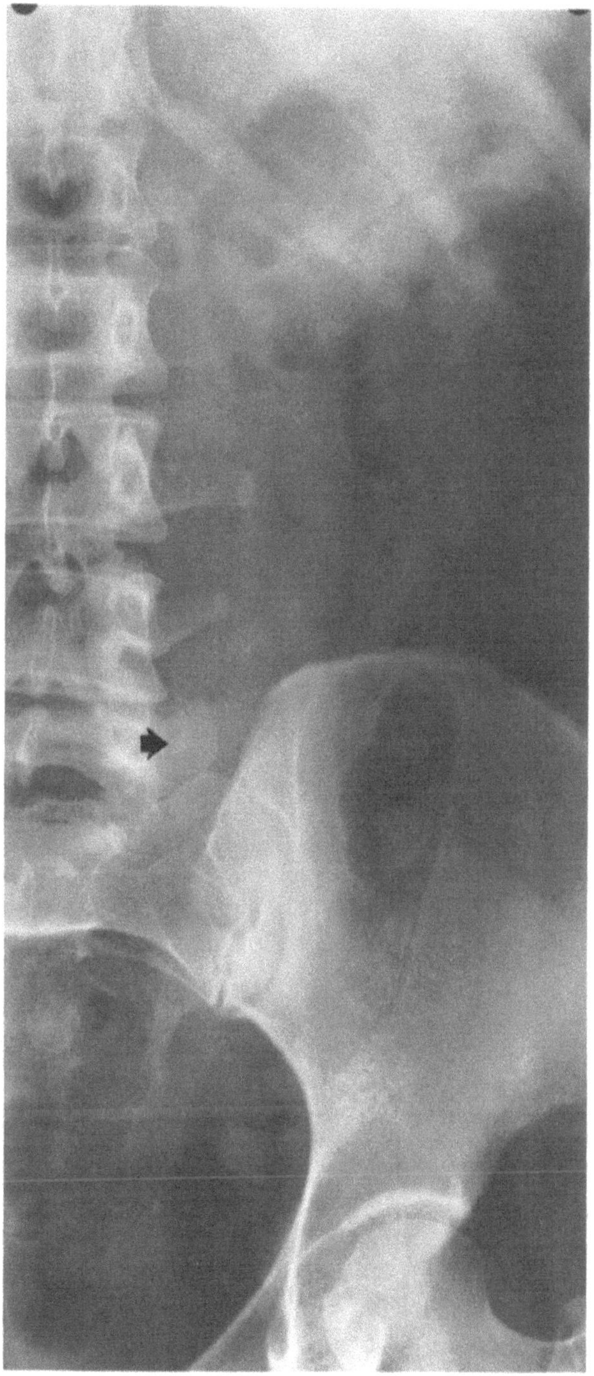

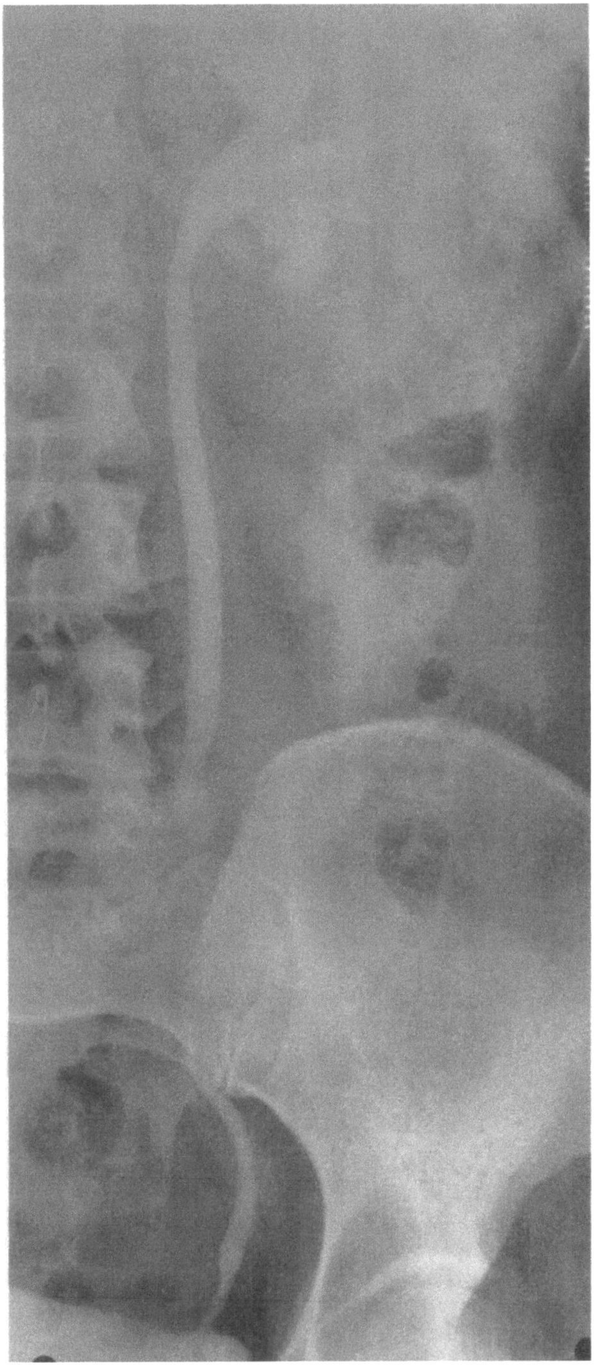

Fig. 2. Patient A.M.: Delayed film of IVU. Moderately obstructed upper ureter points towards area of obstruction

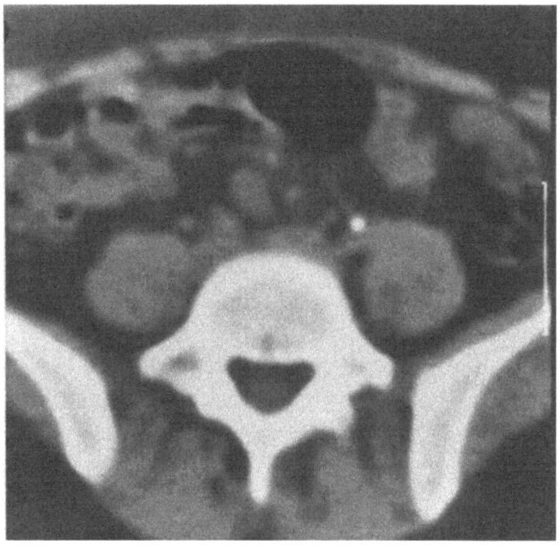

Fig. 3. Patient A.M.: CT-scan showing stone in the left ureter at the area of the 5th vertebral body

Weakly or non-opaque calculi may be difficult to distinguish from other causes of ureteric obstruction, such as tumors or strictures following surgery or radiotherapy. The next line of non-invasive investigation may then be computed tomography, which is capable of detecting ureteric calculi down to a diameter of 1–2 mm, irrespective of level (Fig. 3). The alternative invasive techniques to be discussed are retrograde and antegrade pyelography, the latter after percutaneous puncture of the renal pelvis (Fig. 4). Both techniques may also be employed therapeutically to decompress the collecting system. The retrograde approach may be barred by urethral obstacles such as stricture and prostatic adenoma as well as by stricture or tortuosity of the distal ureter.

There are two further disadvantages to the retrograde approach. Even with the most meticulous technique, micro-organisms may be carried into the obstructed proximal tract. If it proves impossible to maneuver a ureteric catheter past the obstructing stone, infection in the upper tract may introduce an unwanted element of urgency. Even if the maneuver succeeds a second procedure such as loop-extraction has still not been avoided, since there is no guarantee that removal of the catheter will be followed by spontaneous passage of the stone (Butler and O'Flynn 1973). This problem may be circumvened by using special stone extraction catheters (Steffens 1984; Korth 1984), designed both to allow adequate drainage of the upper tract and to permit subsequent extraction of the stone. With an external diameter of Ch. 5 or Ch. 5.4, the draining capacity of these catheters may be inadequate for purulent urine.

The antegrade approach is made easier by proximal obstructive dilatation. The difficulty of manipulating a catheter past the stone is obviated and by dilating the percutaneous track the collecting system can be adequately drained without constraint on the caliber of the catheter. In problem cases final diagnosis may be delayed until after the acute episode and can be considered at leisure. The presence of a nephrostomy tube will not impede possible spontaneous passage of the stone.

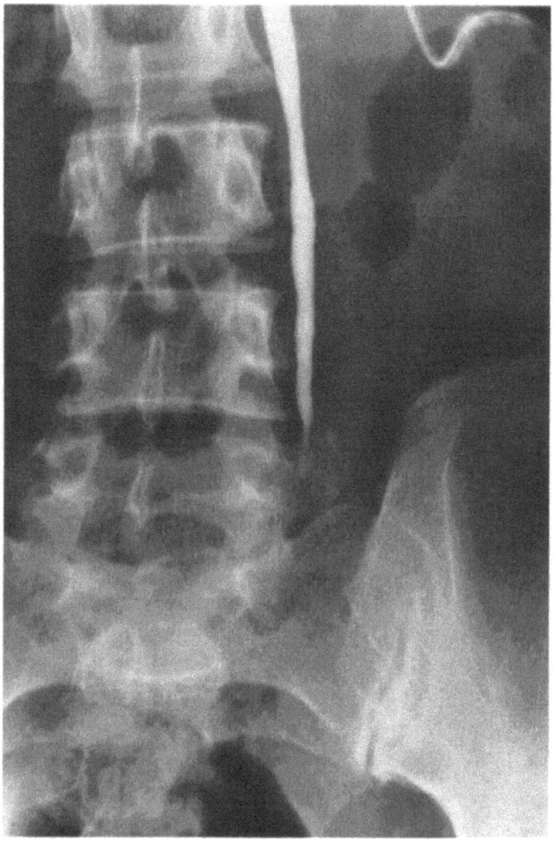

Fig. 4. Patient A.M.: Antegrade Pyelography after percutaneous nephrostomy. Small ureteral stone below the column of contrast dye

Additional clinical and laboratory factors such as temperature, leucocytosis or thrombocytopenia may herald the serious complication of sepsis in an obstructed system and generally demand a more active therapeutic approach. Even so, the first line of treatment should be decompression by ureteric catheter or percutaneous nephrostomy.

V. Spontaneous Passage and Size of Stone

Two measurements are quoted in the literature for the likelyhood of ureteric stones passing spontaneously. SANDEGARD recorded 93% spontaneous passage within 4 weeks for stones up to a maximum of 4 mm in diameter (SANDEGARD 1956). According to UENO a 6 mm stone has only a 35% chance of passing spontaneously within a year and he recommends intervention for any stone greater than 8 mm (UENO et al. 1977).

Since the spontaneous passage rate is definitely smaller for stones located in the upper third of the ureter at the time of first diagnosis than for those in the lower ureter (BANDHAUER 1970) and since patients with the former generally have more pronounced obstruction and worse symptoms (FOX et al. 1965), the majority of authors recommend a more agressive approach to upper ureteric calculi.

VI. Stone Removal

Four different forms of active intervention are now available:
I. Retrograde Techniques
II. Antegrade Techniques
III. Extracorporeal shockwave lithotripsy
IV. Surgery

1. Retrograde Techniques Under X-Ray Control

A wide variety of ureteric catheters have been designed, all for introduction by basically the same cystoscopic approach followed by advancement under X-ray guidance. There are two main techniques: immediate extraction or placement of indwelling catheters to accelerate spontaneous passage.

a) Indications

Although the feasibility of retrograde extraction under X-ray guidance has been demonstrated, e.g. by ZEISS (1959) and DOURMASHKIN (1945), in more than 5000 cases of ureteric and even renal calculi, later studies have attempted, in the light of the likely complications, to restrict the indications to stones in the lower third of the ureter and of a size that could in principle pass spontaneously, yet that have failed to do so despite several weeks of conservative treatment. Most recently, improvements in endo-urologic techniques have led to some relaxation of this rule.

b) Technique

In all X-ray-guided techniques the extraction catheter is first introduced into the ureter under direct endoscopic vision. X-ray guidance is then employed to advance the catheter until its tip reaches past the stone into the proximal ureter. The part of the catheter design to ensnare the stone is opened within the ureter or renal pelvis and the catheter withdrawn to the level of the stone.

Catheters of COUNCIL (1945), JOHNSON (1937) or DORMIA (1982) pattern possess an extraction device consisting of a spindel-shaped basket of spring wire which opens spontaneously to trap the stone (Fig. 5). Stones are extracted immediately under X-ray guidance. Whilst COUNCIL (1945) has recommended

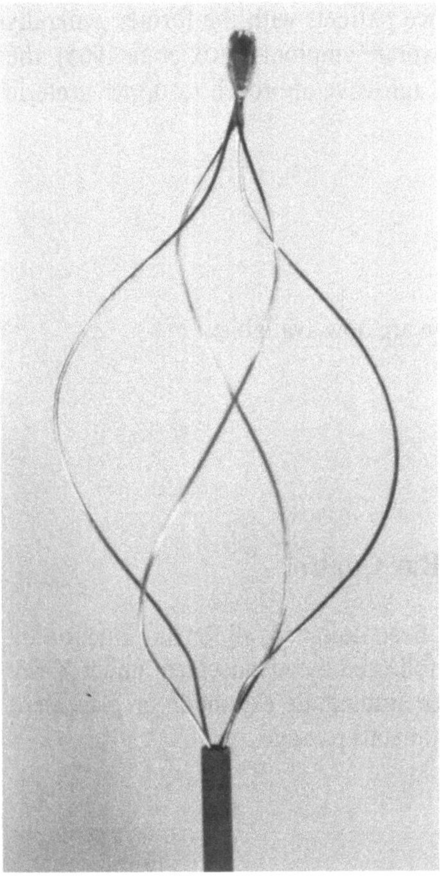

Fig. 5. Dormia stone dislodger opened

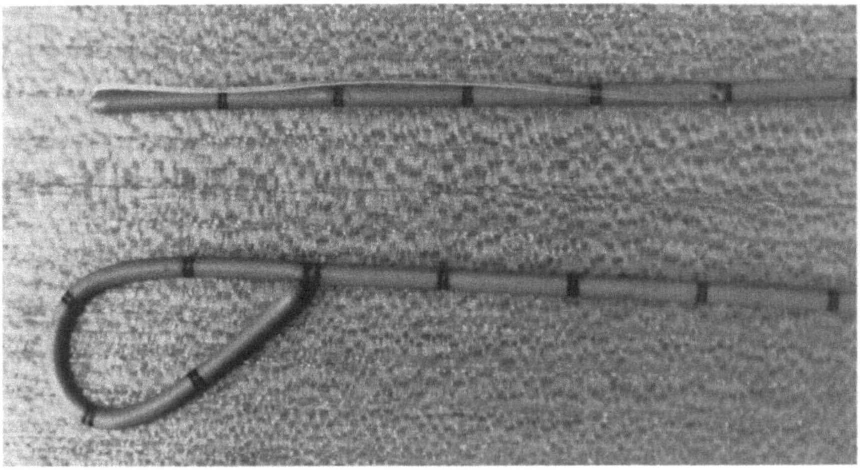

Fig. 6. Zeiss loop opened and closed

closing the basket around the stone, DORMIA (1982) prefers to withdraw the stone with the basket open, so as to avoid accidentally pinching the ureteric wall.

The DAVIS loop extractor although classified as a side loop also follows the basket principle (DAVIS 1854, 1961). Traction on the two ends of a nylon filament running outside a short segment of the catheter pulls the latter into an arch. A basket consisting of the ureteric catheter and the two filaments is thus formed around the stone. Good results have been achieved with extraction catheters of COUNCIL, JOHNSON or DAVIS pattern throughout the Angloamerican area.

In the German-speaking world stone extraction tends to be performed with loop catheters of the ZEISS pattern (Fig. 6). After advancement past the stone this device is formed into a complete loop in the proximal ureter or renal pelvis. The loop is then withdrawn down to or around the stone and stone and catheter left to pass spontaneously over the ensuing days, if necessary accelerated by hanging weights on the catheter. The duration of hospital admission is usually greater than with direct extraction techniques (TSUANG and EVANS 1983). Authors who favor the Zeiss loop type of instrument stress its relatively atraumatic character compared to immediate extraction (KARCHER 1964, BANDHAUER 1977; BORGMANN and NAGEL 1981). Pooled data, however, fails to give a definite advantage to one technique or the other if duration of hospital admission, efficiency, and complication rate are taken into account (Table 1) (DRACH 1978).

The difficulties and hazards associated with retrograde extraction of ureteric calculi include perforation of the ureter as the catheter is maneuvered past the calculus and ureteral avulsion as the stone is extracted. The only protection lies in careful instrumentation and continuous radiological monitoring. Instruments of the basket pattern are frequently rather rigid and the hazard of perforation may be further reduced by using instruments fitted with a soft filiform leader (RUTNER and FUCILLA 1976).

Whatever instrument is used, forced extraction, eventually resulting in ureteral avulsion should never be employed in the attempt to overcome firm resistance. Although extractors of COUNCIL, JOHNSON or DAVIS pattern may be left in situ, most authors regard arrest of the instrument within the ureter as an indication for open surgery (WALSH 1974; DORMIA 1982; HARRISON et al. 1983). Since any technique is associated with complications that may require open surgical exposure, patients should always be informed of this eventuality. For the same reason many authors recommend preparing the patient as for open surgery, although endoscopic extraction under radiological control is itself quite suitable for use under local anesthetic on an outpatient basis, particularly in women.

c) Other Techniques

At the turn of the century and before the introduction of extractors or loop catheters it had already become routine to dilate the ureter to Ch. 20, with the

Table 1. Retrograde stone manipulation under X-ray control

Author	Year	Attempted extractions	Successful retrieval	Severe complications	Secondary surgery
Extraction with basket					
COUNCIL	1945	504	353 = 70%	5	?
PRINCE and SARDINO	1960	298	195 = 65%	6	28
MAHON and WATERS	1973	193	110 = 57%	4	10
WALSH	1974	136	82 = 65%	3	12
CONSTANTIAN	1974	265	238 = 90%	?	?
HENRY and TAMLIN	1975	549	421 = 77%	4	13
FURLOW and BUCCHIERE	1976	661	588 = 89%	?	45
KLOMPUS and OWENS	1978	97	89 = 92%	1	4
TSUANG and EVANS	1983	299	212 = 71%	6	?
HARRISON et al.	1983	205	105 = 52%	7	26
		3207	2393 = 75%	36	138
Loop delivery					
KARCHER	1964	220	143 = 65%	?	34
BANDHAUER	1970	232	146 = 63%	0	?
BOWERS	1973	117	108 = 93%	0	0
KARCHER	1981	1483	1338 = 95%	0	1
BORGMANN and NAGEL	1981	567	481 = 84%	3	69
IPIENS-AZNAR	1982	68	48 = 71%	0	14
TSUANG and EVANS	1983	207	95 = 47%	6	?
		2894	2359 = 82%	9	118

aim of facilitating spontaneous passage (GOTTSTEIN 1927). With the advent of ureterorenoscopy the appropriate metal dilators have experienced a renaissance and the technique of balloon dilatation of the ureter has, for example, been taken up by RUTNER (1983) in his balloon extraction catheter. This instrument has a 4 cm dilating balloon fitted distal to a wire basket of DORMIA pattern. Using this technique RUTNER (1983) has been able to extract stones of up to 8 mm under radiologic guidance. SHIHATA has employed an alternative principle in his coaxial twin-balloon extraction catheter (SHIHATA and GREENE 1983). Finally, however, all these techniques are limited by the size of the stone. Both excessive dilatation of the ureter and subsequent extraction through it of very large calculi must involve uncharted hazards of longterm damage to the ureter.

d) Ureteric Stone Disintegration Under Radiologic Control

In the early seventies FABIANO (1970) and REUTER and KERN (1973) described electrohydraulic litholapaxy of ureteric calculi under X-ray control. Although good stone disruption was achieved, the serious, if fortunately uncommon, complication of ureteric perforation apparently condemned this technique to obscurity (REUTER and KERN 1973; GELLISSEN and REUTER 1974; GOODFRIEND

1984), although PUROHIT et al. (1980) published some further data from animal experiments in 1980. Only the advent of ureterorenoscopy and its direct endoscopic control of stone destruction has restored the technique to a position of significance.

2. Ureterorenoscopy

Transurethral endoscopy of the ureter was at first undertaken with fiberoptic instruments (TAKAYASU et al. 1971). Compared to rigid optical systems these instruments yield a poor quality image and have little or no irrigating power. Their usefulness for the endoscopic treatment of ureteric calculi is therefore strictly limited (BUSH et al. 1982).

In 1977 and 1978, GOODMAN (1977) and LYON et al. (1978) described endoscopy of the lower ureter with pediatric cystoscopes. In 1980 and 1981, TEICHMANN (1980) and DAS (1981) reported the extraction of distal ureteric calculi under direct vision with the same type of instrument. Only with the development by PERES CASTRO of his ureterorenoscope – basically a 12 Fr. pediatric cystoscope extended to a length of 50 cm – did the entirity of the ureter become accessible to endoscopy (PEREZ-CASTRO ELLENDT and MARTINEZ PINEIRO 1980, 1982). At this point ureterorenoscopy became a viable clinical proposition. The various instruments currently available commercially already (Figs. 7a, b) suffice for the effective treatment of ureteric calculi. Despite continuous modification and updating, however, an ideal instrument that would allow inspection of most of the renal collecting system, permit the introduction of two ancillary instruments and comprise the advantages of continuous irrigation has yet to appear on the market.

a) Technique

The procedure is performed on a urological X-ray table under spinal or general anesthesia. Since only about 40% of cases require dilatation of the ureteric orifice or transmural ureter prior to introduction of the ureterorenoscope (Table 2), ureterorenoscopy may be attempted forthwith. If the ureteric orifice or distal ureter cannot be negotiated, these segments will require preliminary dilatation. First a flexible Ch. 3 guide wire is passed up the ureter through a cystoscope. Dilatation is then undertaken with Ch. 9–15 metal or Ch. 6–16 plastic dilators (Fig. 8). Depending on the size of the cystoscope sheath, the larger plastic dilators can only be used under X-ray guidance. Balloon dilatation catheters that can be passed over the guide wire into the ureter are also available (Figs. 9, 10a–d), but are considerably more expensive than the other equipment just described. The ideal solution is a balloon catheter that can be passed up the ureterorenoscope and that permits dilatation and endoscopy in a single sequence. As the instrument is advanced through the ureteric orifice and intramural ureter, segments immediately ahead of the instrument are dilated under direct vision. The introduction of several ureteric catheters for 24 hours

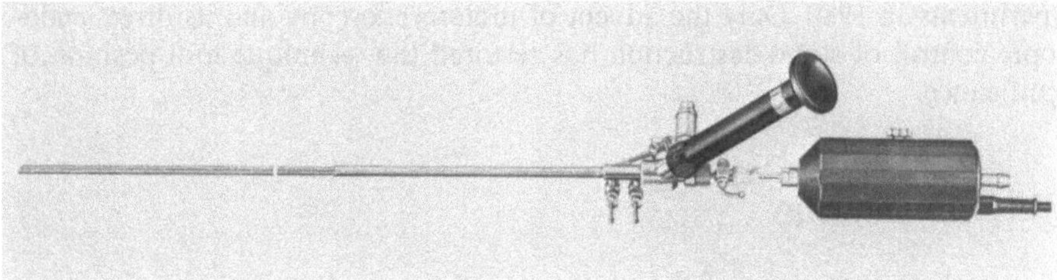

a

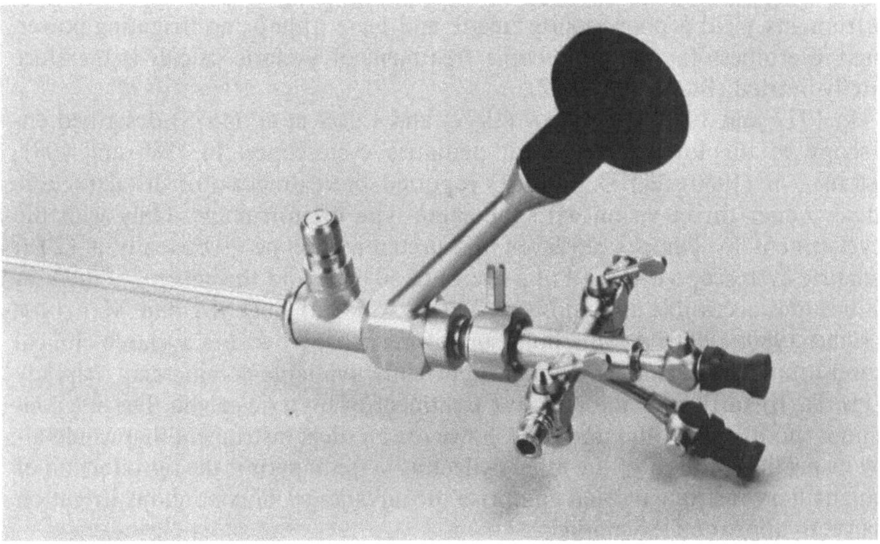

b

Fig. 7a. Perez-Castro Ellendt operating uretero-renoscope. **b** Bichler operating uretero-renoscope

Table 2. Uretero-renoscopy for stone manipulation (Dept. of Urol. Johannes Gutenberg Universität Mainz) n = 103

Not accessable	8%
Dilation of distal ureter necessary	58%
Stone localization	
Proximal ureter	24%
Middle ureter	38%
Distal ureter	38%
Stone fragments after ESWL	22%
Stone removal by	
Ultrasound disintegration	34%
Extraction	34%
Subsequent ESWL	22%
Subsequent PNL	2%
Late complications requiring surgery	
Extended ureteral necrosis	1
Praevesical stenosis	3

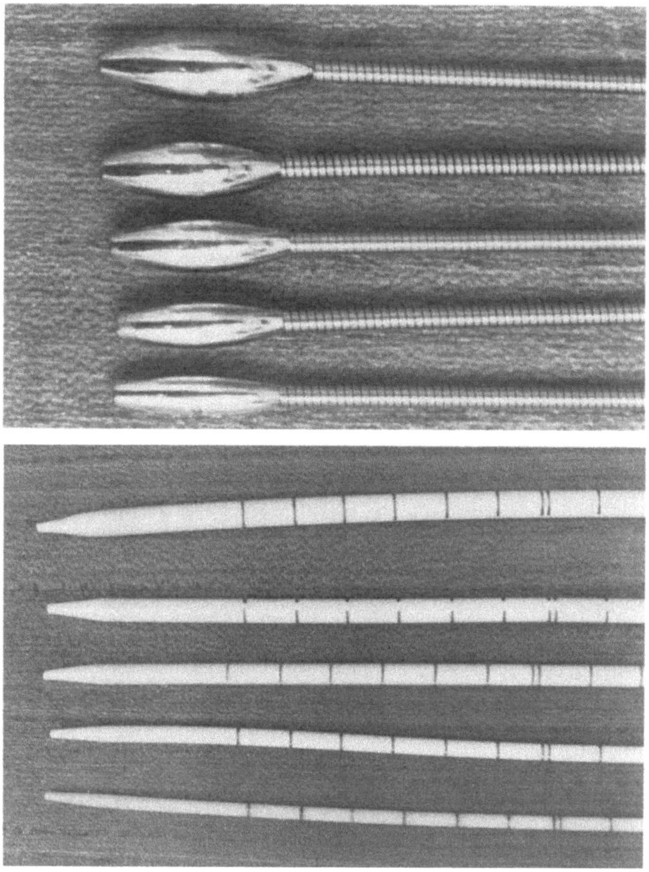

Fig. 8. Metallic and Teflon dilators used for ureteral dilation

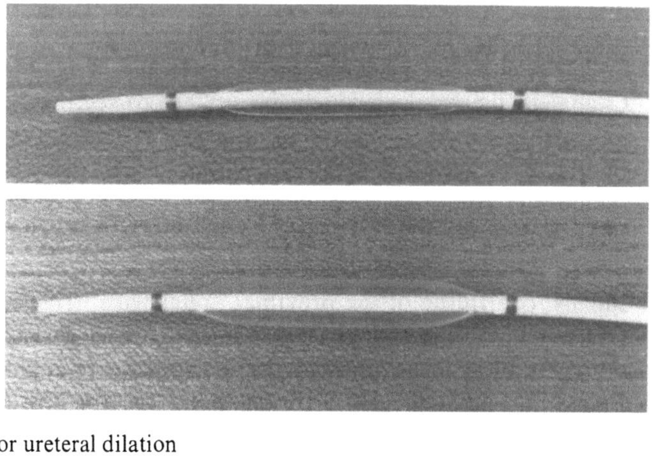

Fig. 9. Balloon catheter for ureteral dilation

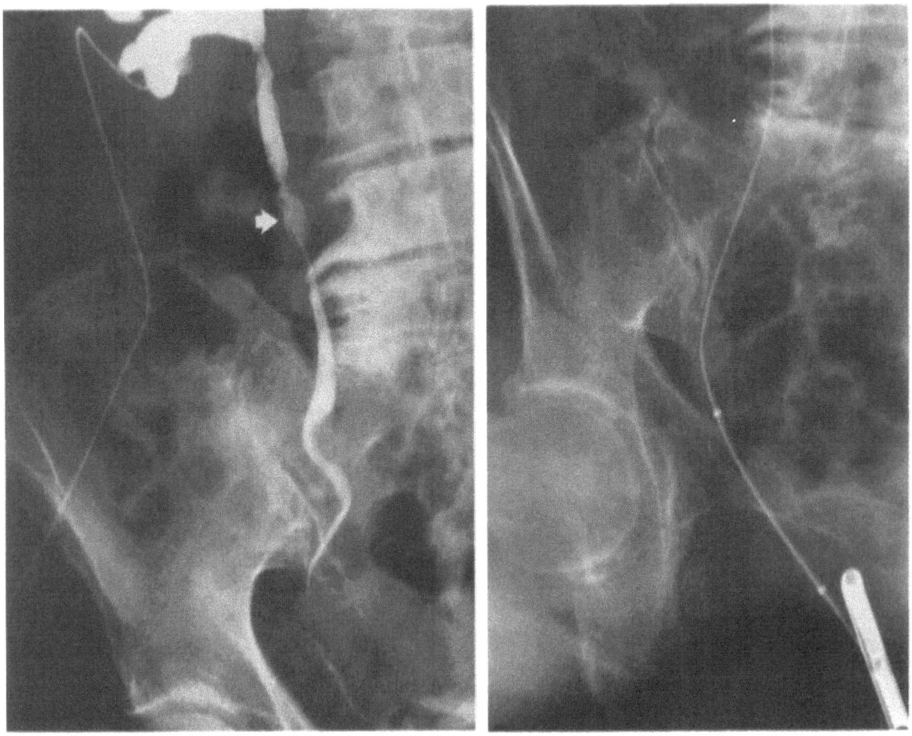

a b

Fig. 10a. Antegrade pyelography after percutaneous nephrostomy in case of ureteral stone (*arrow*). **b** Balloon dilation catheter introduced over guide wire

has also been described as an alternative for negotiating difficult segments, as has limited incision of the ureteric orifice. Under optimal conditions the lumen of the ureter is held continuously in the center of the field of view and the ureterorenoscope is advanced straight ahead under direct vision. There are three sets of circumstances under which orientation may be impaired:

1. Caudal to the level at which the ureter crosses the iliac vessels the ureter loops from dorsal to ventral and it may become impossible to see anything but the ureteric wall as the instrument is advanced.
2. As the tip of the instrument closely approaches the obstructing calculus even quite minor bleeding may obscure the field of view, since the irrigating power of the instrument is very modest.
3. Finally, overfilling of the proximal ureter with irrigating fluid may cause it to distend into loops which impede passage of the rigid instrument.

If any of these three problems occur two principal methods are available for reorientating and advancing the instrument. Injecting contrast medium will provide radiologic evidence of the route up the proximal ureter above the instru-

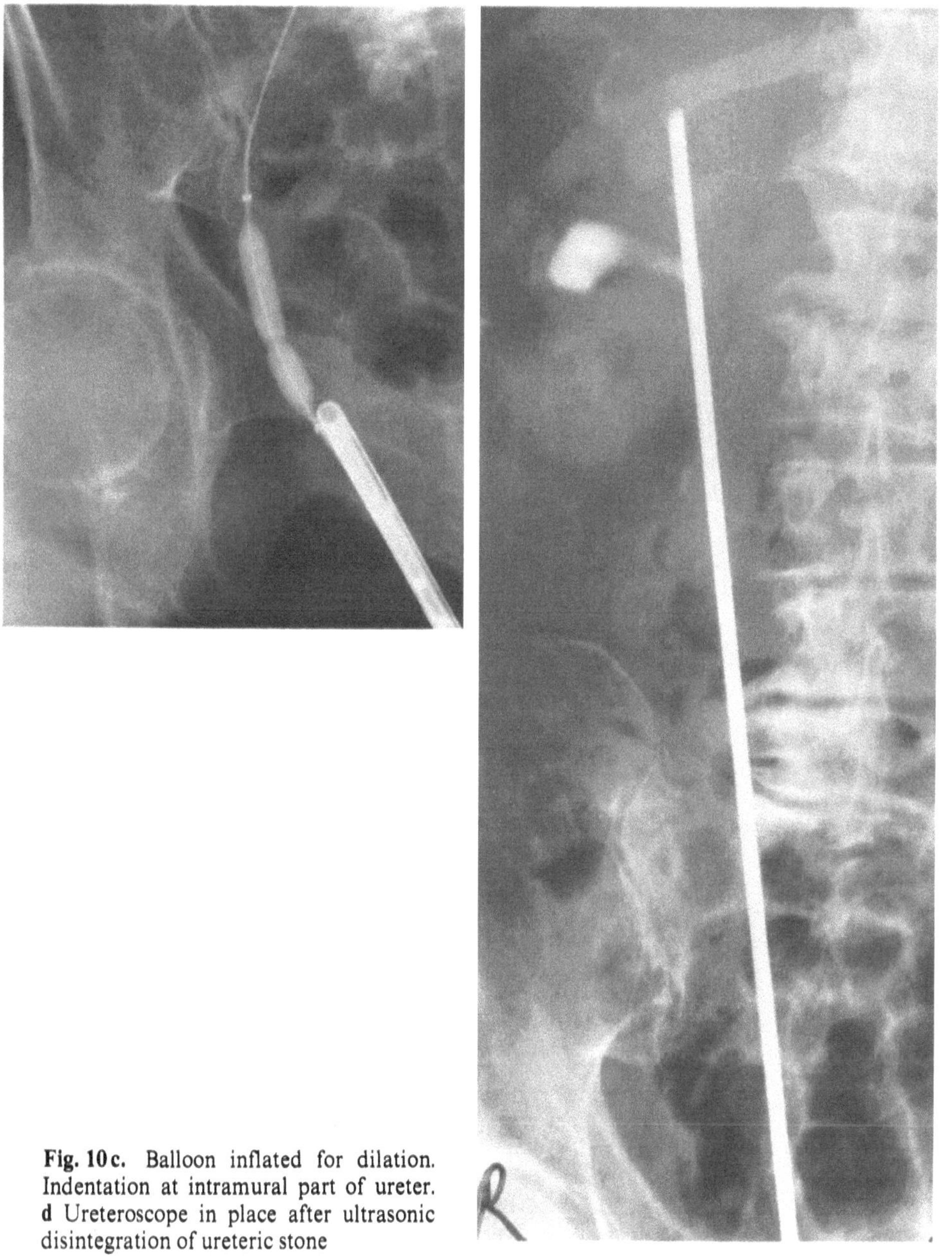

Fig. 10c. Balloon inflated for dilation. Indentation at intramural part of ureter. **d** Ureteroscope in place after ultrasonic disintegration of ureteric stone

ment. If contrast is injected as a bolus, the proximal ureteric lumen often opens up beyond the instrument and the latter can be further advanced under endoscopic vision. Secondly, a guide wire or ureteric catheter (the latter aids drainage of irrigating fluid) may first be inserted under X-ray guidance into the upper ureter (Figs. 11 a–c). Even under poor conditions of visibility and orientation, the instrument can then be advanced along this guide.

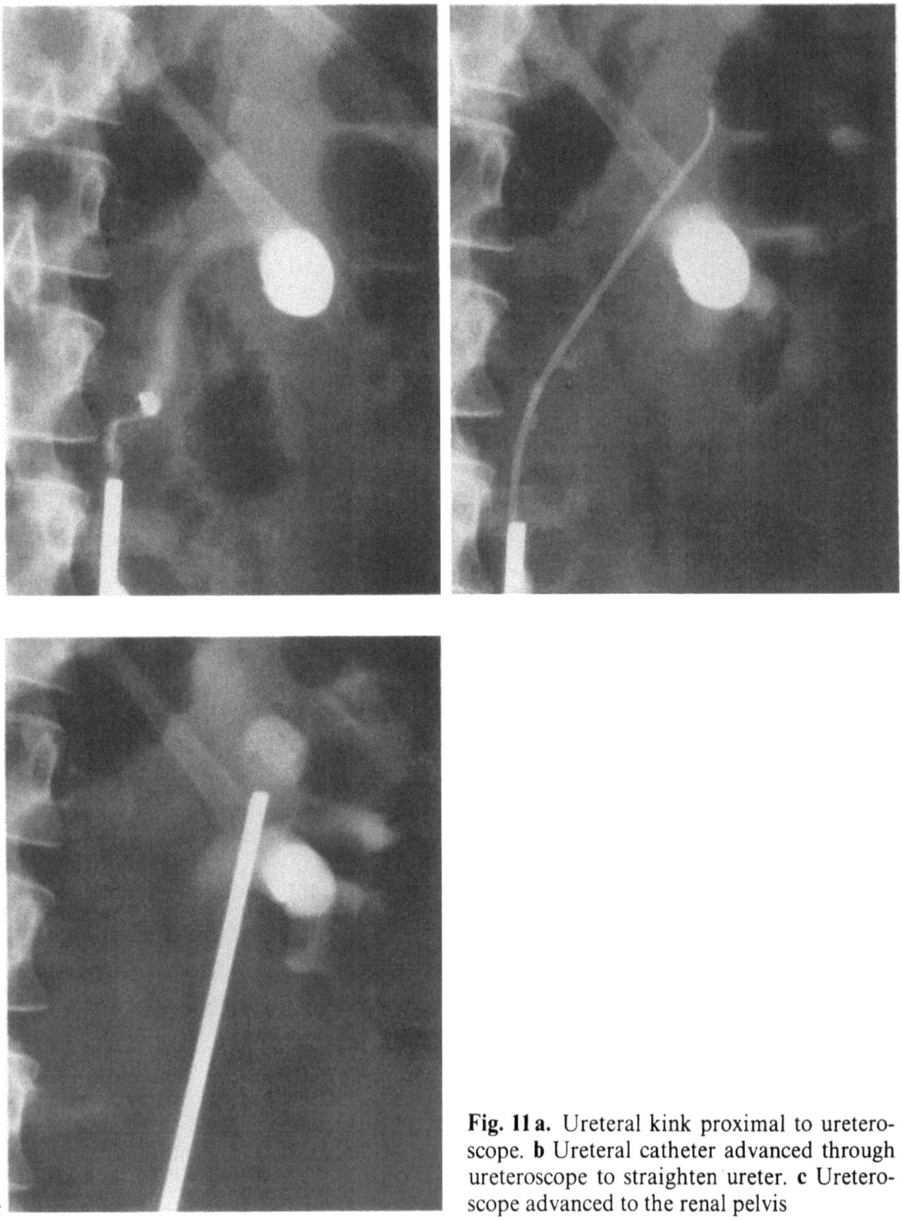

a b c

Fig. 11 a. Ureteral kink proximal to ureteroscope. **b** Ureteral catheter advanced through ureteroscope to straighten ureter. **c** Ureteroscope advanced to the renal pelvis

b) Endoscopy

Even if a continuously irrigating sheath is used, and especially with other instruments of lesser irrigating power, visibility deteriorates markedly as ancillary instruments are introduced, even in the presence of quite minor bleeding. Only rarely in cases of obstructing calculi can a forced diuresis be employed to improve visibility. In the short term improved vision results from manually injecting small volumes of saline under pressure with a syringe attached to the drainage port of the instrument. The irrigating reservoir, however, should never be raised more than 60 cm above kidney level. It is easily overlooked during long procedures that substantial quantities of irrigating fluid leak down into the bladder. As the latter becomes distended it may considerably impede free movement of the instrument. In women therefore it is as well to insert a Ch. 10 bladder catheter beside the ureterorenoscope. If the male urethra will not allow this maneuver, the instrument must intermittently be withdrawn into the bladder and irrigating fluid allowed to drain. Fitting a suction pump to the drainage port greatly accelerates with the procedure.

When the instrument is being introduced into the ureter and later during intraureteric maneuvers the pressure of the irrigating fluid may wash the calculus back up into inaccessible parts of the pelvicalyceal system. Reverse Trendelburg positioning of the patient helps to reduce the frequency with which this complication occurs. Alternatively, a ureteric balloon catheter or a Dormia basket can first be inserted past the stone so as either to block the proximal ureter or to trap the stone in the basket, however, the maneuver is not always successful with impacted stones.

c) Eliminating the Stone

Small calculi can be removed under direct vision in the basket or with forceps. Larger stones will have to be broken up within the ureter.

α) Ultrasound Litholapaxy

Despite reports of successful ultrasound litholapaxy under exclusively radiological control (Goodfriend 1973; Hufman et al. 1983), fragmentation under endoscopic vision is safer (Reuter 1984; Bichler et al. 1984) (Fig. 12a–d). The larger the probe the less problematic is simultaneous evacuation of the debris during disintegration of the stone. The overall duration of the procedure and the risk of implanting debris in the proximal urinary tract may be reduced if large fragments are dealt with by withdrawing the ultrasound drill and inserting grasping forceps. However, this usually means repeated withdrawing of the instrument into the bladder and depositing the fragments there to be voided spontaneously.

β) Electrohydraulic Litholapaxy

Little experience has so far been accumulated of electrohydraulic lithotresis for ureteric calculi (Lyon et al. 1984; Marberger 1984; Matouschek 1984). The technique differs from ultrasound litholapaxy, which may occasionally be undertaken under relatively poor viewing conditions, in that it demands first class visibility. Only then can an adequately safe distance be maintained from the telescope and ureteric perforation be avoided.

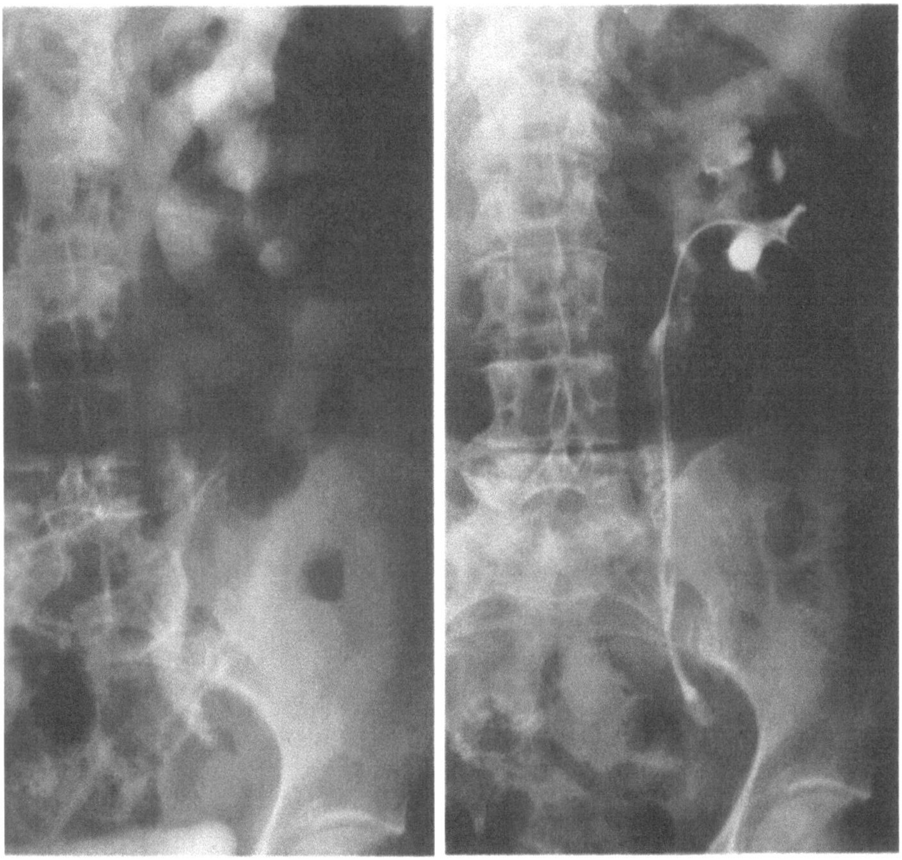

a b

Fig. 12a. Ureteral stone above the iliac vessels. **b** Emergency nephrostomy to relief obstruction

d) Aftercare

If, at the end of an intraureteric procedure, there is any doubt as to the integrity of the ureteric wall, contrast should be injected for radiologic confirmation. A Ch. 6 ureteric catheter is passed up the instrument into the upper tract and in uncomplicated cases may be removed after 24 hours. In cases of perforation the catheter should be left in situ for at least 3–4 days. In uncomplicated cases it is sufficient to demonstrate free drainage by urography after removing the catheter. If there has been a perforation the ureteric catheter may be used to inject contrast. If contrast medium flows freely past the catheter into the bladder, the ureteric catheter is removed.

e) Complications

The complications of ureterorenoscopy include acute pyelonephritis, due to extravasation of infected urine and irrigating fluid under pressure into the renal

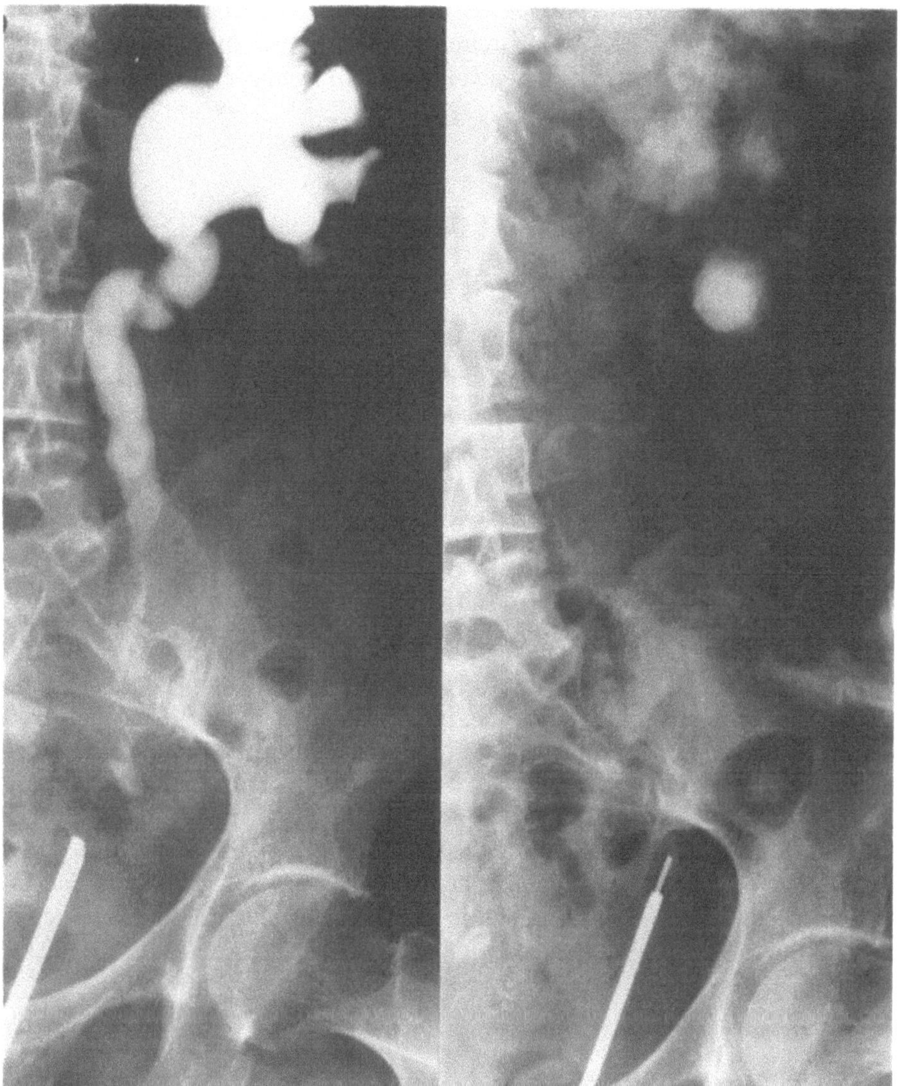

c d

Fig. 12 c. Ureteroscope in place. **d** Ureteroscope with ultrasound probe in place after complete disintegration of ureteral stone

parenchyma, and perforation of the ureter. Injudicious dilatation of the distal ureter can result in lesions eventually requiring reimplantation of the ureter. All complications can be avoided by cautious technique and by abandoning difficult procedures at an early juncture.

Ureterorenoscopic stone clearance generally takes longer than an open surgical approach. Before embarking on the procedure patients should be made aware of the complications just outlined and warned of the possibility of subsequent open surgery. Although the difficulties in dilating the ureter and removing the stone that are encountered at the first sitting may often be overcome on a second subsequent attempt (FORD et al. 1984), perforation during the first attempt prior to succesful stone removal should lead to immediate open ureterolithotomy. Patient and surgeon alike benefit from complete resolution of the problem in a single session.

f) Results

Successful ureteroscopic stone removal is achieved in between 93% – 65% of the procedures reported in the literature; the complication rate including ureteral perforation or avulsion varies between 1% and 12% (HUFMAN et al. 1983; LYON et al. 1984; MARBERGER 1984; FORD et al. 1984; MILLER et al. 1985; REUTER and REUTER 1983). The exact rate of late complications is currently not known but said to be negligible (LYON et al. 1984).

3. Antegrade Removal

Access to ureteric calculi may also be gained by percutaneous puncture of the renal collecting system, although rigid instruments generally allow only limited inspection of the ureter. Flexible instruments of a suitable diameter and length can be used to examine more remote segments of the ureter. The technique of antegrade ureteric stone extraction with loops, baskets and balloon catheters is described in the chapter on "Percutaneous Manipulation of Renal Calculi". Since the success rate of the antegrade approach as a first procedure for ureteric calculi is clearly inferior to that for the treatment of renal stones (LE ROY and SEGURA 1984; CLAYMAN and CASTANEDA-ZUNIGA 1984), some authors recommend an initial retrograde approach to carry the calculus back into the renal pelvis, whence it can be extracted percutaneously (KELLET et al. 1985; MILLER et al. 1985).

4. Shockwave Lithotripsy

In principle ureteric calculi should be just as amenable to shockwave lithotripsy as calculi in the renal pelvis. There are, however, two problems associated with this treatment. Firstly the geometrical arrangement of the treatment couch and the ellipsoid within which the waves are generated will not always allow the patient to be so positioned as to bring the stone into the sencondary focus of the shockwave. Furthermore, stones masked by the wing of the ilium or by the sacrum are fundamentally inaccessible to shockwave treatment. Such cases require prior transfer of the stone from its original level to a more cephalad position in the ureter or renal pelvis. Clinical experience has also shown that calculi impacted in the ureter are less thoroughly broken up than stones floating freely in the renal pelvis (CHAUSSY and SCHMIEDT 1984) (Fig. 13a–d). In practice

Fig. 13a. IVP in case of impacted ureteral stone. **b** Plain film before (*left*) and after (*right*) in situ shock wave lithotripsy. Incomplete disintegration

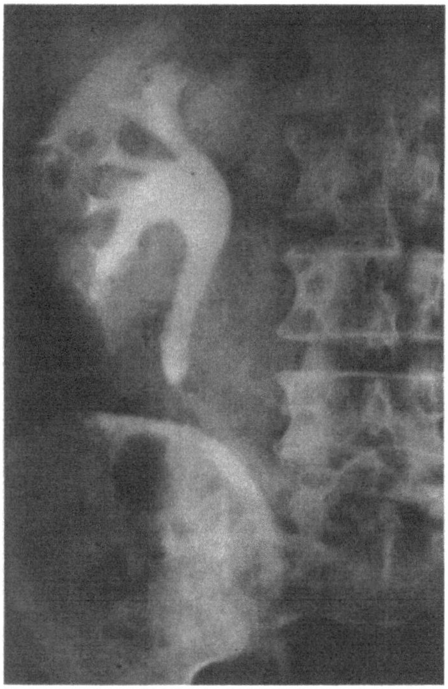

a

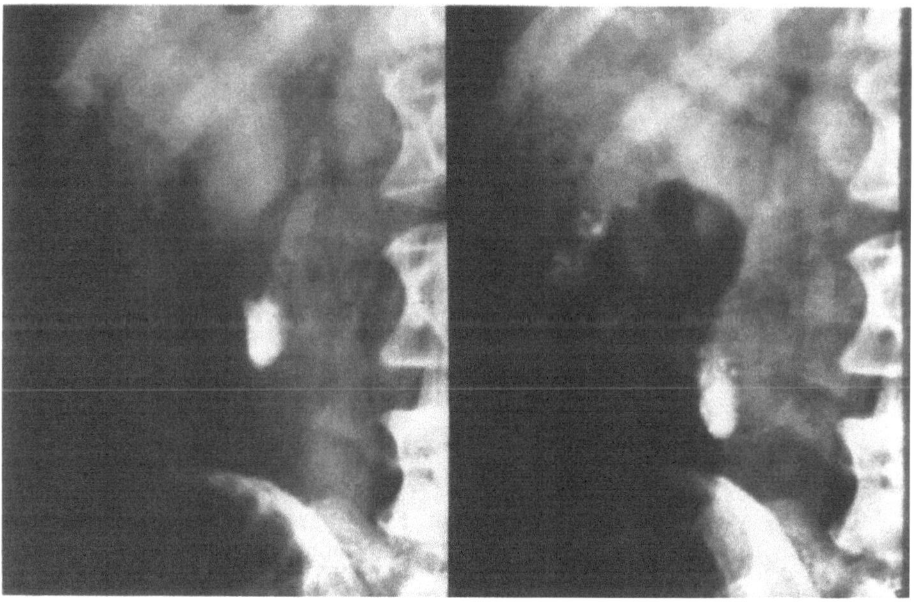

b

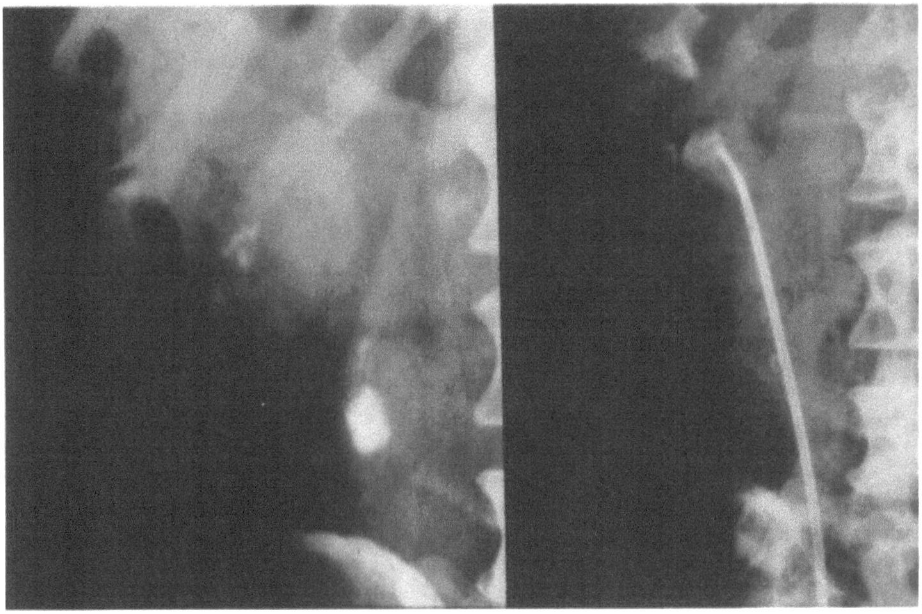

c

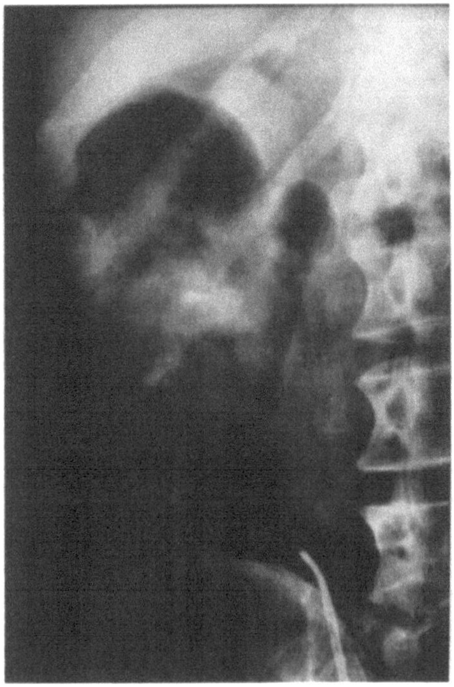

d

Fig. 13 c. Plain film before and after dislocation of ureteral stone into renal pelvis. **d** Plain film after successful shock wave disintegration

both problems are best solved by the so-called "push and smash" technique: Cystoscopy and retrograde catheterisation of the ureter enable the stones to be pushed up under X-ray guidance into the renal pelvis, where they can be shattered by shockwave lithotripsy under the same anesthetic. In the majority of cases the stone can simply be pushed up by the tip of the ureteric catheter, but if this maneuver fails a balloon catheter may be used, the balloon blocking the ureteric lumen distal to the stone and the stone being forced up into the renal pelvis by the sudden injection of a bolus of saline. Even if this procedure remains fruitless, a successful outcome may still be achieved by introducing a ureteric catheter past the stone and up into the lumen of the kidney, the stone then being attacked by shockwave lithotripsy at its original level. If the stone is shown to be well disintegrated on X-ray, the ureteric catheter may be withdrawn the following day.

5. Open Surgery

If all the treatments outlined above are available, surgical ureterolithotomy becomes a rare event (Table 3) (MILLER et al. 1985). At the time of writing there are four recognised indications for open surgical treatment of ureteric calculi:

1. In the presence of congenital or acquired anatomical abnormality of the urinary tract requiring correction in its own right there may be little point in attempting closed treatment of the stone, since the latter is likely to reform so long as the abnormality persists. Thus a distal ureteric calculus in a megaureter or in a ureterocele with a duplex system and upper tract reflux should be treated by open ureterolithotomy and reimplantation of the ureter.

2. Prior urinary diversion or reimplantation of the ureter into the bladder may render modern techniques either impossible to apply or unlikely to succeed. Following ureterocolic anastomosis the risk of sepsis rules out retrograde instrumentation. Shockwave lithotresis can also give rise to intractable problems: the debris may be inadequately cleared and result in further distal obstruction. Similar difficulties attach to urinary diversion by ileal conduit or cutaneous ureterostomy, since only in exceptional cases will these diversions allow rigid instrumentation of the ureter. Finally COHEN ureteric reimplants must be mentioned, since this operation subsequently renders even simple ureteric catheterisation a problem (LAMESCH 1981).

Table 3. Treatment of ureteral stones requiring active removal. (Dept. Urol. Johannes Gutenberg-Universität Mainz) Jan. 1984–Mar. 1985, n=401

ESWL	239	60%
Ureterorenoscopy	95	24%
Loop delivery	45	11%
Surgery	17	4%
Antegrade percutaneous removal	5	1%

3. und 4. If one of the more modern techniques has failed, or if complications ensure that prevent stone extraction in the same session, immediate recourse should be taken to open ureterolithotomy. This is undoubtedly less hazardous to the patient and less tiresome for the surgeon than a second attempt by one of the so-called non-invasive techniques. Individual cases should be managed according to the experience of the operator and the overall condition of the patient.

The choice of surgical approach will depend on the radiological level of the calculus. Stones at the level of the inferior pole may be approached in the same way as the kidney itself, i.e. by a supracostal, transcostal or infracostal 12th rib approach or by modified lumbotomy. Although these incisions are also suitable for stones in the middle third of the ureter, the latter can also be reached through a more lateral muscle splitting incision. Even lower calculi are approached by a standard paramedian approach, extended as required in either direction. The extraperitoneal plane should be adhered to whichever route is chosen, although multiple previous operations make the ureter easier to identify transperitoneally.

The ureter should be displayed and the stone removed by the so-called in situ technique, i.e. the ureter is dissected out only to the extent that allows accurate incision over the stone and proper closure of the ureter. Since escape of the stone into the inaccessible proximal ureter is one of the more tiresome complications, it is worth dissecting right around and slinging the ureter above the stone. Although some authors recommend a transverse ureterotomy because of its lower postoperative leakage rate (GIL-VERNET 1974), most authors employ the more avascular longitudinal technique. It is not strictly necessary to hold the ureteric wall on stay sutures. The stone is carefully wrinkled out with hooks and blunt probes and the distal and proximal ureter sounded in every case, irrigating to remove miniscule calculi not seen on X-ray. By the same technique the patency of the distal ureter can be established beyond doubt. If there is marked inflammatory change at the level of the stone it may be worth leaving an intraluminal splint between renal pelvis and bladder. The ureterotomy is then closed by coapting the margins with absorbable sutures. A watertight closure is not needed, but every ureterotomy should be drained. If the stone should escape during the procedure into the proximal ureter, a fibreoptic endoscope is introduced through the ureterotomy and the stone extracted. If the instrument is not available, intraoperative radiology will reveal the new site of the calculus and the merits of extending the incision or repositioning the patient for a new approach must then be considered.

Because of the detailed dissection required behind the bladder some authors prefer transvesical (BARMEHOUS et al. 1983) or transvaginal (SHAW 1936) ureterotomy for low supravesical or intramural stones. Certainly the latter procedure is undertaken extremely rarely, but in the hands of an expert may offer advantages of perioperative morbidity for the treatment of supravesical stones.

References

Andren-Sandberg A, Isacson S, Silferskiöld I (1980) Intravenous pyelography versus radioisotope renography combined with plain roentgenography of the urinary tract in the follow-up of patients with ureteral calculi. Scand J Urol Nephrol 14:57–59

Bandhauer K (1970) Therapie des Uretersteines. Akt Urol 1:42–47

Barnehous DH, Marshall M, Price SE (1983) Ureterolithotomy for juxtavesicular stone. J Urol 129:944–945

Bichler K-H, Erdmann D, Schmitz-Moormann P, Halim S (1984) Operatives Ureterorenoskop für Ultraschallanwendung und Steinextraktion. Urologe [Ausg A] 23:95–104

Borgmann V, Nagel R (1981) Indikation und Komplikation der Behandlung von Harnleitersteinen mit der Zeiss'schen Schlinge. Therapiewoche 31:3740–3744

Bowers L (1973) Loop catheter delivery of ureteral calculi. J Urol 110:178–180

Bush IM, Guinan P, Lanners J (1982) Ureterorenoscopy. Urol Clin North Am 9:131–136

Butler MR, O'Flynn JD (1973) Management of ureteric calculi – a review of 500 cases. J Irish Med Assoc 66:1–4

Chaussy CH, Schmiedt E (1984) Extracorporeal shock wave lithotripsy (ESWL) for kidney stones. An alternative to surgery. Urol Radiol 6:80–87

Clayman RV, Castaneda-Zuniga W (1984) Nephrolithotomy: Percutaneous removal of renal calculi. Urol Radiol 6:95–112

Constantian HM (1974) Management of ureteral calculi. Series of 574 cases with special emphasis on use of Davis loop extractor. J Urol 112:33–35

Council WA (1945) The treatment of ureteral calculi. J Urol 53:534–538

Das S (1981) Transurethral ureteroscopy and stone manipulation under direct vision. J Urol 125:112–113

Davis TA (1954) Removal of ureteral calculus by a new catheter type extractor. J Urol 72:346–349

Davis TA (1961) Progress report on the Thomas A. Davis stone extractor. J Urol 85:502–505

Dormia E (1982) Dormia basket: standard technique, observations, and general concepts. Urology 20:437

Dourmashkin RL (1945) Cystoscopic treatment of stones in the ureter with special reference to large calculi based on a study of 1550 cases. J Urol 54:245–283

Drach GW (1978) Stone manipulation. Urology 7:286–289

Fabiano A (1970) Die elektrische Lithotripsie von Steinen der Harnwege unter besonderer Berücksichtigung der transvesikalen Uretersteinzertrümmerung. Endoscopy 2:157

Ford TF, Payne SR, Wickham JEA (1984) The impact of transurethral ureteroscopy in the management of ureteric calculi. Br J Urol 56:602–603

Fox M, Pyrah LN, Raper FP (1965) Management of ureteric stone: a review of 292 cases. Br J Urol 37:660–670

Furlow WL, Bucchiere JJ (1976) The surgical fate of ureteral calculi: review of Mayo Clinic experience. J Urol 116:559–561

Gellißen H, Reuter H (1974) Erste Erfahrungen mit der elektrohydraulischen Lithotripsie von Harnleitersteinen. Z Urol Nephrol 66:81–87

Gil-Vernet JM (1974) Transverse ureterotomy. J Urol 111:755–756

Goodfriend R (1973) Disintegration of ureteral calculi by ultrasound. Urology 1:260–263

Goodfriend R (1984) Ultrasonic and electrohydraulic lithotripsy of ureteral calculi. Urology 23:5–8

Goodman TM (1977) Ureteroscopy with pediatric cystoscope in adults. Urology 9:394

Gottstein G (1927) Nephrolithiasis. In: Lichtenberg VA, Voelcker F, Wildbolz H (eds) Handbuch der Urologie IV, II. Springer, Berlin, p 263

Harrison GSM, Davies GA, Holdsworth PJ (1983) 12 year experience using the Dormia basket for the extraction of ureteric stones. Eur Urol 9:93–96

Henry HH, Tamlin EM (1975) Ureteral calculi: review of 17 years of experience at a community hospital. J Urol 113:762–764

Holm-Nielsen A, Jørgensen T, Mogensen P, Fogh J (1981) The prognostic value of probe renography in ureteric stone obstruction. Br J Urol 53:504–507

Hufman JL, Bagley DH, Schoenberg HW, Lyon ES (1983) Transurethral removal of large ureteral and renal pelvic calculi using ureteroscopic ultrasonic lithotripsy. J Urol 130:31–34
Ipiens-Aznar A (1982) Delivery of low ureteric stones with the Zeiss indwelling probe. Br J Urol 54:223–225
Johnson FP (1937) A new method of removing ureteral calculi. J Urol 37:84–89
Karcher G (1964) Beitrag zur transurethralen Uretersteinentfernung unter besonderer Berücksichtigung eventueller Spätfolgen. Urologe [Ausg A] 3:135–138
Karcher G (1981) Entfernung von Uretersteinen mit transurethral-endoskopischen Maßnahmen unter besonderer Berücksichtigung der sogenannten „Dauerschlinge nach Zeiss". Urologe [Ausg A] 20:269–273
Kellet MJ, Wickham JEA, Payne SR (1985) Combined retrograde and antegrade manipulations for percutaneous nephrolithotomy of ureteric calculi: "Push-Pull" technique. Urology 25:391–392
Klompus WH, Owens J (1978) Semi-closed basket extraction of ureteral calculi. J Urol 119:320–321
Korth K (1984) Neue selbstdrainierende Korbschlinge zur Behandlung des Harnleitersteines. Urologe [Ausg B] 24:263–264
Lamesch AJ (1981) Retrograde catheterization of the ureter after antireflux plasty by the Cohen technique of transverse advancement. J Urol 125:73–74
Le Roy AJ, Segura JW (1984) Percutaneous ultrasonic lithotripsy. Urol Radiol 6:88–94
Lundstam S, Wihed A, Suurküla M, Lukes P, Kral JG (1983) Acute radiorenography during attacks of renal colic. J Urol 130:855–857
Lyon ES, Kyker JS, Schoenberg HW (1978) Transurethral ureteroscopy on women: a ready addition to the urological armamentarium. J Urol 119:35–36
Lyon ES, Hufmann JL, Bagley DM (1984) Ureteroscopy and ureteropyeloscopy. Urology 23:29–36
Mahon FB, Waters RF (1973) A critical review of stone manipulation: a 5 year study. J Urol 110:387–388
Marberger M (1984) Die endoskopische Behandlung des Uretersteines. Urologe [Ausg A] 23:308–316
Matouschek E (1984) The lithotrity of stones in the ureter under visual control. Eur Urol 10:60–61
Miller K, Fuchs G, Rassweiler J, Eisenberger F (1985) Treatment of ureteral stone disease: the role of ESWL and endourology. World J Urol 3:53–57
O'Flynn JD (1980) The treatment of ureteric stones. Br J Urol 52:436–438
Perez-Castro Ellendt E, Martinez Pineiro JA (1980) La ureterorenoscopia transuretral. Arch Esp Urol 33:3–18
Perez-Castro Ellendt E, Martinez Pineiro JA (1982) Ureteral and renal endoscopy. Eur Urol 8:117–120
Prince CL, Scardino PL (1960) A statistical analysis of ureteral calculi. J Urol 83:561–565
Purohit GS, Pham D, Raney AM, Bogaer JH (1980) Electrohydraulic ureterolithotripsy. Invest Urol 17:462–464
Reuter HJ (1984) Transurethrale Ultraschallithotripsie im Ureter. Akt Urol 15:28–31
Reuter HJ, Kern E (1973) Electronic lithotripsy of ureteral calculi. J Urol 110:181–183
Reuter MA, Reuter HJ (1983) Die diagnostische und operative Endoskopie von Ureter und Niere. Urologe [Ausg A] 22:103–107
Rutner AB (1983) Balloon-dilatation of lower ureter to facilitate cystoscopic extraction of large ureteral calculi. Urology 21:226–231
Rutner AB, Fucilla IS (1976) An improved helical stone basket. J Urol 116:784–785
Sandegard E (1956) Prognosis of stone in the ureter. Acta Chir Scand [Suppl] 219:1
Shaw EC (1936) Vaginal ureterolithotomy. J Urol 35:289–299
Shihata AA, Greene JE (1983) Ureteric stone extraction by a new double-balloon catheter: an experimental study. J Urol 129:616–620
Steffens L (1984) Behandlung von Harnleitersteinen mittels Schlaufenschlinge nach Steffens. Akt Urol 15:66–69

Takayasu A, Aso Y, Takagi T, Go T (1971) Clinical application of fiber-optic pyeloureteroscope. Urol Int 26:97–104
Teichmann HH (1980) Intraureterale Lithotripsie. Urologe [Ausg A] 19:231
Tsuang MT, Evans AT (1983) Ten-year experience with looped catheter manipulation of ureteral calculi. Urology 21:242–244
Ueno A, Kawamura T, Ogawa A, Takayasu H (1977) Relation of spontaneous passage of ureteral calculi to size. Urology 10:544–546
Walsh A (1974) An aggressive approach to stones in the lower ureter. Br J Urol 46:11–14
Zeiss L (1959) 20 Jahre Zeiss-Schlinge. Urban Schwarzenberg, München Berlin

Treatment of Bladder Stones

R. HAUTMANN

I. Surgical Removal of Bladder Stones

1. Historical Perspective

a) Perineal Lithotomy

Perineal lithotomy was already practiced in India and in Persia some time before the birth of Christ. Ammonius of Alexandria (200 B.C.) was first to introduce the procedure on the European scene: Celsus gives a description in his "De Re Medicina".

"Apparatus minor" was the term applied to the operation in its simpler form and was carried out with just the knife and stone forceps. Since the bladder had to be opened immediately above the prostate, the operation was only considered suitable for boys between the ages of 9 and 14. A detailed description is given in Lorenz Heister's 1710 "General System of Surgery". With the patient's legs drawn right up the operator would introduce two fingers into the rectum in an attempt to grasp the stone and draw it down onto the perineum, where it would be cut straight down onto.

"Apparatus major" was introduced around 1520 by the Italian surgeon Francis of Cremona and entailed approaching the bladder via the previously opened urethra. To this purpose a grooved sound was passed up the urethra into the bladder to serve as a guide for the introduction of knives, forceps and any other instrument which might prove necessary. In the Middle Ages this technique was practiced throughout France by the famous Colot family of lithotomists. Toward the end of the 16th century Jacques Beaulieu (1651–1714), better known as Frere Jacques, introduced lateral perineal lithotomy. This procedure was further developed by William Cheseldam (1688–1752) and involved incising the perineum two fingers' breath medial to the ischial tuberosity.

The lithotomist François Tolet, who worked in Paris at the "Charité des Hommes", was one of the last exponents of this approach. At the end of his reign the art of lithotomy, previously practiced by laymen, was to return to the hands of the medical profession (MURPHY 1971).

b) Suprapubic Lithotomy

The first suprapubic lithotomy was carried out by Pierre Franco (1500–1561). A finger in the rectum elevated the stone to above the pubis, immediately over

which it could be cut down onto if the bladder was first been artificially filled with water. He describes the advantages of this procedure in his book "Lithotomia Douglassiana":
1. Impotence and incontinence are substantially reduced
2. Fistulation is impossible
3. Blood loss is trivial

Cheseldam also used the technique with some success, but the hazards of suprapubic lithotomy (peritonitis, incisional hernia, ruptured bladder) later drove him back to the perineal approach. Suprapubic lithotomy finally became a routine procedure once anesthesia and asepsis had come of age toward the end of the 19th century.

c) Transurethral Lithotresis

Instruments for the transurethral removal of bladder stones began to be developed early in the 19th century. FRANZ VON GRUITHUISEN (1813) designed a hollow metal cylinder equipped with a copper wire snare with which the stone would be drawn up to the mouth of the tube to be tackled with a drill. However, this instrument never saw clinical usage.

Jean Civiale (1792–1867) was the first to carry out transurethral lithotresis. His instrument consisted of a straight tube through which a three-jawed spring loaded forceps, the "trilabe", could be introduced to grasp the stone. Once the stone had been caught and secured by slightly withdrawing the forceps, a drill-like insert was passed down the hollow center of the tube and rotated to break up the calculus. As a rule numerous sessions were required to completely reduce the stone, the fragments being passed during micturition. The Heurteloups lithotrite (1831) represented a considerable advance and soon displaced all other designs. The instrument consisted of two interlocking steel rods with curved ends shaped like a metal catheter. The two jaws could be slid along each other to grasp the stone. Once this was achieved, the end of one jaw would be struck with a hammer to smash the calculus.

In 1834 Francis L'Estrange of Dublin presented his "calculofractor". In place of a hammer he employed a screw which slowly and fairly firmly crushed the stone, with the added advantage that the patient no longer had to be tied down! (ELLIS 1969).

d) Litholapaxy

Litholapaxy means crushing a stone and subsequently evacuating the fragments (ELLIS 1969). This technique was pioneered by the American surgeon Henry Jacob Bigelow (1818–1890).

Both the surgeon Phillip Crampton and the anesthetist Joseph Clover had developed socalled "evacuators", vessels of glass or rubber which could be connected to a catheter via a stopcock. If a vacuum was first generated within the evacuator and the cock then opened, stone debris could be sucked out of the bladder.

Bigelow performed his first litholapaxy in 1876. He used an evacuator consisting of an elastic container in the bottom of which was a metal hood to trap stone fragments. The instrument was connected via a length of rubber tubing to a Ch. 27–31 silver tube. Litholapaxy significantly reduced the number of sessions needed to crush and evacuate a stone and there were fewer injuries to bladder and urethra from the spontaneous passage of sharp fragments. The great disadvantage of litholapaxy remained, however, in common with all other transurethral techniques, that it was essentially a blind procedure in which the operator worked without visual control. Thus less practiced surgeons in particular could never be quite confident of not injuring the bladder. Furthermore such "blind litholapaxy" was incapable of completely demolishing a stone, probably one cause for the high recurrence rate.

It was left to Maximilian Nitze's invention of the cystoscope (1877) to bring the final and decisive improvement, that of litholapaxy under direct vision. Nitze himself had in fact developed his own transurethral lithotrites, although the first viewing lithotrites to enter widespread clinical use were those of Young and Canny-Ryall. The advent of the direct viewing technique enabled correctly performed litholapaxy to become a reliable procedure with its own specific indications.

2. Indications

a) Patient Selection

From reports on large treatment series (BORGMANN et al. 1980; BUELOW and FROHMUELLER 1981; HAUTMANN et al. 1984) a mean age of 70 seems to be the norm for bladder stone patients. Less than 10% of patients are women.

About 40% are high risk cases in the eyes of the surgeon. As one might expect of this age group, cardiac, pulmonary and neurological factors are chiefly responsible and the indications for the surgical treatment of bladder calculi cannot depend on the stone alone. Subvesical obstruction, usually the prime cause of the stone and present in 80.5% (BUELOW and FROHMUELLER 1981) to 95.4% (HAUTMANN et al. 1984; BRUNDIG and SCHNEIDER 1980; JEDINY 1978) of patients, will need equally careful consideration.

Table 1 shows the frequency of various types of subvesical obstruction in the largest series published so far. The figures agree well both with the reviews previously quoted and with other publications. In order of descending frequency the causes are prostatic adenoma (59%), prostatic carcinoma (16%), bladder neck fibrosis (14%), urethral stricture (7%), neurogenic bladder (3%) and foreign bodies (2%).

b) Anesthesia

The type of anesthesia selected will depend on which precipitating disorder is to be treated in the same session. In our own series 80% of patients required

Table 1. Types of infravesical obstruction in 392 male patients on whom ultrasonic litholapaxy was performed (HAUTMANN et al. 1984)

	No.	(%)
BPH	231	(58.9)
Prostatic CA	61	(15.6)
Vesical neck stenosis	54	(13.8)
Urethral stricture	28	(7.1)
Neurogenic bladder	11	(2.8)
Foreign body	7	(1.8)
Total	392	(100.0)

Table 2. Operative procedures in addition to ultrasonic litholapaxy in 187 male patients, performed under the same anesthetic (HAUTMANN et al. 1984)

	No.	(%)
Tur-P	149	(79.7)
Internal urethrotomy	17	(9.1)
Others	21	(11.2)
Total	187	(100.0)

Table 3. Relationship between type (infrared spectroscopy), weight of calculus and operating time in 412 ultrasonic litholapaxies (HAUTMANN et al. 1984)

	No.	(%)	Av. Wt. (gms)[a]	Av. operating time (min)
Uric acid and urates	196	(47.5)	17.4	14
Struvite	62	(15.0)	21.9	19
Calcium oxalate	82	(20.0)	9.2	23
Mixed stones	72	(17.5)	11.5	21
Total	412	(100.0)	15.0	19.25

[a] Calculated

prostatic resection in addition to the destruction of their bladder stone. Approximately 10% of patients required internal urethrotomy in the first instance and a further 10% needed to be considered for a variey of other unspecified operative procedures such as circumcision. Within an overall operative strategy that embraces both elimination of the stone and abolition of the causative subvesical obstacle, 90% of patients will be suitable for regional anesthesia, with about 10% needing a general anesthetic. For around 1% instillation of local anesthetic into the urethra will suffice (BUELOW and FROHMUELLER 1980; HAUTMANN et al. 1984). The duration of operation will be determined not only by the nature of the procedure to relieve obstruction, but equally by the size and chemical composition of the stone (Table 3). 47.5% of our own patients had uric acid or urate stones. 15% had struvite calculi, in 20% most of the material was calcium oxalate and 17.5% had mixed stones. Stones had a mean mass of 15.0 g. Table 3 gives the frequency distribution for the occurrence of various chemical species of stone. This is a subject on which there is wide variation in the figures from one individual report to another (BORGMANN et al. 1980). Depending on composition, size and number of calculi, operation times in our patients varied around a mean of 19.25%. BUELOW and FROHMUELLER (1981), for example, quote almost identical operating times. To this figure for lithotomy *per se* should be added the duration of transurethral bladder neck procedures. As a rough guide the duration of this second part of the operation may be estimated at 1 minute per gram of adenoma tissue.

c) Prerequisites

At least for the transurethral approach the following general requirements must be fulfilled that apply to any transurethral procedure.

1. The urethra must be able to accept the intended instrument.
2. Adequate bladder capacity.
3. Adequate clarity of view within the bladder, i.e. adequate transparency of the bladder contents.

Various minimum volumes are worth considering as limiting bladder capacities for transurethral lithotomy: Whereas ultrasound lithotresis theoretically permits a minimum of 50 ml (shrunken fibrotic bladder) any further reduction in bladder inflation may allow the bladder wall to approach the instrument so closely as not to exceed the minimum distance of 25 mm between objective and object. In shock wave litholapaxy care should be taken to maintain a safe distance between the surface of the stone and the bladder wall. The technique is therefore contraindicated in contracted bladders!

For shock wave litholapaxy the bladder should have a minimum capacity of 150–200 ml.

d) Contraindications

In view of the diversity of operative techniques now available the contraindications are discussed individually with each of the various procedures. Compli cations are dealt with in the same fashion.

e) Conclusion

It may be stated as a general principle that the indications for removing bladder stones are manifold and that they should be interpreted liberally, never more than where a transurethral approach is envisaged. This is merely a logical extension of the trend affecting all other transurethral procedures over the past two decades (MAUERMAYER 1983). For all the same reasons a transurethral approach with simultaneous correction of precipitating obstruction should be regarded as the treatment of choice, an opinion unanimously reflected throughout the most recent world literature (BORGMANN et al. 1980; BUELOW and FROHMUELLER 1981; HAUTMANN et al. 1984).

II. Techniques of Litholapaxy

1. The Ultrasonic Lithotrite

a) Definition of Ultrasound

Sound of higher frequency than the upper limit of the human ear (16,000 to 18,000 cycles per second or 16 to 18 kHz) is called ultrasound. The frequency band usually employed in clinical practice is 26–27 kHz. The chief properties of ultrasound are largely determined by its short wavelength. This frequency range differs from the audible spectrum in the high energy density that may be achieved. Furthermore, ultrasound can be collimated to a beam comparable to a light beam. The resulting concentration of high energy densities onto a small cross-sectional area is precisely the property that permits the application of ultrasound for the destruction of bladder stones.

b) The Effect of Ultrasound on Urinary Calculi

The phenomena were investigated by MULVANEY in 1953. By 1967, TAKAHASHI and OUCHI had succeeded in constructing an instrument capable of shattering stones, but it was experimental. Clinical pioneer work at the Aachen Urology Clinic in the years 1970 to 1977 that resulted in the first production of an ultrasonic lithotrite (LUTZEYER et al. 1970). As a result of this work the following facts have been established:

1. No absolutely ultrasound resistant stones have so far been recorded.
2. Comparisons of penetration rates for stones of varying chemical composition soon revealed that organic stones such as cystine and uric acid are the easiest to reduce, followed by phosphate and carbonate calculi. Calcium oxalate is the most resistant to ultrasound.
3. The outer mantle of a stone is more easily broken up than is the inner core.
4. Small diameter probes (2.3 mm) were effective. Stones might at least theoretically be destroyed within the lumen of narrow organs such as the ureter.
5. No significant heat can be shown to be generated by the probe (TERHORST and CICHOS 1971).

By his animal studies on the effects of ultrasound on the bladder GASTEYER (1971) has also been able to exclude any possibility of thermal damage to the bladder, since there is no detectable heating of the probe tip. Even if some heat were generated it would be unlikely to be of any significance under normal irrigating conditions.

c) The Instrument

The following equipment is needed for ultrasound litholapaxy:

1. The lithotrite (Fig. 1). This consists of a commercially available cranked cystoscope with ultrasound transducer and probe.

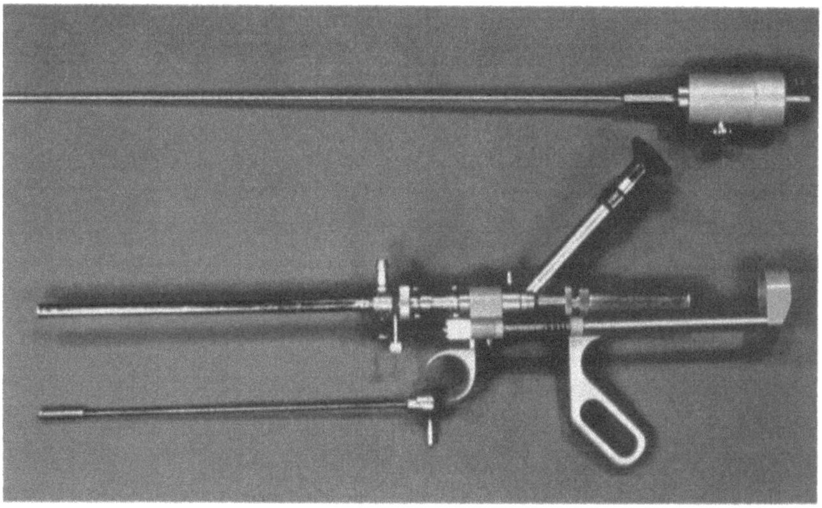

Fig. 1. Commercially available cranked cystoscope (center), ultrasound transducer and probe (*above*) and obturator (*below*)

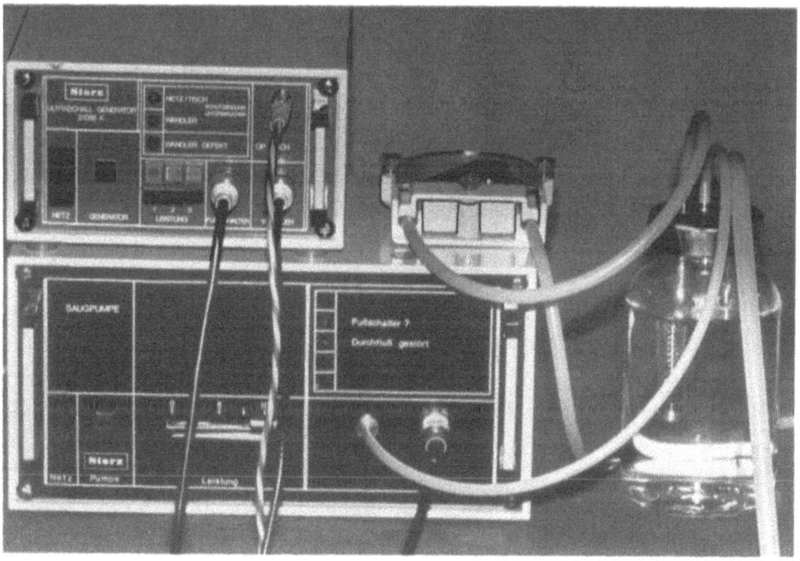

Fig. 2. Ultrasound generator (*above*) with evacuator pump (*below*) and collecting trap (*right*)

2. The ultrasound generator
3. The evacuator pump and receiver (Fig. 2).

The piezoelectric ultrasound transducer is driven at a frequency of 23 kHz and has a power output of approx. 30 W. The attached tubular probe has an outside diameter of 3.5 mm and resonates at 26.5 kHz. The external end of the probe is connected to a pump which continuously evacuates stone swarf and irrigation fluid infused via the cystoscope sheath. During the procedure the entire probe may be advanced down the cystoscope sheath to expose the drill tip and bring it into contact with the stone.

A variety of instruments based on the ultrasound principle have been in use for several years and with varying success.

According to FLACHENECKER and GMINDER (1982) the differences in effectiveness between individual commercially available instruments depends on the quality of force transmission from ultrasonic hammer tip to stone. Probably resonant frequency drift in the ultrasonic resonator results in mismatch between high frequency generator and transducer. The drift in turn would be produced by changes in load and temperature during the procedure as well as by variations in the properties of the metal shaft. These problems have led FLACHENECKER and GMINDER (1982) to introduce a new type of high frequency generator equipped with a frequency scanner which automatically selects the optimum operating frequency. At the beginning of every operating cycle a frequency band around 27 kHz is swept and the frequency for optimum coupling of generator and transducer locked on too.

Stones are broken up under direct vision and the instrument controlled by a foot switch, affording independent or coupled control of ultrasound drill and evacuator pump. A bayonet lock allows the removal of telescope and transducer from the sheath, the latter being introduced with an obturator in the usual fashion.

The probe itself only comes into contact with the calculus via an interposed hammer tip having slight axial play and equipped with a crown of slightly inward pointing teeth. The function of the teeth is to increase the local pressure at the point of contact between stone and drill and thus to ensure the production of fine, easily evacuated swarf. Evacuated material collects in a separate receiver, whence it is available for analysis.

d) The Technique of Ultrasound Litholapaxy

The sheath is introduced either blind with an obturator or under direct vision. Initial full cystoscopy provides spatial orientation, allowing calculi to be located and diverticula to be detected. The drill and its transducer are now inserted and the evacuator switched on. Although the irrigation inlet is under manual control, drainage is provided by the evacuator pump and will operate every time the transducer pedal is partly depressed. With this automatic continuous irrigation and evacuation in progress the hammer tip is now brought into contact with the smoothest available surface of the stone. The calculus is sucked against the end of the sheath and may thus be maneuvered against the bladder wall. The operating pedal is now depressed further to energise the transducer.

At first the stone may rotate around the tip of the probe. The appearance of clouds of debris despite proper function of the evacuator is a sure sign that the stone is beginning to break up. Whenever possible, pieces should by this process be chipped from the periphery of the stone rather than attacking its center. Although the drilling of holes straight into the center is impressive for operator

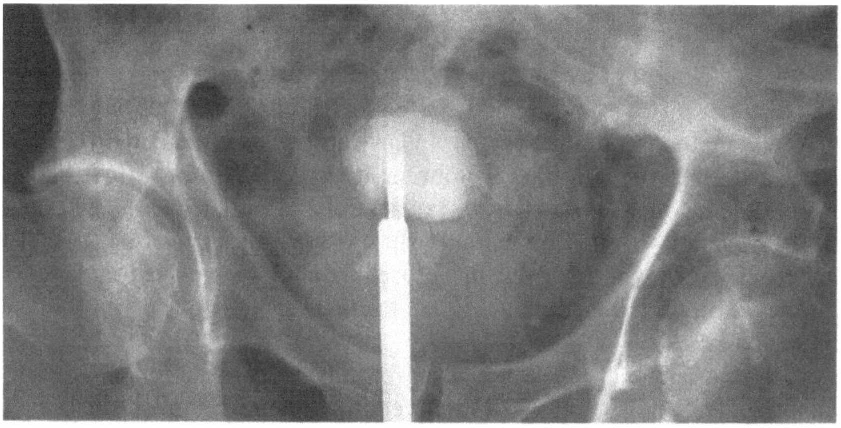

Fig. 3. Pelvic X-ray of a 62 year old patient. The ultrasound probe has been advanced up to a stone. In the course of the procedure contact with the calculus is maintained by progressively extending the drill out of the sheath

and spectator alike and is fairly unlikely to lead to the drill actually seizing, continuous irrigation and evacuation will soon cease, with the possible consequence of overheating and damage to the transducer (Fig. 3).

If a central attack is nevertheless decided on, the calculus frequently breaks into several fragments before one or more drill holes have been made to any depth. The individual fragments may then be broken up and evacuated in succession. When small fragments are being drilled and evacuated they may tend to fly off sideways away from the drill tip. Operation of the evacuator pump alone easily clears these particles from the base of the bladder.

Indeed the procedure can be considerably curtailed if telescope and ultrasound unit are from time to time withdrawn from the sheath and an Ellik evacuator or bladder syrinage is used to wash out the bladder. Use of a Ch. 23.5 sheath allows surprisingly large chunks of stone to be evacuated, thus avoiding the time-consuming process of drilling them down to sand-grain size.

Ultrasound energy seems not to inflict any injury on the bladder wall. Nevertheless contact between the probe or its hammer tip and the bladder wall should be avoided, to minimize petechial hemorrhage and edema. At the end of litholapaxy the entire bladder is carefully inspected for residual fragments and copiously washed out. Large stone fragments have a way of coming to rest behind trabeculae, in diverticula or under a large median lobe, and it is this material that is apt to cause recurrences, particularly where bladder neck obstruction has not been relieved and incomplete emptying persists.

We always catheterize the bladder for at least 24 hours postoperatively. If there has been a subsequent TUR of the prostate this question is in any case obviated. In particular, a catheter should always be left in situ wherever there is an untreated disorder of bladder emptying or marked hematuria (LUTZEYER et al. 1972).

e) Technical Reliability of the Lithotrite

In the first clinical procedures (LUTZEYER et al. 1970; THIEL and RATHERT 1977) the hammer probe snapped and fell into the bladder. Once this had been traced to faulty material it did not reoccur in any subsequent operation. In the event of such a mishap the end of the probe or its hammer tip must first be located within the bladder cavity under X-ray control and can then easily be evacuated with the pump. If only the hammer tip has separated and if only small fragments remain to be removed the procedure may be finished with the same probe. Extra care should, however, be taken to avoid contact with the bladder mucosa (THIEL 1977).

Table 4 lists our experience using prototypes over the past 10 years. The high incidence (34% and 17% repectively) of technical problems with the first two series of a hundred cases were generally in line with expectation. Whilst these difficulties could only be moderately reduced with the first prototpye, our experience over the last few years with a second prototype has been excellent. Technical failures have occurred in less than 1% of procedures (HAUTMANN et al. 1982).

f) The Complications of Ultrasonic Litholapaxy

One complication which may occur is diffuse hemorrhage, especially where the bladder mucosa had already been damaged preoperatively by inflammatory processes or rough calculi. In our experience the problem tends to settle after 1–2 days. The exact complications due to ultrasonic litholapaxy itself are hard to determine, since, as already mentioned in section 2a above, the procedure is nearly always coupled with some other operation carrying a higher complication rate of its own. For this reason Table 5 lists only those operative compli-

Table 4. Incidence of apparatus failure (needing help from the engineer) in 412 ultrasonic litholapaxies (HAUTMANN et al. 1984)

No. of procedures 1971–1981	Engineer and/or technician aside	Failure rate (%)[a]
1st Prototype		
1–100	Yes	34
101–200	No	22
2nd Prototype		
201–300	Yes	17
301–412	No	1

[a] Help of engineer necessary

Table 5. Intraoperative complications in 412 ultrasonic litholapaxies (HAUTMANN et al. 1984)

	No.	(%)
Bladder perforation		
Intraperitoneal	2[a]	(0.5)
Extraperitoneal	2	(0.5)
(no surgical revision)		
Bleeding	1	(0.25)
Coagulation and transfusion necessary		
Total	5	(1.25)

[a] Contract bladder (65 cc, 80 cc), Prototype of sheath, Bladder tumor

cations directly related to ultrasound litholapaxy per se. Although on theoretical grounds perforation of the bladder is never expected (and should never occur), we have nevertheless had two cases. In both of them it was not the ultrasound energy input but the nature of the territory (contracted bladder, carcinoma) and the use of a preproduction prototype sheath designed to grip the stone which led to this mishap. Only one of our 412 patients suffered hematuria to an extent requiring cystoscopy and blood transfusion.

Unanesthetized patients occasionally complain of pain if ultrasound is applied to the bladder mucosa for a period of time. Pain may also occur if the drill tip seizes in the stone and proper irrigation cannot be maintained (which should not be allowed to occur) (THIEL 1977). Postoperative cardiovascular or pulmonary emergencies have been excluded from Table 5, since they represent only indirect complications of the operation itself: indeed they are more probably due to the concomitant transurethral resection of the prostate than to ultrasonic litholapaxy.

g) Conclusion

Our ten year experience with a vast number of patients has led us to regard ultrasound litholapaxy as the treatment of choice. The procedure has the following signal advantages:

1. All the anesthetic and cardiovascular hazards of open operation are avoided.
2. The stone is broken up progressively and under direct visual control.
3. Simultaneous evacuation of debris obviates time consuming irrigations.
4. The ultrasound insert slides within the sheath, thus facilitating detection and destruction of calculi.
5. The patient is not imperilled by any risk to the bladder wall.
6. Any type of stone may be broken up, particularly small calculi close to the wall or within diverticula.
7. The patient spends a considerably shorter time in hospital.
8. Ultrasonic litholapaxy is technically undemanding, although a knowledge of the basic principle of transurethral surgery remains *de rigeur* (THIEL and RATHERT 1977).

2. Electrohydraulic Litholapaxy

When, in 1950, L.A. Jutkind developed his Urat I apparatus in the Soviet Union it became possible for the first time to shatter bladder stones by electrohydraulic shock waves.

a) Definition of Electrohydraulic Shockwaves

The heat suddenly liberated by an underwater electric spark discharge results in rapid vaporisation of water around the tip of the probe. The resulting sudden evolution of a gas phase leads to a substantial density gradient and socalled "hydraulic shockwaves". The waves in turn are a sum of fundamental frequency and numerous harmonics of varying amplitude. If one component of the shockwave corresponds to the resonant frequency of the calculus, the latter will burst or break up (ROUVALIS 1970).

b) Principle of the Operation

A series of hydraulic shocks are thus required to break up bladder calculi. The fragments are then evacuated with a bladder syringe or Ellik evacuator attached to the sheath. Careful attention to correct procedure will protect the bladder mucosa from the direct effects of electrohydraulic discharge (RANEY 1976; REUTER 1969, 1970; ROUVALIS 1970; TESSLER and KOSSOW 1975; BUELOW and FROHMUELLER 1981; BORGMANN et al. 1980).

c) Instrumentation

The power unit consists of a pulse generator to provide electrical discharges of variable frequency and power.

The lithotrite, a Ch. 10 probe, is introduced transurethrally via a standard cystoscope. The probe has a central and an encasing cylindrical electrode, the discharge passing between the two at the tip of the probe.

A Ch. 23.5 operating cystoscope is generally used to pass the lithotrite probe.

d) Technique of Electrohydraulic Lithotresis

General or spinal and epidural anesthesia is just as suitable for electrohydraulic as for ultrasound litholapaxy. In occasional cases local urethral anesthesia may even be adequate.

The patient should be prepared as for transurethral resection of the prostate and is placed in lithotomy position. The bladder is first inspected via the Ch 23.5 cystoscope.

The lithotrite probe is now advanced up to the stone. An optimal effect is achieved if the probe lies perpendicularly in contact with the surface of the stone. Stones are operated on under direct vision, as in ultrasound litholapaxy. To test the hardness of the stone one or two short burst of test discharges are fired, maximally one second in duration and at least 10 seconds apart. Ajustments may then be made to the power output of the instrument. Depending on bladder capacity it is essential to ensure a filling of at least 150–200 ml fluid.

Lithotresis is easiest for stones with a rough surface and haredst where the surface is smooth. The explanation is that a smooth surface tends to reflect hydraulic pressure waves and reduce their effectiveness (ALBRECHT et al. 1972; RANEY 1975; ROUVALIS 1970; BORGMANN et al. 1980; JEDINY 1978).

e) Reliability

In the literature reports on large series accord the method a reasonable to high degree of reliability, at least in the technical sense (BORGMANN et al. 1980; BUELOW and FROHMUELLER 1981; BATON et al. 1972; ROUVALIS 1970; BRUNDIG and SCHNEIDER 1982; KIERFELD 1969; JEDINY 1978). Reports on smaller series, by way of contrast, suggest a far worse track record (PELANDER and KAUFMANN 1980). In this respect there is little to choose between electrohydraulic and ultrasound litholapaxy: in both cases the success rate would appear to depend chiefly on a degree of experience on the part of the operator which can only be gained by performing the procedure a number of times.

Precautions and Hazards

The hazards of electrohydraulic lithotresis are easily avoided by adopting appropriate precautions! Electrical safety procedures should be strictly adhered to, i.e. both instrument and operating table must be properly grounded. Any hint of instrument malfunction should lead to the procedure immediately being abandoned. The objective of the telescope should never be allowed to come too close to the tip of the probe, since it may otherwise loosen or crack.

The dangers cannot be overemphasized of allowing the probe to touch the bladder wall. At the beginning of the operation there is no doubt little risk of this mishap, but as the stone fragments become smaller it occurs more easily (MAUERMAYER 1983).

f) Complications

The majority of users of electrohydraulic litholapaxy report sporadic moderate to severe postoperative macroscopic hematuria analogous to that occuring in the ultrasonic technique and due to mucosal damage. Furthermore most authors agree that urate-phosphate and carbonate calculi are easy to shatter whilst oxalate and urate stones are far harder, chiefly because they have a smooth surface.

g) Contraindications

Because of the danger of perforation, the presence of ulceration in the bladder mucosa represents a contraindication to electrohydraulic lithotresis. Attention must be drawn at this point to a number of animal studies, principally those of TIDD (1976). Fortunately the corresponding clinical hazards seems not to occur.

Narrow-necked diverticula containing stones also present a contraindication to electrohydraulic litholapaxy. Generally speaking these stones cannot be completely broken up under direct vision (BORGMANN et al. 1980).

Coexistant urethral stricture should first be treated by internal urethrotomy to provide adequate access to the bladder. Adenomata with large intravesical extension will tend to obscure the view into the retroprostatic recess. Like ultrasound, electrohydraulic litholapaxy should nevertheless be undertaken to destroy the calculus *prior* to any bladder neck correction.

Intrarenal vesicoureteric reflux with urinary tract infection represents a relative contraindication to electrohydraulic stone therapy (Borgmann et al. 1980).

h) Conclusion

The experience of a number of authors over large clinical series has allowed correctly applied Urat I litholapaxy to become established as a low risk technique of stone therapy. By analogy to ultrasound litholapaxy the technique may be combined with transurethral treatment of subvesical obstruction in a single sitting. As the underlying physical principles would lead one to expect, a potential for damage to the bladder wall and subjacent gut has been demonstrated in suitable animal experiments. In clinical practice, however, this serious complication is so rare (Buelow and Frohmueller 1980; Alfthan and Murtomaa 1972) as to virtually never occur (Angeloff 1972; Mitchell 1977; Raney 1975, 1976; Tessler 1975; Borgmann et al. 1980). The group of Pelander and Kaufmann (1980) stand alone in presenting poor results.

Borgmann et al. (1980) have summarized the *advantages* of electrohydraulic lithotresis as follows:

1. Open surgery and its attendant hazards are avoided.
2. Stones are broken up progressively and under direct vision.
3. The Urat probe may be slid back and forth within the cystoscope sheath, thus facilitating the detection and breaking up of stones.
4. Any type of stone may be destroyed, especially small stones lying close to the bladder wall.
5. No serious harmful effects have been reported, in particular no problems of excessive heating.

The same authors cite as a disadvantage of the Urat I instrument the lack of any available pediatric equipment. The problem lies in the thickness (Ch. 10) of the probe with its requirement for a large sheath (Ch. 23.5).

Jediny (1978) has reported otherwise. In the years 1960 to 1977 his Kiev group operated on 2000 bladder stone patients, among them 17 children, of whom albeit 16 were girls aged 2–6 and one a boy aged 14. All the calculi were solitary and had a maximum diameter of 30 mm. In all the children electrohydraulic cystolithotresis was performed under general anesthesia. The Ch. 24 panendoscope, which is the standard instrument in Kiev, could of course only be used in the girls, on whom urethral dilatation to Ch. 24 was first performed. The boy was operated on with a pediatric instrument.

Finally, electrohydraulic lithotresis becomes impossible where the stone is of such a size as to prevent the normal safety clearance being maintained between the surface of the stone and the bladder wall. Thus a shrivelled bladder represents a contraindication.

Although the theoretical dangers of electrohydraulic shockwaves are greater than those of ultrasound, the two techniques are, in clinical practice, quite comparable.

3. Microexplosion Cystolithotresis

This technique has been under development since 1977 by the group of WATANABE et al. in Japan and of XUI et al. in China. The basic principle entails producing a simple explosion, the shockwaves from which are ultimately responsible for the disintegration of the stone, just as they are in electrohydraulic litholapaxy.

a) Definition and Physical Principles of Microexplosion Cystolithotresis

Any explosive intended to destroy stones within the body must on the one hand be of adequate power to keep the quantities small and on the other not so sensitive as to be detonated by simple maneuvers.

The workers just mentioned chose lead azide, which detonates at 350 °C liberating 0.35 calories per milligram weight. The reaction follows the formula:

$$Pb(N_3)_2 = Pb + 3\,N_2 + 108\ \text{Kcal}$$

This explosive power is of the same order of magnitude as in industrial explosives, e.g. dynamite. Spontaneous ignition does not occur at normal temperatures.

Once again the physical energy required for lithotresis is provided in the form of a shockwave. Surrounding tissue damage is thus not due to the detonation itself but to the expansion of any gas bubbles generated and to flying stone fragments. It is therefore essential that air is never allowed to surround the stone, since there would otherwise be rapid energy transfer across the gas/solid tissue interface. For a detailed description of shockwave behavior the reader is referred to the whole extracorporeal lithotresis literature (KONDO 1981; XUI et al. 1981; WATANABE et al. 1977a, b, 1978, 1983).

b) Experimental Studies

WATANABE and his colleagues were able to produce satisfactory lithotresis both of artificial and of natural human and animal stones in animal experimental systems. High speed photography was able to demonstrate underlying physical processes analogous to those observed for extracorporeal shockwave apparatus. A stone of 10 mm diameter for example requires 2 mg explosive charge and a 20 mm one 5 mg lead azide.

Particular attention focussed on the surrounding tissue, i.e. the bladder. Minimum safety clearances emerged of 5 mm in gel and 7.5 mm in water. Once again, it could be shown that the shock-wave passes through water and tissue without causing damage until encountering material of more solid consistency, where the wavefront breaks up.

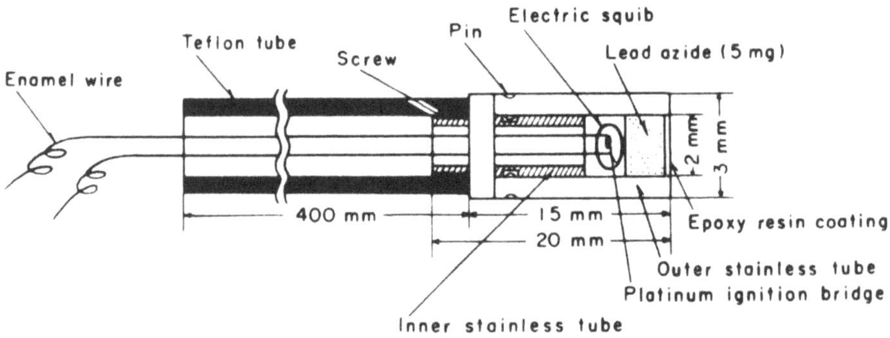

Fig. 4. Explosive catheter, reprinted with kind permission of WATANABE et al. (1980)

c) Instrumentation

2 to 10 mg of lead azide are loaded into one end of a cylindrical explosion chamber made of stainless steel 3 mm in diameter and up to 20 mm long. The opposite end contains a platinum ignition gap. The entire chamber is fitted into a flexible polyurethane sheath which thus acts as a detonator catheter (Fig. 4). The lead azide charge is ignited by connecting a 3 Volt battery across the platinum electrodes.

The lithotrite consists of a specially designed cystoscope fitted at its end with a forceps in which the stone can be gripped and withdrawn toward the outlet of the bladder. The bladder is filled with at least 200 ml water to ensure the calculus is completely surrounded with fluid. The detonator catheter is now introduced and automatically comes to point at the center of the stone. Since 1981 WATANABE has treated three and XUI over twenty patients by this technique under general anesthesia. All the stones concerned, some of them quite sizeable, disintegrated 2–6 detonations being needed per stone. The authors concede that large stones had first had drill holes made in them with the ultrasound lithotrite to facilitate detonation. The stone fragments are subsequently broken up with a conventional viewing lithotrite (e.g. Young's punch) and washed from the bladder by Ellik evacuator or bladder syringe.

d) Clinical Experience and Complications

Of the twenty-three cases (3 WATANABE, 20 XUI) reported to date, none were noted to suffer a lesion of the bladder wall or significant hematuria.

e) Conclusion

At first sight this technique seems more than a little adventurous. Nevertheless, the underlying energy transfer is no different to that occurring in extracorporeal lithotresis, except it is generated by true explosion rather than by electrical discharge. In view of the already substantial number of techniques available for litholapaxy, the procedure is likely to remain a curiosity. The practicability of applications involving the ureter and upper urinary tract, as proposed by WATANABE (1983), remains to be seen. Whilst the surrounding bony pelvis renders extracorporeal lithotresis impossible in the bladder local internally generated shockwaves are still effective. The supreme advantage of the extracorporeal technique, i.e. its lack of invasiveness, is, however, lost. The principal disadvantage of microexplosion cystolithotresis is indeed its invasive nature.

4. Viewing Litholapaxy

The limitations of viewing litholapaxy are fully appreciated by anyone who has crushed a number of stones under direct vision. Most viewing lithotrites have the disadvantage in common that even a slight quantity of blood in the urine or irrigating fluid impedes orientation within the bladder. Irrigating arrangements are either absent or inadequate.

Two basic types of viewing lithotrite are available:

1. Instruments using the principle of longitudinal coaxial sliding of one element on another. These lithotrites follow the design of blind instruments, whose jaws slide axially, a construction having the advantage of great mechanical rigidity but the disadvantage of providing the worst possible view, frequently only one jaw being in the field of view at a time. Thus it is often difficult or even impossible to get hold of a calculus with instruments of this type. Figure 6b shows plainly why lithotrites of this design are so strong: in the example shown this feature is accentuated by the provision of a closing screw which will crush the hardest of stones.

2. Lithotrites having coaxially rotating elements. Each of two tubes ends in a jaw and rotation of the tubes on one another opens and closes the forceps. This group of instruments, based on the Lichtenberg-Heywalt lithotrite, has the advantage of always keeping both jaws within the operator's field of view, thus considerably simplifying the gripping and crushing of stones. The price to be paid is that of limited mechanical strength. Large stones are either difficult or impossible to deal with. The "ideal calculus" for this instrument should be less than 1.5–2 cm in diameter (MAUERMAYER and HARTUNG 1976) (Fig. 5).

In 1976 MAUERMAYER and HARTUNG had the idea of combining the longitudinal slide principle of the instruments listed under paragraph 1. with the virtues of the resectoscope. The well known failure of viewing lithotrites to provide adequate irrigation and maintain visibility in the presence of any significant bleeding is thus corrected by incorporating precisely the design features of the resectoscope that allow a clear view even where hemorrhage is brisk. The direct viewing instrument described by MAUERMAYER and HARTUNG (1976) as the "punch lithotrite" has the following convincing advantages:

1. The instrument is of only Ch. 24 circumference.
2. Despite this the jaws are 5 mm deep and open to a total of 15 mm.

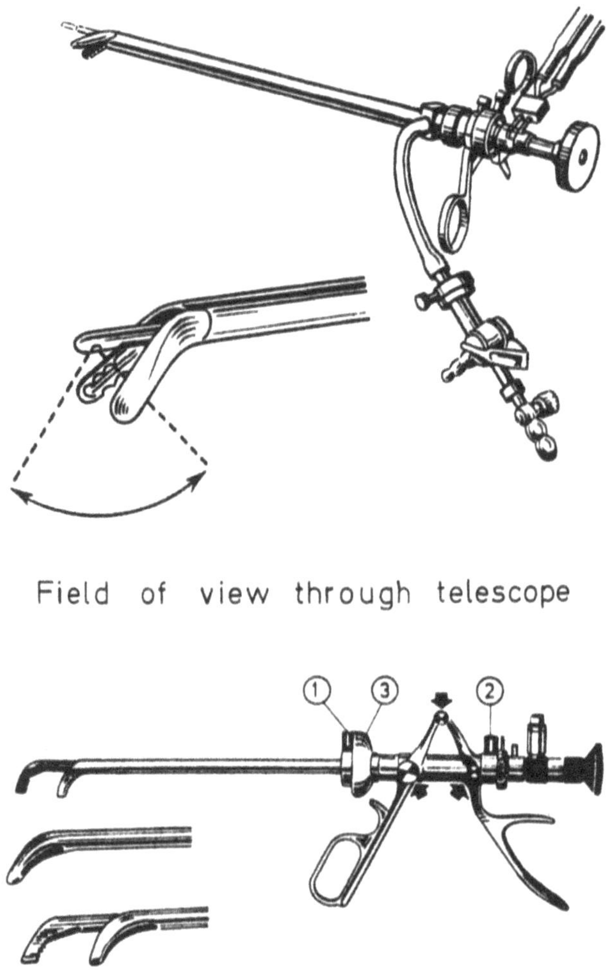

Fig. 5. *Above:* Young pattern lithotrite by LICHTENBERG-HEYWALT. In this type of instrument the stone is continuously held in the field of view. The instrument is, however, of limited mechanical strength (MAUERMAYER 1975). *Below:* Instrument of coaxial sliding pattern. These much more robust instruments have the disadvantage that the stone is only in view when the jaws are in certain positions (MAUERMAYER 1975)

3. The instrument is of rigid mechanical construction. The mechanical advantage of the operating grip and the construction of the jaws are such that extremely hard concretions may be broken up.
4. The irrigating system is that used in resectoscopes and therefore maintains a clear field even in the presence of heavy bleeding.
5. The Urat I apparatus may be used without a change of sheath. Larger calculi can therefore be broken up initially by electrohydraulic means and then further reduced to evacuatable size with the punch.
6. Stones can be picked up from within small diverticula or pseudodiverticula, since only a small part of the instrument is a hazard to the bladder mucosa.

7. By using a shrouded obturator of the LEUSCH pattern the instrument may be passed blind: the sharp edge of the sheath end is then covered and unable to traumatize the urethral mucosa.
8. Where necessary, e.g. where the urethral lumen is such that preliminary internal urethrotomy is needed, the instrument may be handled just like a resectoscope with 0° telescope and be passed under direct vision.
9. The maker has fully integrated this instrument into a modular program so it can be used in combination with the complete range of diagnostic telescopes, with coagulating electrodes or with biopsy forceps.
10. Stone debris can be evacuated with or without direct vision. In the latter case the entire lumen of the instrument is available for the removal of larger fragments.
11. Ease and simplicity of dismantling have been carefully designed into this instrument. It is convenient to clean and is suitable for ethylene oxide or autoclave sterilization.

Components of the Instrument (Fig. 6)

1. Sheath obturator after B. LEUSCH
2. Stone punch sheath (Ch. 24)
3. Punch insert with jaws
4. 0° operating telescope
5. Direct viewing telescope
6. Bridge for passing Urat I electrode
7. Insert for 0° telescope for instrumentation under vision
8. Bladder syringe for evacuating stone debris

Operating Technique (MAUERMAYER and HARTUNG 1976)

1. Passing the instrument:

The Ch. 24 sheath may be passed either blind like any resectoscope or, equally, under vision through a 0° telescope insert.

2. Litholapaxy:

α) Pure Punch Litholapaxy

Stones up to just over cherry size are ideally gripped and crushed between the jaws of the punch. Stone fragments corresponding to the insert lumen may at this stage either be left in the bladder or extracted by removing the inner part of the forceps. By this technique even very hard calculi are rapidly dealt with, since the instrument has the irrigating power of a conventional resectoscope. Once all calculous material has been broken up by punch the debris may be removed using the evacuator pump. Residual pieces may be removed by sliding the operating insert out of the sheath.

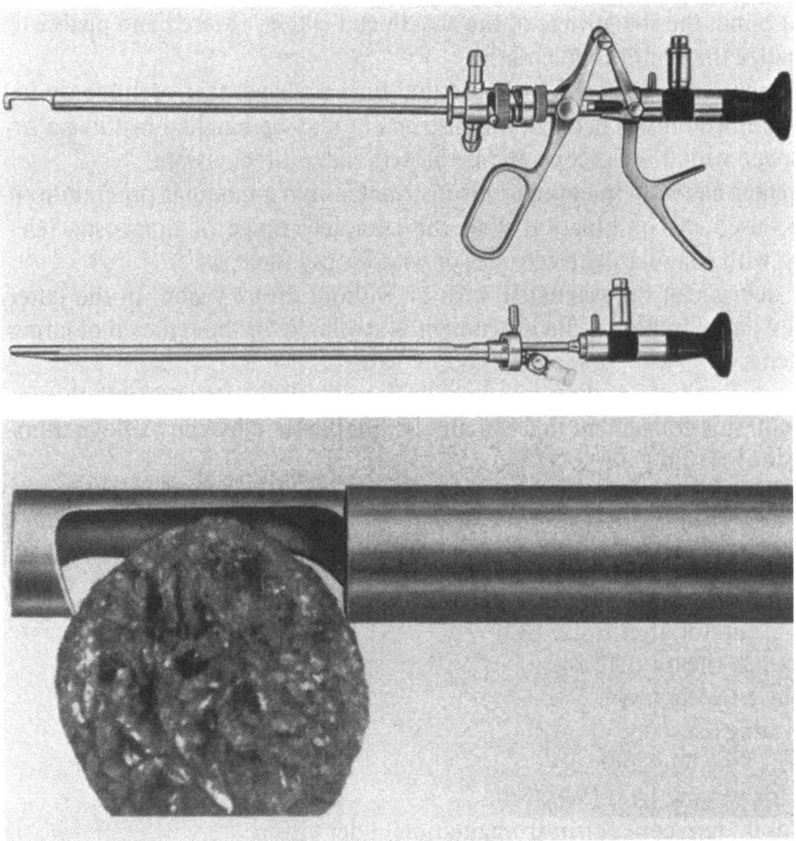

Fig. 6. The stone punch

β) Combined Shockwave- and Punch Litholapaxy

The convexity of plum sized stones is usually no longer adequate to allow them to be gripped in the punch jaws. To nibble to pieces and evacuate them by this means alone would become extremely laborious. Instead, a bridge insert is fitted to the sheath, through which a Urat I electrode can be passed. The stone is then initially shot to pieces as already repeatedly described, until the fragments are of suitable size to be broken up in the punch. This combination, without change of sheath, of Urat I and punch has proved of particular value for large bladder stones and considerably curtails litholapaxy prior to TUR of the prostate. The fact that the various maneuvers can be carried out without changing the sheath should also reduce urethral trauma.

5. Blind Litholapaxy

The world literature of the last ten years contains only few new publications on blind litholapaxy (MAUERMAYER 1975; HADLEY et al. 1977). MAUERMAYER (1975) has, however, pointed out that this is not, in itself, the reason why modern day urologists hardly ever use the technique. Modern anesthesiology has rendered suprapubic cystotomy and retropubic prostatectomy relatively low-risk procedures. Furthermore, the new techniques of ultrasound and shockwave, described in previous paragraphs, have dramatically altered what one may expect to achieve under direct vision. The consequence has been a relative eclipse of blind litholapaxy. Both MAUERMAYER (1975) and HADLEY et al. (1977) insist that the blind technique is in fact easy to learn. Blind lithotrites are so designed as to largely obviate any risk of pinching the bladder and to facilitate grasping the stone. One serious problem of the technique is how to pass it on to younger colleagues, since it is a fundamentally blind technique. The principle is illustrated in Fig. 7.

MAUERMAYER (1975) has given the following basic description of the art of blind litholapaxy:

"The size of the stone should be known from radiographs and preliminary cystoscopy. By the same token, the extent to which a prostatic adenoma protrudes into the bladder (endovesical growth) is also known. Thus the suitability of the stone for blind litholapaxy can largely be assessed before the procedure. The configuration of the adenoma is important because an excessively deep retroprostatic recess may make it difficult to grasp the stone.

The best information will come from preoperative cystoscopy, at which position, size and number of calculi can finally be determined. The depth of the recess is also easy to assess. Before removing the cystoscope 200 ml of irrigating fluid are run into the bladder. Passing the lithotrite occasionally causes difficulty because the sharply curved end will not always find its own way through the bulbar urethra. Pressure on the perineum usually solves this problem. The closed lithotrite is first used to palpate the base of the bladder and seek out the stone, a process which may be helped by a degree of Trendelenburg. There are two basic ways to hold the lithotrite and grasp the stone:
1. The "funnel" technique
2. The "sugar-tongs" technique

1. This way of holding the lithotrite is the less hazardous and more often used. The lithotrite is pressed somewhat into the floor of the bladder, thus forming a depression – or funnel. Gentle shaking rolls the stone to the lowest point in the bladder, where it may easily be felt to make contact with the lithotrite. Next the jaws are opened: gently advancing and withdrawing the male jaw eases the stone between them. Once the stone has been grasped, the jaws are locked on and the instrument gently moved around to make sure no bladder mucosa has been picked up. The screw mechanism is now progressively tightened to close the jaws. The entire process is repeated in rapid succession. Initially the fragments are large, but a scale on the handle of the instrument will show a progressive reduction in size until only gravel is left in the bladder.

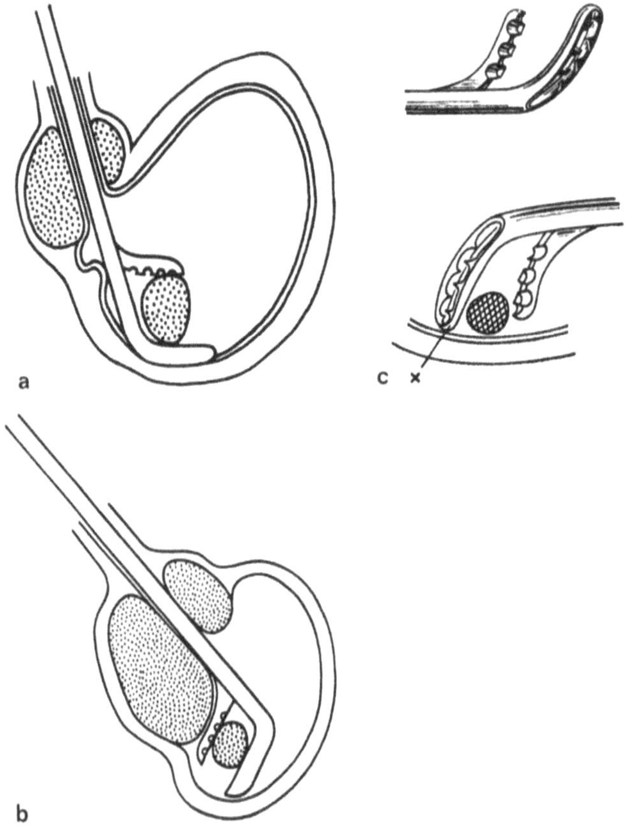

Fig. 7a, b. Holding the blind lithotrite in "funnel" and "sugar-tongs" techniques **c.** The bladder mucosa can only be pinched and traumatized if the bladder is inadequately distended and unfolded. Even in the sugar-tongs technique the mucosa is protected by the pronounced overhang of the male jaw (×) (MAUERMAYER 1975)

2. The sugar-tongs technique is only needed where a stone lies in a deep retroprostatic recess not accessible to the funnel technique. In fact we prefer prior resection of the adenoma in the same sitting for these cases, although the requirements on hemostasis are then most stringent.

Evacuating the debris takes only a few minutes, if one uses a sheath of adequate caliber. We have found instruments with a separate drain port on the external end most useful, since a vacuum bottle may then be attached. The base of the bladder is first scrutinized with the electrotome in situ and the bladder filled with irrigating fluid. The sheath aperture is placed over the heaviest debris deposit and the electrotome withdrawn. If a finger is kept over the end of the sheath the irrigating fluid and part of the debris will be evacuated. The process is repeated, the site of residual debris being determined at each check inspection. The entire process takes only a few minutes."

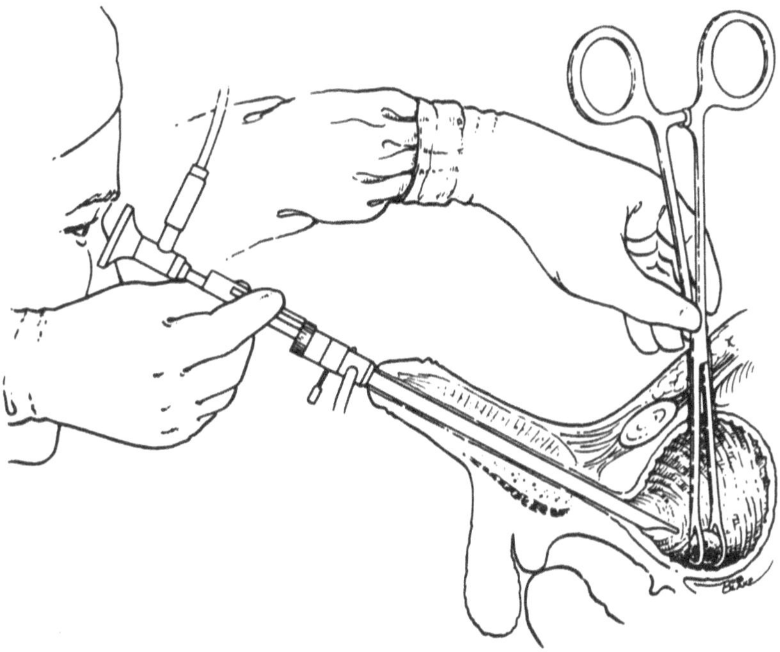

Fig. 8. Combined transurethral and suprapubic technique for the removal of bladder calculi (LINDSEY et al. 1975)

MAUERMAYER (1975) reports that between 1966 and 1973, 140 out of 181 patients with a previously diagnosed bladder stone could be treated by blind litholapaxy. The stones measured 20 to 40 mm. 91.2% of male patients underwent TUR of the prostate in the same session. Stones larger than 40 mm were removed at suprapubic cystotomy. In his extensive 1977 review HADLEY reports comparative results for viewing litholapaxy, blind litholapaxy and cystolithotomy in an even larger series to which identical indications had been applied. Although blind litholapaxy is in some respects a medico-historical curiosity, in the hands of experienced operators it nevertheless remains a mature procedure.

6. Combined Transurethral and Suprapubic Litholapaxy

In 1975, LINDSEY et al. described a combined transurethral and suprapubic approach for the removal of bladder stones (Fig. 8), clearly a precursor of percutaneous techniques. The formation of bladder stones is a particularly well recognized problem in patients with longterm urethral catheters. Once the existence of a bladder stone has been proven transurethrally and if there is no change of mechanical or other litholapaxy by the transurethral route these authors establish either a percutaneous or a formal suprapubic cystostomy and dilate the track progressively, until a standard spongeholding forceps can be passed. Only local anesthesia is required for this maneuver. With adequate dilatation of the cystostomy track, the stones are either removed intact or broken up and extracted piecemeal by the same route. With simultaneous cystoscopy through a standard cystoscope the procedure can be carried out under direct vision. Although the author is unable to envisage any clear indication for such a technique, it must still be mentioned, if only for the sake of completeness.

7. Unusual Transurethral Techniques

Proctoscope
Stone basket

a) The Stone Basket

In 1983, HUNTER et al. reported the successful treatment of bladder calculi by the combined use of electrohydraulic litholapaxy and a "stone basket". In order to avoid the theoretical and only true practical danger of Urat I, they developed the insert shown in Fig. 9. A PTFE net is attached to the end of the lithotrite

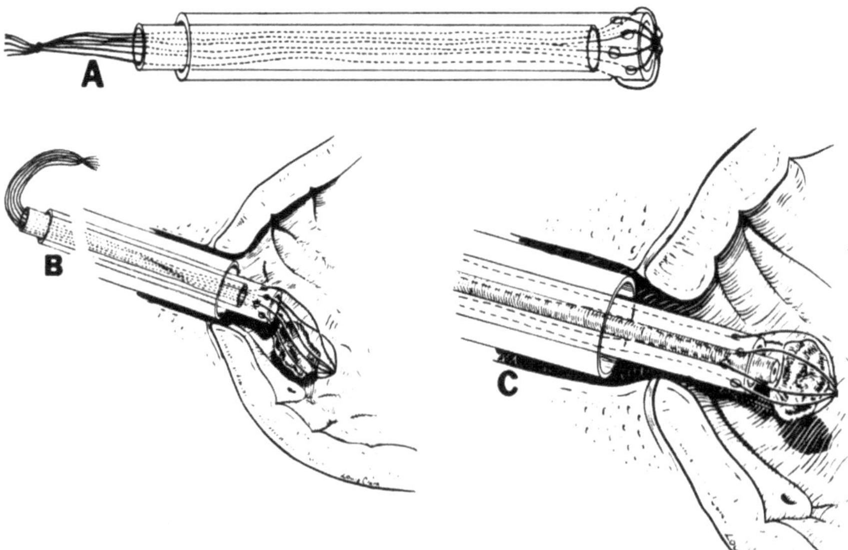

Fig. 9 A. Basket closed: inner catheter pushed forward as monofilament is pulled snug **B** Basket open: inner catheter withdrawn to a distance that determines the size of the basket; the whole is advanced as a unit and the inner strands and catheter used to open the basket and snare the stone **C** Manipulation: The inner catheter has been removed and a lithotrite electrode introduced to attack the stone; the basket catheter serves as a conduit for the aspiration of fragments and for irrigation (HUNTER et al. 1983)

insert and into this net the stone is maneuvered and drawn up to the aperture of the lithotrite sheath. The calculus can thus be held entirely surrounded by irrigating fluid and well away from the bladder wall. The lithotrite electrode is now passed down the lumen of the instrument to point at the center of the netted stone and lithotresis proceeds in the usual fashion. Although there has been adequate clinical experience, only three cases have been reported (HUNTER et al. 1983).

b) The Proctoscope

Extensive urethral dilatation and subsequent urethral passage of a proctoscope through which the stone could then be removed with stone forceps was first described in 1978 by GOTTESMANN and FLANAGAN. The technique is, of course, only appropriate for female patients, in whom the urethra can normally be dilated to Ch. 40 or 45. With careful technique the female urethra can apparently be dilated up to a diameter of 4 cm or about Ch. 150. The authors decided on this approach in a paraplegic incontinent patient whose entire bladder was filled with stones of up to 2 cm diameter. The procedure was tolerated without complication and resulted in only insignificant hematuria. Once again, the technique is mentioned purely for the sake of completeness.

8. Suprapubic Cystotomy

Some centuries ago suprapubic cystotomy was the standard approach to a bladder calculus. Since this book aims to stress the literature of the last decade and since no significant change in the technique of suprapubic surgery can be expected to have come about in this period of time, the following considerations make no reference to current literature.

Ever since their inception, the transurethral techniques listed above under I–VIII have tended to supplant suprapubic cystotomy: the old addage that a stone should always be smaller than the mouth of the lithotrite is no longer true. Nevertheless, the presence of a stone larger than 4 or 5 cm should lead one to think seriously in terms of a suprapubic approach. The size of associated adenoma should also be taken into account when deciding between a transurethral and a suprapubic operation. How often the urologist finds himself dealing with bladder stones, his personal experience and the technical equipment at his disposal will of course also play a considerable part. The relative indications for open surgery versus one of the above methods I–VIII cannot therefore be presented in a cut and dried fashion. The trend is, however, unmistakable: modern transurethral and endoscopic techniques have swung the balance massively against suprapubic procedures.

The following features and indications are in favor of open rather than transurethral surgery:

1. Relative or absolute urethral insufficiency (e.g. stricture)
2. Extreme disproportion of urethra to instrument (e.g. in children)

3. The combination of bladder diverticulum, prostatic adenoma and bladder calculus constitutes an indication for cystotomy, at least wherever the diverticulum is to be excised.
4. Stone size may constitute a relative indication for cystotomy.

In the hands of a practiced operator lithotresis is generally unlikely to take more than a quarter of an hour. In this period of time even 3 to 5 cm stones will have been broken up to the point where successful litholapaxy is achieved. If either the inexperience of the surgeon or limitations in his equipment make litholapaxy unlikely to succeed in under 30 minutes, an open procedure is to be preferred. Perusal of the rather scanty world literature of the last ten years generally confirms this basic approach to suprapubic cystotomy. NIENDORF et al. (1977), LEACH and FITZPATRICK (1981), JEFFERY (1983), WILLIAMS (1977), and likewise KUMAR (1974) have all reported on outsize bladder calculi and give stone size in itself as the indication for cystotomy. In some cases the stone was of such a circumference as to have to be delivered from the open bladder by obstetric forceps (JEFFERY 1983) as previously described by WILLIAMS et al. (1977)! The authors of the recent publications just quoted are all in agreement with the fundamental indications set out under 1–4 above.

9. Pregnancy and Litholapaxy for Bladder Calculi

If urolithiasis in general is rare during pregnancy, this is even more true of bladder stones. In his 1961 review of the world literature COPE found a grand total of 30 cases. In his more recent publication EGWUATU (1980) was able to add a single case. Of the thirty known cases six had been diagnosed prior to labor. Thus the other 24 only became apparent at that point. COPE (1961) and ARMON (1977) both report on two cases of bladder calculi presenting an obstacle to vaginal delivery. As in any other case, the indications for treating bladder calculi in pregnant women will depend on size and consistency of the stone and on the experience of the individual surgeon in using the equipment at his disposal. EGWUATU has performed suprapubic cystotomy at the time of Cesarian section. Under more favorably conditions and where stones are known to be present before the onset of uterine contraction, transurethral litholapaxy should, however, remain the treatment of choice.

10. Conservative Treatment

Longterm catheterisation and its inevitably associated significant bacteriuria are a well established cause of bladder stone formation. More recently (SOLOMON et al. 1980; KUTSCHER and VINSON 1979) there have been reports of bladder stone formation associated with intermittent catheterisation. In SOLOMON's four and VINSON's three cases, stones were formed around pubic hair carried into the bladder on the end of the catheter. These hairs were ideal crystallisation nuclei in the damaged neurogenic bladder. The preventability of this complication must be emphasized, as the authors stress.

11. Drug Therapy for Bladder Calculi (Cystolitholysis)

This is not the appropriate place to discuss the overall justification for attempting drug induced dissolution of bladder calculi in the face of a broad spectrum of simple, available surgical procedures. The few reports in the literature that suggest any hope of chemical stone dissolution are briefly mentioned:

Stones of pure uric acid could theoretically be dissolved by classical neutralization techniques (Uralyt-U, TERHORST 1974). This approach is of course open to criticism on the grounds that it does nothing to relieve the causative obstruction, the transurethral treatment of which could so easily be combined with litholapaxy. Even in uninfected urine (!), what is more, litholytic treatment is liable to take at least 6–8 weeks. This treatment remains, in practice, of theoretical value only.

MULVANEY et al. (1975) have reported successful stone dissolution in cystinurics with acetylcysteine and HAUTMANN et al. (1977) report similar success with mercaptopropionylglycine.

Both these treatments are subject to the same reservations in terms of subvesical obstruction previously mentioned in relation to uric acid lithiasis. Any attempt at a complete literature survey should also mention the study of YOKOYAMA et al. (1977) in which the dissolution of xanthine bladder calculi is discussed and in which literature on the biochemistry of the process is reviewed.

Generally speaking, however, drug therapy of bladder calculi has to be regarded as obsolete.

12. Stones in Conduits

BERGMANN et al. (1978) described a group of 296 patients with conduits, of whom 14 had stones. They rightly pointed out that the extreme dilatation of these patients' urinary tracts no doubt permitted a number of silent stones to pass spontaneously. In one patient stone formation was found to have taken place around intestinal staples which acted as a foreign body within the conduit.

DRETLER (1972) and ASSADNIA (1972) have also described the formation of stones around either suture material or metal clips within conduits.

It is common ground to all authors that stones which would normally require transurethral treatment are liable to pass spontaneously from conduits. The only exception is a report by HOEKSEMA et al. (1979) on a giant conduit stone of 6 × 9.5 cm which had to be excised from the conduit by a parastomal retroperitoneal approach.

References

Albrecht D, Nagel R, Kölln CP (1972) Electrohydraulic waves (Urat I) for the treatment of vesical calculi. Int Urol Nephrol 4:45

Alfthan O, Murtomaa M (1972) Experiences with the clinical and experimental use of the Urat-I Lithotriptor. Scand J Urol Nephrol 6:23

Angeloff A (1972) Hydroelectrolithotrypsy. J Urol 108:867

Armon PJ (1977) Obstructed labour due to a vesical calculus. Br Med J 2(6085):498

Assadnia A, Lee CN, Petre JH, Lyons RC (1972) Two cases of stone formation in ileal conduits after using the staple gun for closure of proximal end of isolated loop. J Urol 108:553

Baton JM, Malin JM jr, Glenn JF (1972) Electrohydraulic lithotrypsy. J Urol 108:865

Bergmann SM, Sears HF, Javadpour N (1978) Complication with mechanical stapling device in creation of ileoconduit. Urology 12:71–73

Borgmann V, Salim SA, Nagel R (1980) Ergebnisse der elektrohydraulischen Lithotrypsie von Harnblasensteinen mit dem Urat I. Akt Urol 11:421–425

Brundig P, Schneider HJ (1980) Zystolithotripsie. Ihre Ergebnisse in Beziehung zur Steinart. In: Schneider HJ (ed) Wissenschaftliche Beiträge der Friedrich-Schiller-Universität Jena 1980: IV. Jenaer Harnsteinsymposium Friedrich-Schiller-Universität Jena 1980, S 247

Bülow H, Frohmüller HG (1981) Electrohydraulic lithotripsy with aspiration of the fragments under vision – 304 consecutive cases. J Urol 126:455–456

Celsus (1846) De Medicina. Trans C Etangs (Paris)

Cope E (1961) Obstructed labour due to vesical calculus. J Obstet Gyn Br Comm 68:476

Dretler SP (1972) Urinary tract calculi and ileal conduit diversion. Am J Surg 123:480

Egwuatu VE (1980) Bladder calculus with pregnancy. J Urol 123:954–955

Ellis H (1969) A history of bladder stones. Blackwell Scientific Publications, Oxford and Edinburgh

Flachenecker G, Gminder F, Lutzeyer W (1982) A new high-frequency generator for the ultrasonic lithotrite. The XIX International Congress of the Société Internationale d'Urologie San Francisco, September 5–10, 1982 (Abstract)

Gasteyer KH (1971) Eine neue Methode der Blasensteinzertrümmerung. Die Ultraschall-Lithotripsie. Der Urologe [Ausg A] 10:30

Gottesman JE, Flanagan MJ (1978) Removal of bladder stones in females. Urology 11:636

Hadley H, Barnes R, Rosenquist R (1977) Tactile Litholapaxy – safe and efficient. Urology 9:263–265

Hautmann R, Terhorst B, Stuhlsatz HW, Lutzeyer W (1977) Mercaptopropionylglycine: Progress in cystine stone therapy. J Urol 117:628–630

Hautmann R, Terhorst B, Rathert P, Gminder F, Lutzeyer W (1980) Ultrasonic litholapaxy of bladder stones – 10 years of experience with more than 400 cases. In: Brockis JG (Hrsg) Urinary calculus. 2nd International Urinary Stone Conference. PSG Publishing Company Inc. Littleton Massachusetts (in press)

Hautmann R, Terhorst B, Rathert P, Gminder F, Lutzeyer W (1982) Ultrasonic litholapaxy of bladder stones – 10 years of experience with more than 400 cases. The XIX International Congress of the Société Internationale d'Urologie San Francisco, September 5–10, 1982 (Abstract)

Hoeksema J, Zamora S, McKiel C, Guinan P (1979) Case profile: Giant ileal conduit stone. Urology 14:192–193

Hunter PT, Finlayson B, Demler JW, Hawkins I, Nanni GS (1983) New monofilament basket for bladder calculi. Urology 21:388–389

Jediny GY (1978) Elektrohydraulische Zystolithotripsie bei Kindern. In: Schneider HJ (ed) Wissenschaftliche Beiträge der Friedrich-Schiller-Universität Jena 1978: V. Jenaer Harnsteinsymposium Friedrich-Schiller-Universität, Jena 1978, S 248

Jeffery JT (1983) Successful delivery of huge bladder stone with obstetric forceps. Urology 21:162–163

Kaneko H, Watanabe H, Takahashi T, Watanabe K, Akiyama K, Kondo K, Furue K, Oinuma S (1979) Studies on the application of microexplosion to medicine and biology. IV. Strength of wet and dry urinary calculi. Jpn J Urol 70:61

Kierfeld G (1968) Lithotripsie von Blasensteinen durch hydraulische Schlagwellenwirkung. Verhandlungsbericht der deutschen Gesellschaft für Urologie 22. Tagung. Berlin, S 263
Kierfeld G, Mellin P (1969) Blasensteinzertrümmerung durch hydraulische Schlagwellenwirkung im Tierexperiment. Urologe [Ausg A] 8:99
Kondo K (1981) Studies on the application of microexplosion to medicine and biology. IV. The pressure profile of blast wave in air by detonation of a lead azide charging chamber. Jpn J Urol 72:662
Kumar AV (1974) A case of giant vesicoprostatic calculus following retropubic prostatectomy. J R Coll Surg Edn 19:48
Kutscher HA, Vinson RK (1979) Bladder calculi formation during clean intermittent catheterization. Urology 14:357–358
Leach GE, Fitzpatrich TJ (1981) Giant vesical calculi in the female. Urology 17:274–275
Lindsey CM, Hawes SP, Anderson EE (1975) Removal of vesical calculi in patients with suprapubic cystostomy diversion – modified endoscopic technique. Urology 5:259–260
Lutzeyer W, Terhorst B, Cichos M (1970) Die Zerstörung von Harnsteinen durch Ultraschall. I. Experimentelle Untersuchungen. Urol Int 25:47
Lutzeyer W, Terhorst B, Cichos M, Pohlmann R (1972) Die Zerstörung von Harnsteinen durch Ultraschall. II. Ultraschall-Lithotripsie von Blasensteinen. Urol Int 27:458
Mauermayer W (1975) Die blinde Lithotripsie. Eine medizinische Kuriosität oder ein ausgereiftes Verfahren? Akt Urol 6:257
Mauermayer W (1983) Litholapaxy. In: Mauermayer W (ed) Transurethral Surgery. Springer, Berlin Heidelberg New York, p 359
Mauermayer W, Hartung R (1976) Der Stein-Punch, ein neues Prinzip zur Sicht-Lithotrypsie. Urologe [Ausg A] 15:164
Mitchel ME, Kerr W (1977) Experience with the electrohydraulic disintegrator. J Urol 117:159–160
Mulvaney WP (1953) Attempted disintegration of calculi by ultrasonic vibrations. J Urol 70:704
Mulvaney et al. (1975) Bladder calculi in cystinuric patients, value of acetylcysteine. J Urol 114:107
Murata S, Watanabe H, Watanabe K, Takahashi T, Akiyama K, Oinuma S, Yoshikawa M (1978) Studies on the application of microexplosion to medicine and biology. III. Amino acids in urinary calculi. Jpn J Urol 69:33
Murphy JT (1972) The history of Urology. Charles C Thomas Publisher
Niendorf DC, Factor DE, Shapiro SR (1977) Case profile: Giant-vesical calculus: Urology 10:66–67
Ouchi T, Takahashi H (1967) Disintegration of urinary calculi by means of ultrasonic vibration. XIV. Kongreß der internationalen Gesellschaft für Urologie Band 2, Joby, Paris, p 316
Pelander WM, Kaufman JE (1980) Complications of electrohydraulic lithotresis. Urology 16:155–157
Raney AM (1975) Electrohydraulic lithotripsy: experimental study and case reports with stone disintegrator. J Urol 113:345
Raney AM (1976) Electrohydraulic cystolithotripsy. Urology 7:379–381
Reuter HJ (1969) Electric lithotripsy: a new method for transurethral treatment of bladder stones. Endoscopy 1:63
Reuter HJ (1970) Electronic lithotripsy; transurethral treatment of bladder stones in fifty cases. J Urol 104:834
Rouvalis P (1970) Electronic lithotripsy for vesical calculus with Urat I. An experience of 100 cases and an experimental application of the method to stones in the upper urinary tract. Br J Urol 42:486
Solomon HM, Koff SA, Diokno AC (1980) Bladder calculi complicating intermittent catheterization. J Urol 124:140–141
Terhorst B (1974) Blasensteinbehandlung durch Ultraschall. Deutsches Ärzteblatt 8:519
Terhorst B, Chichos M (1971) Harnsteinzertrümmerung. Biomed Tech (Berlin) 16:106
Tessler AN, Kossow J (1975) Electrohydraulic stone disintegration. Urology 5:470–474

Thiel D, Rathert P (1977) Ultraschall-Lithotripsie von Blasensteinen: Katamnestische Untersuchung an 107 Patienten: Von der Fakultät für Medizin der Rheinisch-Westfälischen-Technischen-Hochschule Aachen zur Erlangung des akademischen Grades eines Doktors der Medizin, genehmigte Dissertation

Tidd MJ, Wright HC, Oliver Y, Wallace DM, Porteous M (1976) Hazards to bladder and intestinal tissues from intravesical underwater electrical discharges from a surgical electronic lithoclast. Urol Res 4:49

Watanabe H, Oinuma S (1977) Studies on the application of microexplosion to medicine and biology. I. Development of special explosive for the experiments. Jpn J Urol 68:243

Watanabe H, Watanabe K, Shiino K, Oinuma S (1980) A prototype apparatus for microexplosion cystolithotripsy. Tohoku J Exp Med 132:243

Watanabe H, Watanabe K, Shiino K, Oinuma S (1982) Microexplosion cystolithotripsy. The XIX International Congress of the Société Internationale d'Urologe, San Francisco, September 5–10, 1982 (Abstract)

Watanabe H, Watanabe K, Shiino K, Oinuma S (1983) Microexplosion-cystolithotripsy. J Urol 129:23–28

Watanabe K, Watanabe H, Takahashi H, Akiyama K, Kaneko H, Kondo K, Uchida M, Oinuma S, Shiino K, Tanaka I (1980) Studies on the application of microexplosion to medicine and biology. V. Development of experimental apparatus for microexplosion and histological change in dog bladder wall by blast in air. Jpn J Urol 71:15

Williams JP, Mayo ME, Harrison NW (1977) Massive bladder stone. Br J Urol 9:51

Xui M, Chang J, Xui Z, Cheng W, Bao Z, Schi Z, Wang J (1981) Microexplosion of bladder stone. Chin Med J [Engl] 61:341

Yokoyama et al. (1977) Bladder, calculi, xanthine stone in xanthinuric boy, biochemical case study and review of the literature. J Urol 118:651

Treatment of Urethral Stones

H.-J. SCHNEIDER

I. Prevalence

The urethra is probably the rarest site for urinary stone formation (SCHREYER 1974). Among a series of 50,000 stones only 0.9% and 0.4% were from the urethra of men or women respectively (Table 1).

Urethral stones occur most frequently in children and in the elderly. The occurrence, causes and complications of this rare condition are usually presented in the European and North American literature as case reports (DE BRUYNE et al. 1983; DE CARVALHO 1977; DEODHAR and KHOPE 1983; SHAH 1983). In the Near and Far East the disease is far more common, occurring mainly in children as part of the picture of endemic bladder stone disease (BRIDGES et al. 1982).

II. Pathogenesis

A distinction is made in the literature between primary stones, arising in the urethra, and secondary stones lodging there during spontaneous passage from the upper urinary tract or bladder (SCHREYER 1977). Although the latter are undoubtedly far more common, it is impossible to accept the view of FLOCKS et al.

Table 1. Occurrence of urethral calculi in a series of 50,000 stones, according to age and sex (SCHNEIDER and HIENSCH 1979)

Age	Men	Women
– 10 years	2.3	0.6
– 20 years	0.9	0.2
– 30 years	0.9	0.3
– 40 years	0.6	0.3
– 50 years	0.6	0.3
– 60 years	0.7	0.3
– 70 years	1.0	0.5
– 80 years	1.6	0.7
– 90 years	6.3	1.5

(1969) that urethral stones are never primary in origin. Upper tract calculi may indeed come to rest above points of physiological constriction or in the intervening wider segments of the urethra (prostatic urethra, bulb, navicular fossa), but the underlying cause is nearly always a pathologic outflow obstruction (MAYOR and ZINGG 1973).

Calculi able to pass the bladder neck will generally also fit through a normal urethra (FRIEDLAND et al. 1983). Concretions arrested above the level of a stricture or in a diverticulum may interfere with micturition only slightly. They can then grow by apposition to monstrous proportions. Diverticular stones of the female urethra have been recorded that virtually filled the vagina and stones of similar size have been described in men and in children (SINHA and RINTOUL 1982).

Urethral calculi are usually solitary and only rarely multiple. Their shape varies according to site and origin. Stones of the rarer primary group arise in abscess cavities, in fistulous tracks and above all in diverticula (DALENS et al. 1982; GINSBERG and FINKELSTEIN 1983; PASTARMADJIEFF et al. 1982). Typical hour-glass calculi occur after surgery for benign prostatic hypertrophy, yet they are occasionally seen in children (CHARMA and CHAUD 1982).

SRINIVAS and DOW (1983) have described transitional cell carcinoma in a stone-bearing diverticulum of the urethra.

The commonest cause of socalled primary urethral calculi is the encrustation of foreign bodies. The latter may be just hair, following urethral reconstruction with scrotal skin, but a variety of articles get introduced during masturbation. Some foreign bodies that find their way into the bladder become secondarily encrusted and lodge there. MIEDEMA and REDEMAN (1982) found a vascular clip in the nucleus of a calculus and we have seen two calculi formed around non-absorbable ligature material. Our patient, a woman, had undergone surgery seven years previously for ovarian cysts and presented to us with unheralded acute retention of urine.

Primary urethral calculi and foreign body encrustations tend to consist of struvite and carbonate-apatite: they are typical infective calculi.

III. Symptomatology and Diagnosis

The entry of a bladder calculus into the urethra during micturition results in sudden painful interruption of the urinary stream. If the urethra is only partly occluded, the effect may range from a marked reduction in stream to the dripping of urine from the meatus amid considerable pain. Larger calculi lodged in the sphincteric region can interfere with the bladder neck mechanism to the point of incontinence (ZINGG and MAYOR 1973).

Pain and disturbed micturition may be followed by signs of inflammation, since arrest of a calculus for any length of time almost invariably leads to local urethritis, with urethral discharge, hematuria and pyuria, especially in a first-catch specimen. Once there is suppuration, edema will rapidly ensue in the skin of the penis and scrotum.

The diagnosis can usually be made on the history and on palpation. Large stones are easy to feel, but if the findings are uncertain, bouginage or urethroscopy should be undertaken. The majority of calculi are radioopaque and are clearly seen on a plain KUB film (SCHREYER 1974). Urethrography is the investigation of choice for detecting and precisely locating radiolucent calculi and diverticulum stones. The calculi appear as smooth filling defects of varying outline.

The presence of a urethral calculus should be considered, despite a negative history, in any patient with continuing urethritis refractory to treatment (LUTZEYER 1977).

Complications arise from chronic inflammation and local pressure effects on the urethra. Periurethral abscess, fistula or stricture may result.

IV. Treatment

The details of treatment will depend on site and size of the calculus and on local secondary disease process (Table 2).

Stones in the navicular fossa can be grasped and extracted with forceps after dilatation or meatotomy. Careful urethral dilatation (DASGUPTA and GUPTA 1981) or internal urethrotomy of strictures will allow smooth surfaced calculi to be similarly delivered by forceps or snares from the middle or proximal urethra. Great care and adequate lubrication are essential, if mucosal injury and stricture formation are to be avoided (SHAH 1983).

Calculi in the prostatic urethra can often be pushed back into the bladder, either with sounds or under direct vision. There, they may be broken up and subsequently evacuated. Many units are equipped for and expert at percutaneous ultrasound or shockwave lithotresis. The technique is suitable for urethral calculi at virtually any site. The stone is broken up under direct vision without injury to the mucosa and is evacuated in a single step.

Larger stones accompanied by more severe inflammation should be removed by operative urethrotomy (FLOCKS et al. 1969). The urethra is opened on its scrotal aspect over the palpable stone. Temporary suprapubic cystostomy is recommended to facilitate healing (MARBERGER 1983).

Stone bearing diverticula should always be resected at the time of stone removal.

Table 2. Eventual fate of urethral stones in 88 men and women (SCHNEIDER and HESSE 1976)

Fate	Number	Male : female ratio
Spontaneous passage	52	1.9 : 1
Instrumentation	26	25 : 1
Open surgery	10	4 : 1
Total	88	3.2 : 1

References

Bridges Ch, Belville WD, Buck AS, Dresner ML (1982) Urethral calculi. J Urol 128:1036–1037
Dalens B, Vanneuville G, Vincent L, Fabre JL (1982) Congenital polyp of the posterior urethra and vesical calculus in a boy. J Urol 128:1034–1035
Dasgupta HK, Gupta V (1981) Tube-bouginage technic in the management of urethral stone (case reports). J Postgrad Med 27:187–188
De Bruyne R, Braeckman J, Petit R (1983) Urethral lithiasis. Acta Urol Belg 51:334–339
De Carvalho HA (1977) Giant urethral calculus: A case report. J Urol 118:334–335
Deodhar SD, Khope S (1983) Giant prostatic urethral calculus: A case report. J Postgrad Med 29:49–50
Flocks RH, Culp DA, Bauer KM (1969) Urologische Operationslehre. Schattauer, Stuttgart New York, S 348–349
Friedland GW, Filly R, Goris ML, Gross D, Kempson RL, Korabkin M, Thurber BD, Walter J (1983) Uroradiology, an integrated approach. Churchill Livingstone, New York Edinburgh London Melbourne, vol I, p 507
Ginsberg P, Finkelstein LH (1983) Urethral diverticulum with calculi: report of a case. J Am Osteopath Assoc 82:588–590
Marberger M (1983) Klinik und operative Therapie der Steinerkrankungen: In: Hohenfellner R, Zingg EJ (Hrsg) Urologie in Klinik und Praxis, Bd II. Thieme, Stuttgart, S 748–780
Miedema EB, Redman JF (1982) Case profile: radiolucent urethral calculus with hemostatic clip nidus. Urology 19:328
Pastarmadjieff L, Rabe F, Schuelke J (1982) Urethraldivertikelstein. Ein kasuistischer Beitrag. Zentralbl Gynakol 104:886–889
Schneider H-J, Hesse A (1976) Zur Epidemiologie des Harnsteinleidens. Therapiewoche 26:5881–5899
Schneider H-J, Hienzsch E (1979) Epidemiologie der Urolithiasis. Internat. Urologenkongreß, Paris (Kongreßbericht)
Schreyer H (1974) Erkrankungen der unteren Harnwege und Genitalorgane. In: Vogler E (Hrsg) Radiologische Diagnostik der Harnorgane. Thieme, Stuttgart, S 654ff
Shah PJR (1983) Multiple urethral calculi – an unusual cause of acute retention of urine. Br J Urol 55:573–574
Sharma LK, Chand G (1982) The "dumb-bell" vesicouretheral calculus in childhood. Indian J Pediatr 19:799–800
Sinha A, Rintoul RF (1982) Giant calculus in urethral diverticulum. Br J Urol 54:62
Srinivas V, Dow D (1983) Transitional cell carcinoma in a urethral diverticulum with a calculus. J Urol 129:372–373
Zingg E, Mayor G (1973) Klinik der Harnsteine. In: Alken CE, Staenler W (Hrsg) Klinische Urologie. Thieme, Stuttgart, S 224–225

Extracorporeal Shockwave Lithotripsy (ESWL) in the Treatment of Kidney and Ureter Stones

CH. CHAUSSY and E. SCHMIEDT

I. Introduction

Writing a handbook article on a clinical picture, the therapeutic guidelines of which are currently undergoing a dramatic change, is not without risk. All that can be undertaken in this situation is a attempt to appraise future techniques for the treatment of kidney stone disease.

It remains uncontested that despite all analytical investigations into the pathogenesis of stone disease kidney stones are to be seen as a symptomatic manifestation of a multifactorial metabolic dysfunction. Thus stone removal techniques must be sought in a "symptomatic therapy", based on an approach which involves as little invasiveness as possible in order to prevent or minimize complications.

This means that progress towards an ideal therapy must necessarily constitute an advance in nonsurgical treatment. For the surgical urologist this will entail a change in traditional views. To our mind, however, there is no alternative but to accept and integrate these new therapeutic approaches. Failure to recognize this situation involves the danger that what is properly a "urologic clinical picture" will be shifted as a result of disinterest to other medical fields. This, it must be said, would not be in the best interest of the patient.

A forerunner of this development was certainly percutaneous litholapaxy as developed and refined for routine use by ALKEN (ALKEN et al. 1981). Although this technique represented a decisive step away from surgical stone removal, it was nevertheless invasive in nature. At least theoretically extracorporeal shockwave lithotripsy (ESWL), which evolved almost simultaneously, promised to provide a completely noninvasive method for the treatment of kidney stones (CHAUSSY et al. 1976, 1978a; EISENBERGER et al. 1977b; FORSSMANN et al. 1977).

In the following we shall attempt to give a summary of the experience we have gained with this technique and to present some guidelines and comments with regard to the limitations of this new technique. We do so, however, at a time when four other centers in Germany have begun work with ESWL. The first impressions would indicate that the Munich results are reproducible in the main. However, the figures cited below refer only to the Munich results.

1. Method

2. Fundamentals

Nonmedical research in the field of short-time physics opened up the possibility of destroying concrements over a distance by subjecting them to the action of high-energy shockwaves. However, the technique was initially limited by the expensive and clinically unsuitable means of generating the waves. Not until a method was found of generating shockwaves by a reproducible spark discharge across an underwater gap were the prerequisites met for developing the technology and apparatus required to begin experimental work with a view towards possible clinical applications.

At this time, when physicists at Dornier System proposed the use of shockwaves produced outside the body as a means of treating urinary stones noninvasively, only studies on the effect of shockwaves on brittle materials had been carried out. The technology was adapted to medical purposes and the still unknown biological effects assessed in six years of research in close cooperation with Dornier System (CHAUSSY 1982; CHAUSSY et al. 1980b).

3. Shockwaves – Ultrasonic Waves

Basic differences in the physical properties of ultrasonic waves and shockwaves, which are often ignored, should be pointed out. Figure 1 shows the different pressure-time diagrams of ultrasonic and shock waves. Whereas a shockwave consists of a single pressure pulse with a steep onset and slow decay, ultrasound exhibits a sinusoidal pressure curve with a train of compressions and rarefactions. In addition, the two types of wave display fundamentally different frequency patterns. While ultrasound is characterized by a well-defined frequency, shockwaves consist of a spectrum of low and high frequencies.

This also results in different attenuation behavior of the two wave types as they pass through tissue. During passage through tissue high-frequency wave

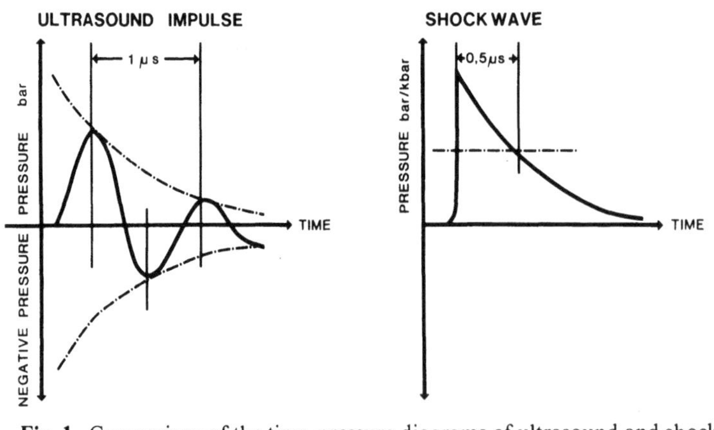

Fig. 1. Comparison of the time-pressure diagrams of ultrasound and shockwaves

portions are attenuated much more strongly than the low-frequency components. Shockwaves, which contain a greater low-frequency portion than ultrasonic waves, thus undergo less damping. As a result, shockwaves are able to penetrate into tissue far deeper than ultrasound. Cell damage observed after protracted exposure to ultrasound can also be explained in terms of the strong attenuation of ultrasonic waves as they pass through tissue, with the mechanical energy of the high-frequency portions being converted into heat and causing thermal damage. This is not to be expected in shockwave therapy, even when high energies are used.

II. Shockwave Generation and Focussing

In shockwave therapy high-energy shockwaves are produced extracorporeally, transmitted into the body and focussed on the stone.

The shockwave is generated by discharging the energy stored in a capacitor within several nanoseconds across an underwater electrode gap. The result is an explosive vaporization of the surrounding fluid, with the associated expansion of volume giving rise to the shockwave.

Under normal circumstances, the wave would propagate spherically in all three dimensions, making precise application of its intrinsic energy impossible. Thus a means of focussing the waves is indispensable for clinical applications.

Shockwaves are focussed by generating them at one of the two foci of a rotationally symmetric semiellipsoid (Fig. 2). At each point on the ellipsoid's wall on which the shockwave impinges a new wave is generated. Owing to the geometric properties of an ellipsoid all of the waves reflected from the ellipsoid wall converge at the second focal point. Thus this point represents the area of maximum energy density in which the kidney stone must be located. The procedure is also advantageous in that stress to tissue lying outside the focus but in the path of the shockwaves is extremely low.

Since the waves are focussed, it is necessary to position the stone precisely and reproducibly into the focal area. An experimental series lasting nearly one and a half years was carried out using an ultrasound locating system arranged within the ellipsoid. After this set-up proved unsatisfactory, the problem could only be solved by integrating an elaborate x-ray locating system in the apparatus.

For three-dimensional localization of the stone two independent x-ray image conversion systems are required (Fig. 3). To this end, the central beams of the two x-ray systems are arranged in such a way that they intersect at the second focus (f2) of the semiellipsoid. The concrement is positioned exactly in the focus when the two axes of the central beams intersect within it. The central beam is represented by a cross-hair in the center of the respective monitors, and the stone to be disintegrated must be moved so that it lies in the cross-hairs of both imaging systems.

Following technical adaptation and integration of the individual elements, various experimental models were constructed, with which the safety and ef-

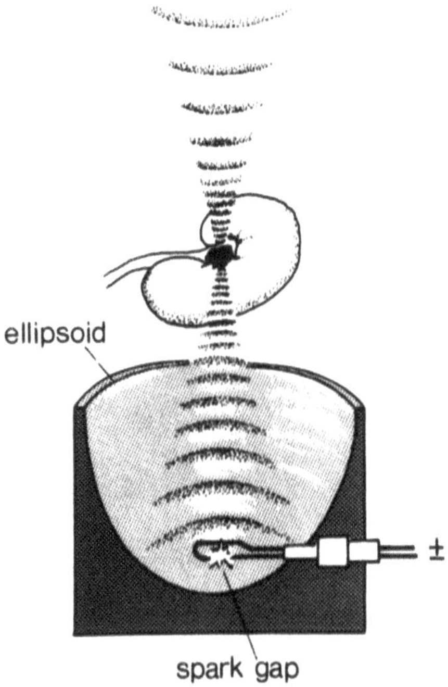

Fig. 2. Schematic representation of the pressure during exposure to focussed shockwaves. The density of the grains roughly corresponds to the magnitude of pressure as the wave passes through tissue. The focussing results in a well-defined area of high pressure in the stone region

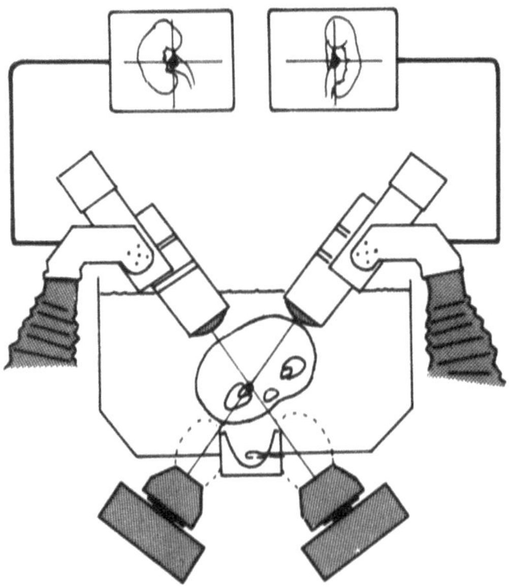

Fig. 3. Arrangement of the central beams of the x-ray localization system. The concrement is positioned in the focus when it is located along the axis of both systems. The adjustment is accomplished by moving the patient above the ellipsoid

fectiveness of this new therapeutic form was substantiated in six years of experimental work (CHAUSSY 1982; CHAUSSY and SCHMIEDT 1983; CHAUSSY et al. 1976, 1977, 1978a, b, 1979, 1980a, b, 1983; EISENBERGER et al. 1977a, b; FORSSMANN et al. 1977). In view of the fact that this represents a new technology in human medicine, a brief summary of the most important experimental results is due, especially since it throws light on the question of clinical safety (CHAUSSY 1982; CHAUSSY et al. 1980b).

1. By exposing kidney stones of various composition to shockwaves it was possible to break them up into pieces capable of being discharged spontaneously.
2. Repeated exposure of human erythrocytes resulted in lowgrade but nevertheless clinically acceptable hemolysis. After exposure of isolated organs such as kidneys, liver, intestine and bones no pathological changes were observed.
3. These results were borne out by the exposure of rats to shockwaves. Although exposure concentrated on the chest did lead to alveolar ruptures, no traumatization of tissue could be demonstrated in the abdominal region after exposure to shockwaves.
4. After exposure of human lymphocytes no cytolysis could be found. Furthermore, no influence on the proliferation rate of mixed lymphocyte cultures was found, so that as far as can be judged from in vitro experiments impairment of cell-proliferative processes may be ruled out.
5. Once an experimental stone model in dogs had been developed (CHAUSSY et al. 1977) successful stone disintegration by means of extracorporeally generated shockwaves and spontaneous discharge of the partial concrements could be demonstrated in vivo. No pathological changes were detected in the kidney region or in neighboring organs.

1. Equipment

In order to ensure unhindered transmission of the shockwaves into the body, the patient must be surrounded by a suitable transmission medium. Owing to the similarity in physical properties between body tissue and water, the most straightforward means of providing this medium is to immerse the patient in a water bath.

Figure 4 shows the patient support. The support is cut away in the back to permit unobstructed transfer of the shockwaves to this area. Thus the fixed points for the patient positioning are the pelvic and shoulder girdles. The patient is strapped onto the support in order to prevent undesirable movement due to buoyancy. The support is constructed in such a way that it can be adjusted for the individual, not only in terms of body length, but also about the longitudinal axis of the body. This possibility must be employed chiefly for positioning stones which are located near the spine so that they can be visualized outside the radiologic shadow of the vertebral column.

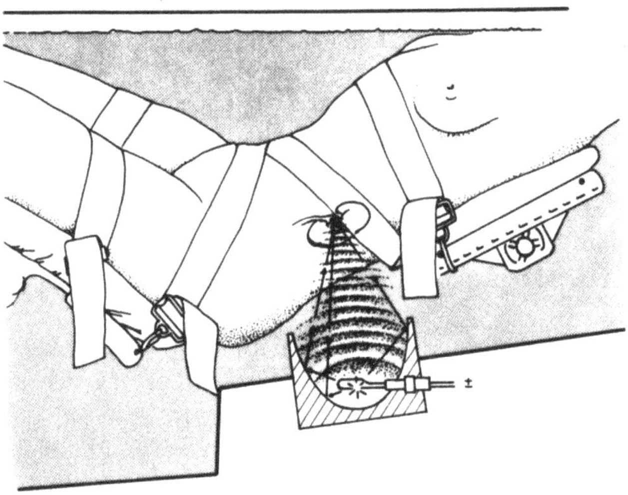

Fig. 4. The patient support and the arrangement of the shockwave reflector, showing the path of the focussed shockwave

2. Stone Localization

In order to bring the stone into the focus of the ellipsoid and of the shockwaves the patient must be moved above the ellipsoid in all three spatial planes. The patient is first anesthesized and strapped onto the support. The support is then moved manually over the water bath. From this "home" position all movements can be carried out by means of a remotecontrol hydraulic system.

The patient is lowered over the ellipsoid until the stone appears on one of the monitors of the image-conversion system. The stone is manipulated into the cross-hairs of this monitor, in other words so that it is located along the axis of the first image-conversion system. By means of an automatically controlled series of movements it is possible to move the stone along this axis until it is also centered under the cross-hairs of the second monitor. Because of the way in which the two systems are arranged the stone is now positioned at the intersection of the two x-ray systems and thus in the area of maximum energy density. The therapeutic procedure may now begin.

3. Respiratory Mobility

It is a well-known phenomenon that in patients who have not been operated on previously respiration-dependent movements of the stone occur. These must be taken into account during positioning. Since the actual focus of the shockwave covers an area of about 1.5 cm^3 and respiratory-related stone displacements seldom exceed 1 to 2 cm, this problem is easily solved. The stone is positioned under fluoroscopic control in the center of the cross-hairs so that the maximum displacement of the stone caused by breathing remains within the focal area. If the concrement is large, however, re-adjustment is required, and disintegration is then carried out stepwise.

4. Procedure

The preparations for ESWL include routine examinations for conventional surgical stone removal and anesthesia. No further measures are necessary aside from the administration of carminatives. To this end the administration of Saab has proven expedient.

5. Trial Runs

In order to simplify the procedure on the day of treatment and provide more effective consultation for the patient a "trial run" is performed. The patient is placed in the apparatus on the day before treatment, and the essentials of the procedure are explained to him. Then the patient is placed on the support, which is adjusted to his body size. The support is moved over the ellipsoid and the stone centered under the cross-hairs of the monitors. The adjustment data are noted, and the image-conversion setting is documented by means of a multiformat camera.

6. Anesthesia

Before induction of the requisite anesthesia, a KUB roentgenogram is made of the kidney region with the patient in the supine position in order to exclude the possibility of strong shadowing by intestinal gas. It has been shown both in experimental studies and in clinical use that shockwave treatment in the presence of intestinal gas does not cause any traumatization of the intestinal sections involved. However, in the presence of excess shadowing caused by air pockets reliable radiologic location of the stone is no longer possible once disintegration has commenced. For this reason treatment is postponed in cases of excessive air accumulation. Often the situation changes within an hour to permit treatment.

Shockwave therapy is painful and requires some means of abolishing pain. As studies with volunteers have shown, individual shockwave pulses would be tolerable, but certainly not the series of shockwaves the patient is exposed to during treatment. The pain is not restricted to the skin area being treated, but is described as visceral pain. Thus, attempts to eliminate pain by means of local infiltration of anesthetics into the skin have proved unsuccessful.

Peridural anesthesia has proved to be the method of choice in 75% of all cases. The peridural catheter, which is sealed water-tight with surgical incision tape, affords the possibility of easily administering additional anesthetics should the procedure be delayed.

In cases where this regional technique is contraindicated, whether for medical or psychological reasons, treatment can always be performed under intubation anesthesia. This technique is also preferred for high-risk patients, since it permits better monitoring.

7. Shockwave Exposure

After being strapped onto the support, the patient is moved in the tub to the home position above the ellipsoid, and the support is adjusted in accordance with the prerecorded data. Fine adjustment for precise localization of the stone is accomplished as described above.

Lithotripsy is then carried out in series of 100 individual shockwave pulses. The desired voltage applied to the electrodes can be set and read off on a voltmeter. The shockwaves are usually generated with 18 kV. Only in the case of large stones and cystine stones is it advantageous to work with voltages of up to 23 kV for the first 100 to 200 individual pulses. The result is more rapid disintegration of the stone structure and an increase in the effective stone area exposed to the shockwaves, making subsequent routine treatment more effective. This initially higher voltage, however, can be disadvantageous, since it gives rise to large fragments which distribute themselves outside the focal area, thus necessitating repeated readjustment.

8. ECG Triggering

The individual shockwaves are ECG-triggered. In this way extrasystoles, which have been observed when the shockwaves are not released in synchronization with the heart, can be avoided. By scanning the R wave of the ECG the shockwave can be triggered in such a way that it occurs during the absolute refractory phase of the heart and thus does not lead to impairment of cardiac function. Since the occurrence of therapy-related arrhythmias is effectively prevented in this way, we shall give only a brief review of the theories which attempt to explain how the extrasystoles arise.

1. Triggering of the extrasystoles by mechanical alteration of a secondary wave, which is generated as the primary wave passes through the body and which could reach the cardiac apex via the diaphragm.
2. Reflective triggering by a boundary layer situated in the area of exposure.

The elimination of this phenomenon by ECG triggering at the same time extended the range of indications to include patients suffering from cardiac conduction disorders.

9. Readjustment During Treatment

After each series of 100 individual pulses a radiological check is again performed, and readjustment is carried out if necessary. The progress of stone disintegration can usually be observed on the monitors, as shown in Fig. 5a. In as-

Fig. 5a–f. Radiological follow-up of a right pelvic stone. **a** AP roentgenogram (KUB) prior to treatment. **b** 0 pulses. **c** After 150 pulses. **d** After 400 pulses. **e** After 600 pulses. **f** Final AP film after treatment

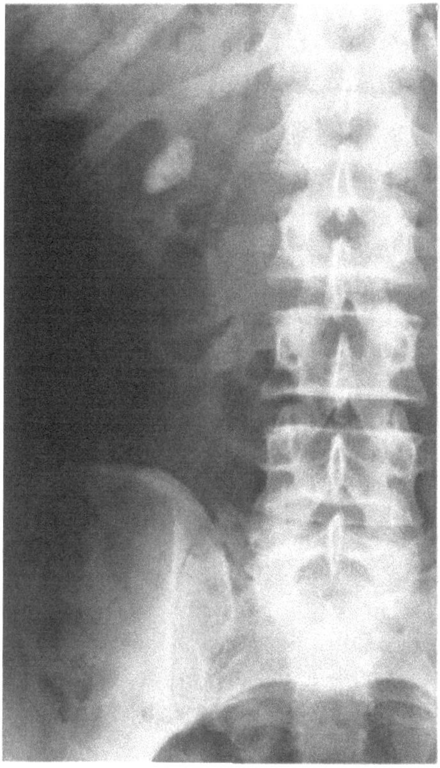
a

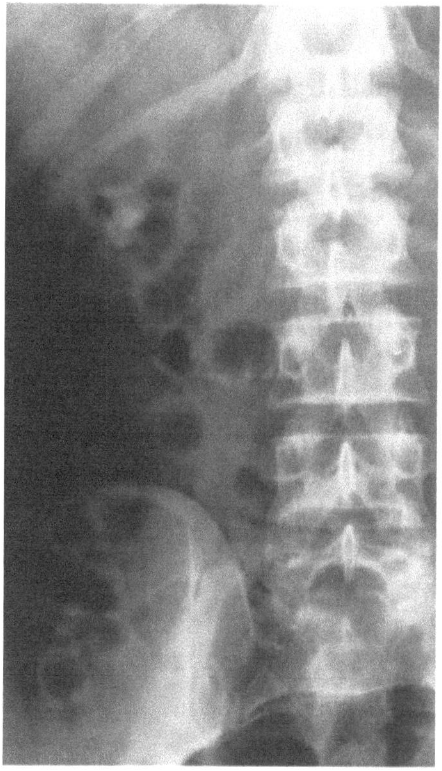
f

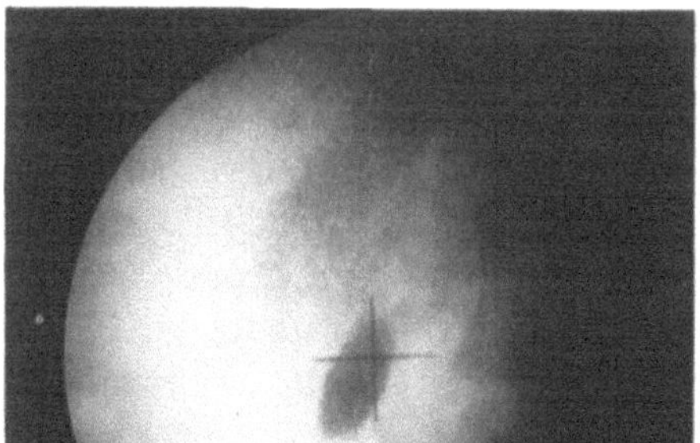
b

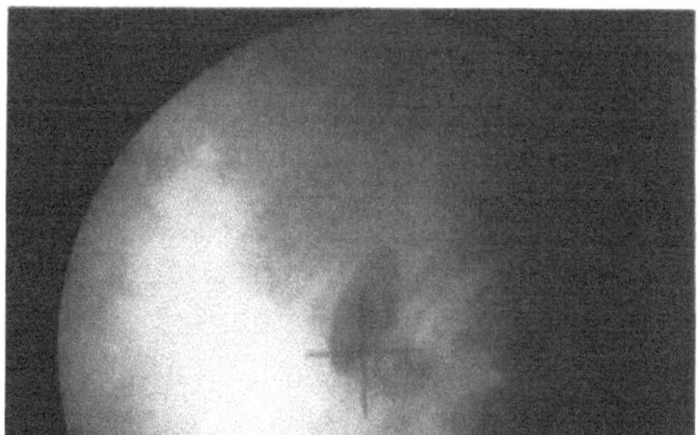
c

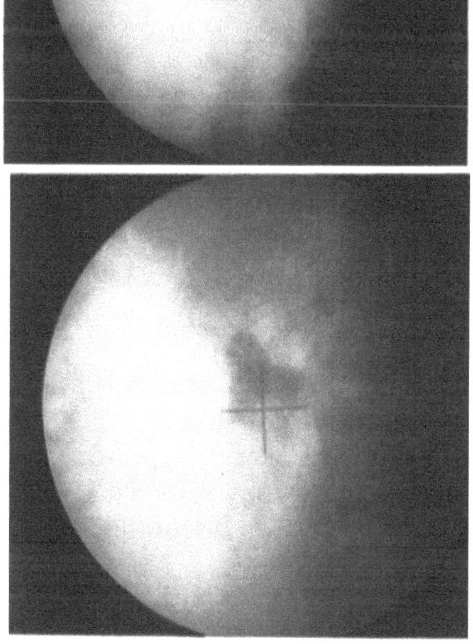

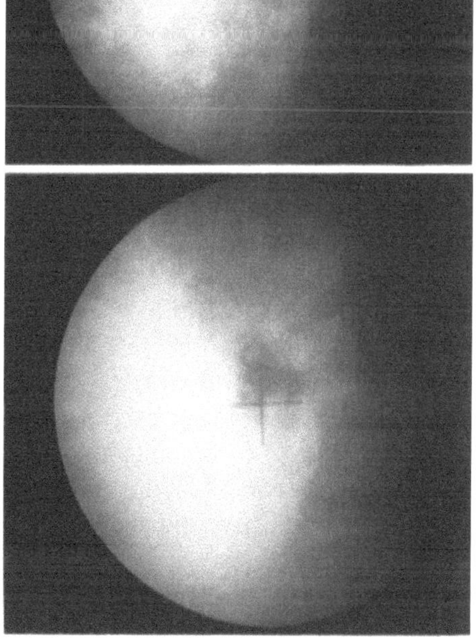

sessing the images it should be borne in mind that no appreciable acceleration of the fragments occurs when the stone is broken up. For this reason the initial effect of the shockwaves is usually evident only as a slight blurring of the previously sharply defined countour of the stone. In most cases the stone mass itself remains at the original site until the end of the session and can be recognized on the monitor as a conglomeration of numerous smaller concrements.

An average of 978 ± 34 individual pulses are required per session. The average length of treatment has been 54 ± 25 minutes, with the shortest treatment being 10 minutes and the longest 185 minutes.

X-ray exposure during therapy has amounted to 125 1 ± 53 sec, including patients with multiple stones and partial staghorn stones. After the session a KUB roentgenogram is made to ensure that the stones have been completely disintegrated.

III. Subsequent Treatment After ESWL

Treatment after ESWL is oriented along the lines of therapy for ureteric stone patients. No further medication or procedures are necessary. Once the peridural anesthesia has abated, the patient is mobilized and urged to exercise and drink plenty of fluids (2½ – 3½ l/day). In the first five days after treatment we administer 5 × 2 tablets of Eupaverin.

Surprisingly, colic is very rare during stone discharge. Thus, spasmolytic measures were necessary in only 16% of the patient collective, and intravenous analgesics had to be administered to combat severe pain in only 8%. Gradual stone discharge is monitored sonographically and radiologically, although the patient is not kept in the hospital until all of the fragments have been discharged. If there are no complaints and urinary congestion can be ruled out by sonography, follow-up care can be on an outpatient basis. In the routine use of ESWL about 35% of the patients are free of stones when they are released from the clinic, so that for many patients complete passage of the stone can proceed without clinical control.

1. Results

From February 1980 to February 1984 a total of 1140 ESWLs were performed on 1000 patients. Despite a considerable extention of the indications, which will be gone into below, the same results were achieved that were obtained initially under restrictive criteria for the use of ESWL. Thus a follow-up performed three months after treatment revealed that 90% of the patients were free of stones. In 9.3% residual concrements could be demonstrated radiologically, usually in a dilated lower calyx (Fig. 6). Since the great majority of these patients were free of complaints and infection, and the fragments appeared to be small enough for spontaneous discharge, further treatment was foregone. Only in 2% of this collective did the remaining stone fragments cause further symp-

RESULTS

free of stones	90,0 %
residual stones	9,3 %
surgery	0,7 %

IODINE 131 - HIPPURANSTUDIES

before treatment	after treatment	
	3 - 6 month	12 - 18 month
100 %	106 %	110 %

Fig. 6. Clinical results after extracorporal shockwave lithotripsy (ESWL) and follow-up test of renal function (131-iodo-Hippuran clearance). The values express function of the treated kidney as a percentage of the value before therapy

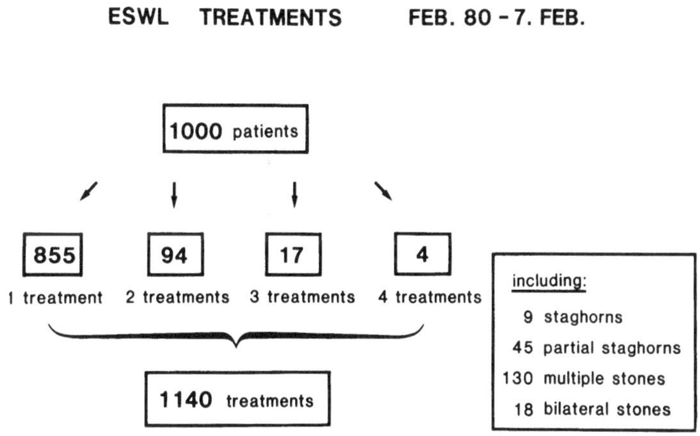

Fig. 7. Treatment and patient figures with a list of multiple treatments

toms so that a second treatment had to be carried out after three months. In all of these cases complete removal of the stones was possible so that with the inclusion of this group no stones could be radiologically detected in a total of 92% of the patients treated.

A total of seven patients had to undergo surgery following ESWL in the initial 18 months of use. In these cases insufficiently disintegrated fragments had lodged in the ureter during discharge, causing long-term obstruction. Judging retrospectively on the basis of present experience, surgery could have been avoided by means of a second ESWL.

As a consequence of the extended range of indications 12% of the patients had to undergo two to three consecutive treatments before they were completely free of stones (Fig. 7).

In patients suffering from bilateral nephrolithiasis treatment was carried out in each case in consecutive sessions so as to preclude the possibility of bilateral obstruction.

In a large portion of the staghorn and partial staghorn patients the therapeutic strategy was geared from the outset to multiple treatments so that in the first session the pelvic parts of the stone were destroyed. Four to five days later, after the fragments had been discharged, the residual concrements were exposed.

In principle, multiple stones can be successfully disintegrated during a single session, so that a considerable portion of the patients with multiple calculi were free of stones after a single treatment. Nevertheless, here too a second ESWL was carried out if the total number of individual pulses exceeded 1500, because of multiple readjustments.

2. Auxiliary Procedures

In order to attain the aforementioned success rate with a broader range of indications, auxiliary procedures to facilitate discharge of the stone were necessary in about 10% of the cases. Figure 8 shows the measures carried out in our patient collective. It can be seen that a delay in passage through the intramural section of the ureter was particularly marked in patients with a prostate adenoma. However, it proved possible in most cases to clear the prevesical section of stones by transuretheral manipulation, e.g. with a ureteroscope and sling. This was not possible in two patients, and a percutaneous nephrostomy was performed. In both cases the stones were discharged spontaneously within 14 days.

In 47 cases percutaneous nephrostomy (PN) was required following ESWL, in 80% of these cases in association with infected hydronephrosis. It was striking that in 52% of these patients a sterile urine culture was found prior to treatment.

BEFORE ESWL	
PERCUT. FISTULA	3
URETHROTOMIA INTERNA	6
TUR - PROST.	3
AFTER ESWL	
URETERAL INSTRUMENTATION	40
PERCUT. FISTULA	47

31.1.84

Fig. 8. Auxiliary procedures needed before and after ESWL

This indicates that in some cases an infection was reactivated by disintegration of the stone. In the remaining 20% the indication for PN was given by a dilation of the pyelocaliceal system due to delayed discharge of stones.

3. Renal Function

In a collective of 100 patients we undertook a study to determine the extent to which shockwave treatment leads to an impairment of renal function, using the bilateral 131-iodo-Hippuran clearance as an index (Fig. 6). It was possible to follow 50 of these patients over a period of two years. It was found that two years after treatment a significant enhancement in renal performance to 110% of the initial value had been achieved. Although this improvement is probably due to the elimination of a stone-related obstruction, it does show that impairment of renal function by shockwave therapy can be ruled out.

IV. Indications

For reasons that can well be understood, very strict criteria were applied to the selection of patients for shockwave lithotripsy at the beginning of clinical use (Chaussy 1982; Chaussy and Schmiedt 1983; Chaussy et al. 1980a, b; 1981; 1982a, b; 1983). Thus only about 20% of a nonselected collective of stone patients were accepted. However, as more experience was gained, many of the initial contraindications for ESWL (Fig. 9) were eliminated or at least moderated. The resulting extended range of indications is discussed below.

1. Infected Stones

Transient obstruction during discharge of concrement can result in pyelonephritis or even urosepsis. At first, we therefore excluded patients with infected kidney stones from shockwave treatment. It soon proved, however, that administration of antibiotics one to two days prior to treatment permits successful

1. Infected stones
2. Size > a cherry
3. High-risk patients
4. Ureter stones
5. Obstruction
6. Translucent stones

Fig. 9. Initial contraindications to ESWL (1980)

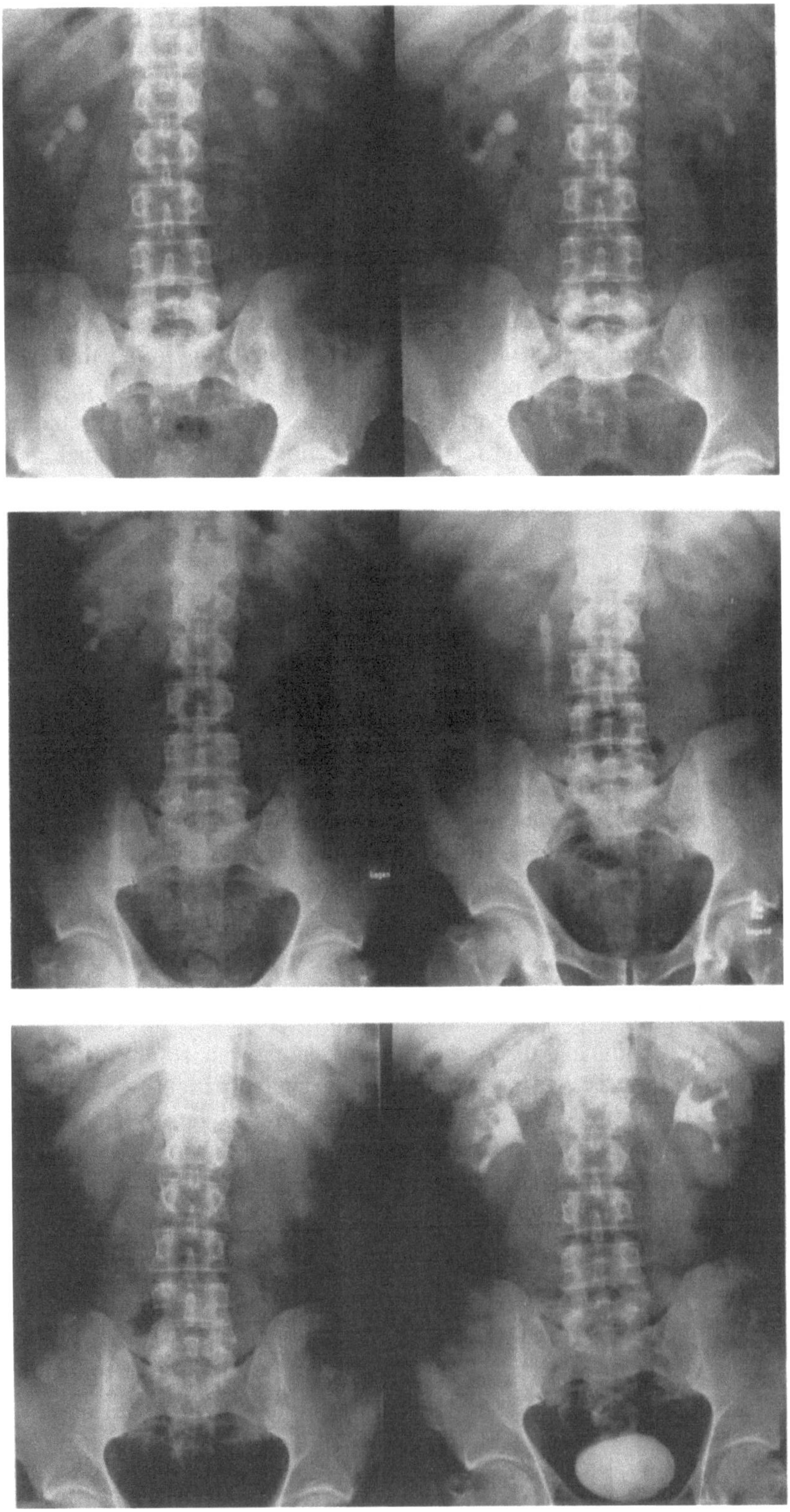

a

b

c

Fig. 10

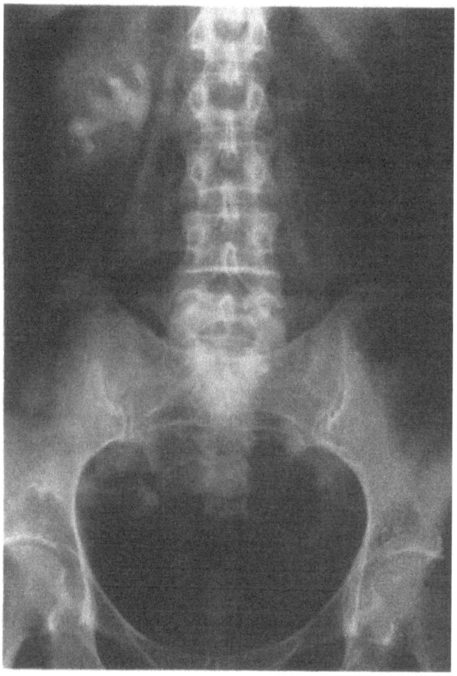
a

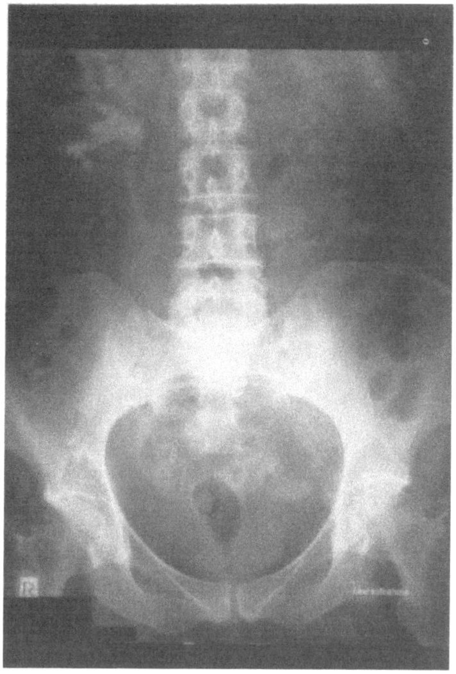
b

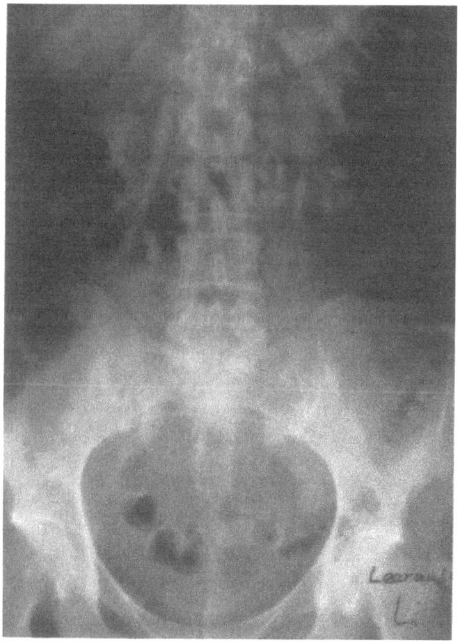
c

Fig. 11. **a** KUB roentgenogram of a total staghorn stone before treatment. **b** Immediately after treatment with discharge of concrements beginning in the proximal ureter. **c** Roentgenogram taken after seven days shows absence of stones

Fig. 10. **a** *Left:* Bilateral lithiasis before treatment. *Right:* Situation after ESWL on the left side with the pyelocaliceal system filled with debris. **b** *Left:* Elimination of stones on left side, situation after ESWL on the right side. *Right:* Ureteral "stone street" on left side two days after treatment. **c** *Left:* Situation after discharge of all stone particles. *Right:* Unhindered drainage in the subsequent infusion urogram

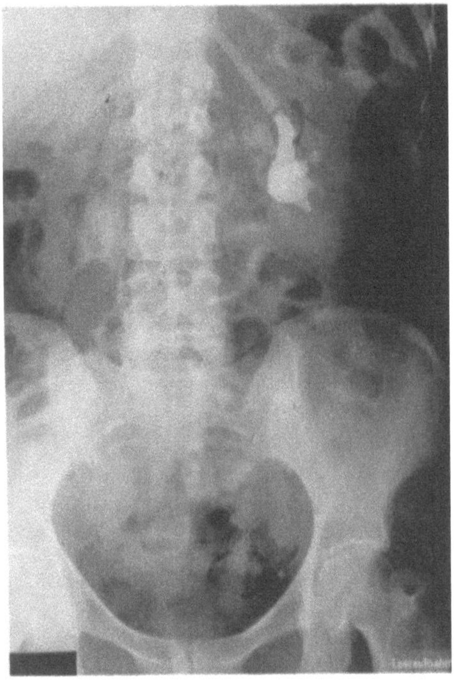
a

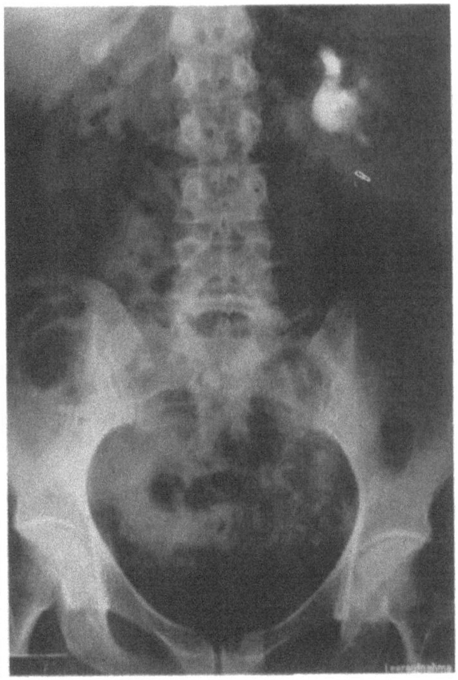
b

Fig. 12. **a** Left staghorn stone before treatment. **b** Situation after ESWL of the lower calyx group. **c** Roentgenogram during percutaneous litholapaxy of the stone part located in the renal pelvis. **d** Situation after ESWL of residual caliceal concrement with nephrostomy performed. **e** Absence of stones following removal of the nephrostomy

therapy without complications – even in cases of infected stones. In addition, it was found in a few cases that through the simple insertion of a 9-French nephrostomy tube it was possible to await the unhindered, uncomplicated passage of the fragmented concrements. Thus the presence of urinary-tract infection no longer constitutes a reason for excluding a patient from ESWL.

2. Stone Size

Since theoretically the transport of even the smallest particles, represents a quantitative problem, we initially accepted only concrements of approximately cherry size. Once experience had shown that stone discharge presented no substantial difficulty, even in the case of sizable concrements, we began accepting calculi for ESWL ranging up to partial staghorn stones. It was also found that treatment in multiple sessions could in some indications eliminate such stones without risk (Figs. 10a–c).

Initial experience in urgent medical indications (Multiple prior operations) with the treatment of total staghorn stones has shown that it is also sometimes

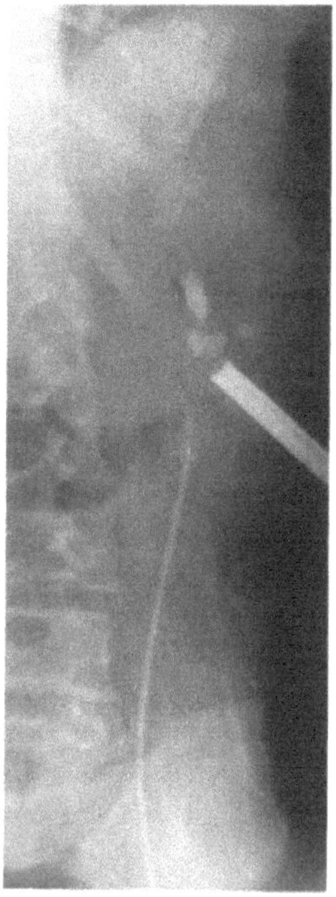
c

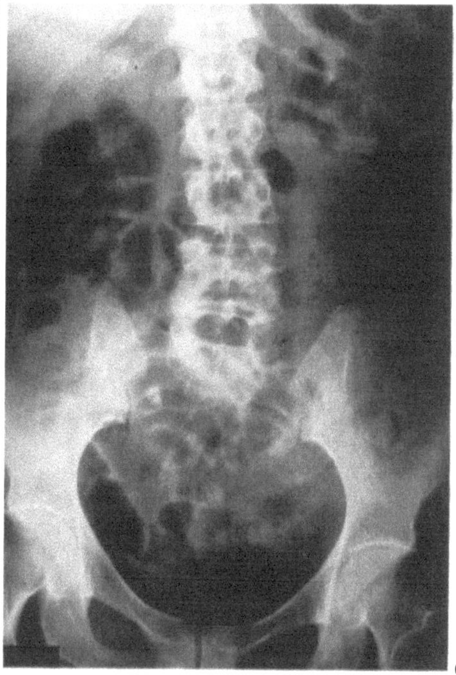
d

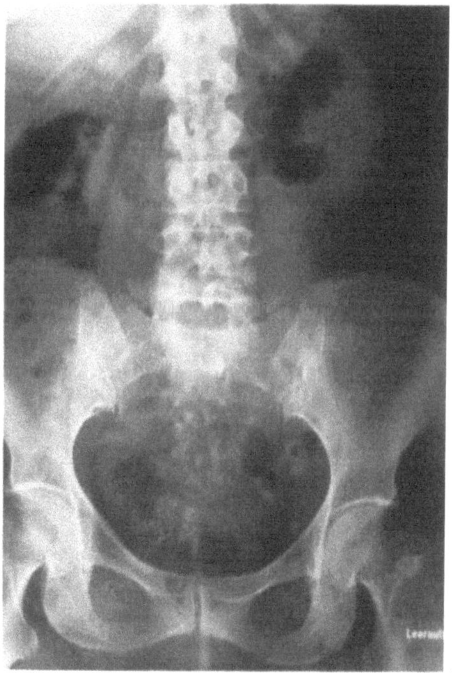
e

Fig. 12c–e

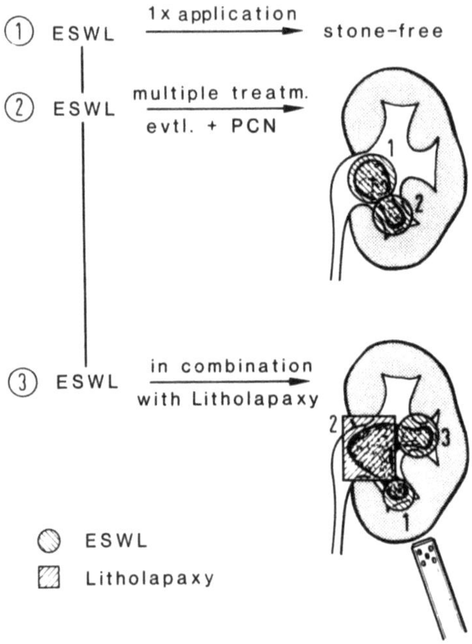

Fig. 13. Strategy for the treatment of partial staghorn stones

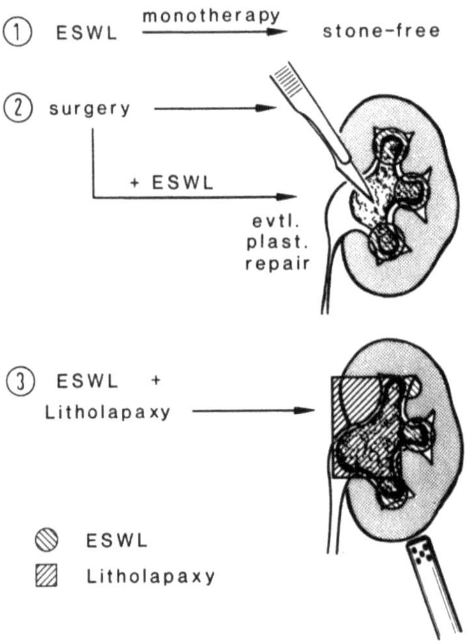

Fig. 14. Strategy for the treatment of total staghorn stones

possible to treat staghorn stones by a combination of lithotripsy and percutaneous nephrostomy and, in some cases, litholapaxy (Figs. 11a–c, 12a–e).

In the following the strategy for the treatment of partial and total staghorn stones will be elaborated.

Whereas for simple staghorn calculi a single therapeutic session generally suffices to disintegrate the stone completely, in the case of more voluminous stones the therapeutic goal may be attained by means of fractionated therapy (Fig. 13). Usually the portions of the stone in or near the renal pelvis are first exposed. After a period of about three to five days, in which a considerable part of the disintegrated concrements are discharged, the remaining caliceal portion of the stone is treated in a second session.

Another alternative, which, however, is seldom used for partial staghorn stones, is to establish a percutaneous nephrostomy after initial disintegration of the lower caliceal portion. The voluminous pelvic portion can then be removed by percutaneous litholapaxy and any residual caliceal fragments by subsequent shockwave therapy.

Similar strategies are applied to total staghorn stones (Fig. 14). In addition to the possibility of removing total staghorn stones by single and multiple-session ESWL the possibility should be mentioned of eliminating residual stones postoperatively by means of shockwave treatment. In cases where a lithotripter is available this approach permits elimination of the total staghorn stone without causing undue trauma to the parenchyma and makes multiple nephrotomies for the removal of poorly accessible caliceal portions superfluous.

We are making increasing use of the approach in which the stone is treated in several sessions with the alternating application of ESWL and percutaneous litholapaxy (Figs. 12a–e).

3. High-Risk Patients

Although in the initial clinical phase reserve was understandably excercized with regard to the acceptance of high-risk patients, it was patently clear from the nature of such cases that a noninvasive method of stone removal is especially desirable. Owing to cardiovascular changes which occur during immersion into and emersion from the water bath, complicated anesthesiologic monitoring is required under intubation anesthesia. In accordance with this postulate an increasing number of patients who are considered at risk or inoperable could be treated.

Routine sonographic follow-up examinations revealed a perirenal hematoma in six patients. It is therefore advisable to perform a global check of the coagulation values before treatment and to exercise reserve in the indication of ESWL if any abnormalities of coagulation are found.

4. Ureteric-Stone Patients

At the beginning we had four ureteric-stone patients who had to undergo surgery after unsuccessful shockwave therapy. Their histories showed that the

ESWL FOR URETERAL CALCULI FEB. 80 - 31. JAN. 84

	PATIENT	SURGERY REQUIRED	SUCCESSFUL
1980	2	2	-
1982	25	-	25
1983	73	2	71
	100	4	96

Fig. 15. Statistical breakdown of the results obtained to date in the treatment of ureteric stones

stone had been located at the same site for several months. On operating we found in all of these cases that the stones had been broken up but were embedded in a sheath of tissue, probably as a result of inflammation, and that the individual stone fragments could not free themselves from the packed configuration for spontaneous discharge.

Realizing that this constellation, which is not amenable to treatment by ESWL, occurs after the stone has been located in the ureter over an extended period, we subsequently accepted ureteric-stone patients in whom the stone had entered the ureter no more than six weeks previously. Figure 15 shows the current results in the treatment of ureteric stones. They indicate that the treatment of ureteric-stone patients is also possible, provided that this time factor is taken into consideration. However, it must be emphasized that this pertains only to stones in the upper two thirds of the ureter, since treatment of the stone below the iliac crest is not possible owing to the arrangement of the apparatus and the location of the stone within the bony pelvis.

Figure 16 is a schematic representation of the current strategy for the treatment of ureteric stones. It should be mentioned that in acutely infected cases the urinary congestion is first relieved by a percutaneous nephrostomy and the pyelonephritis is treated with antibiotics. Only then, usually about one week later, is ESWL performed. If fragmentation is successful, complete elimination of stones can generally be achieved within two to three days. Figures 17a + b show a typical example.

5. Obstruction and Noncontrastive Stones

Once it was established that stones having insufficient contrast density can be localized and treated after administration of contrast medium, obstruction distal to the stone constitutes the only remaining clear contraindication to ESWL (Fig. 18). In the majority of these cases we are also of the conviction that surgical stone removal and concurrent plastic correction represents the optimum therapy today, not least of all as a causal therapy to prevent further stone growth.

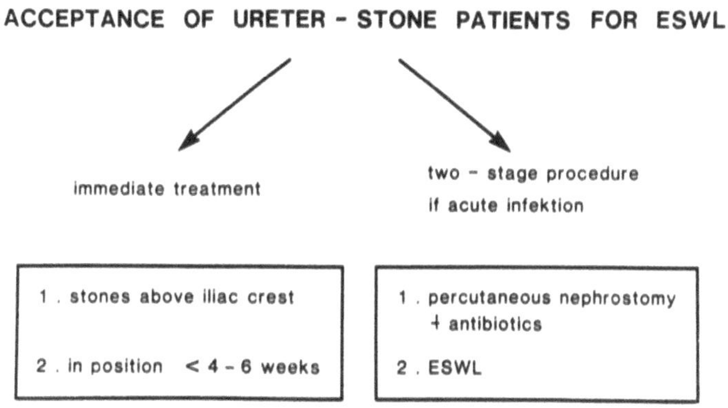

Fig. 16. Strategy for the treatment of ureteric stones

a 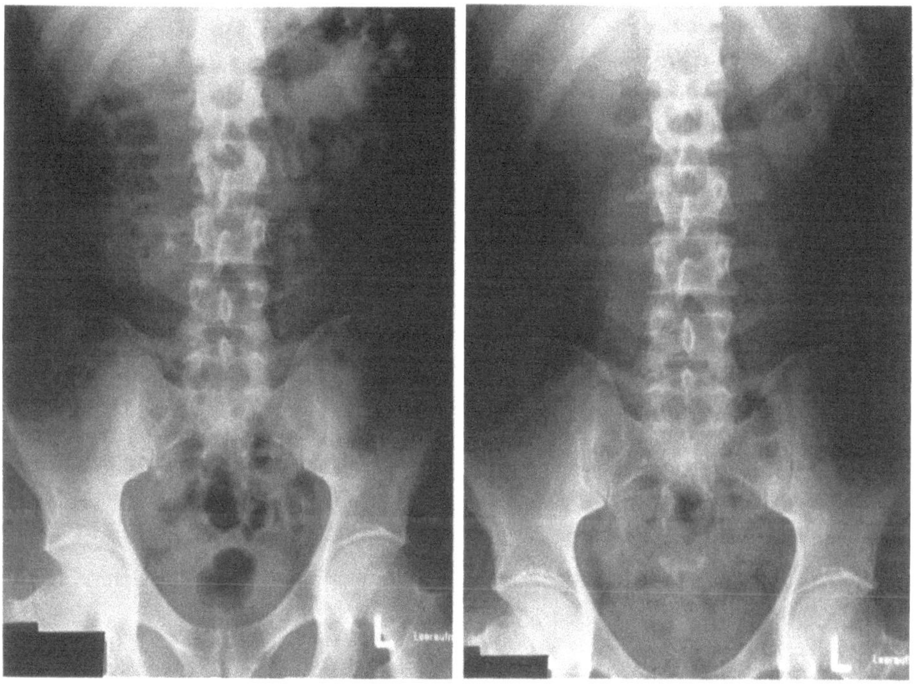 b

Fig. 17 a, b. Radiologic follow-up of a ureteric stone after ESWL. **a** Ureteric stone on right side before treatment. **b** Three days after treatment without residual concrements

However, we have on occasion deviated from this established guideline. In several cases of multiple prior operations due to malignant stone growth, in which the risk of nephrectomy was assessed to be high, it has been possible to aspire the fragments resulting from ESWL through a percutaneous nephrostomy. Although this procedure makes it possible to use ESWL in some cases, it is not recommended as a primary therapeutic technique in cases of obstruction.

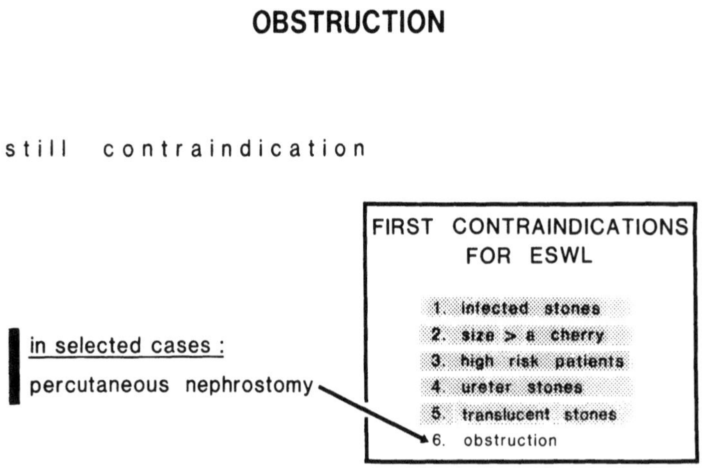

Fig. 18. The initial exclusion criteria. Contraindications 1–5 have meanwhile been eliminated

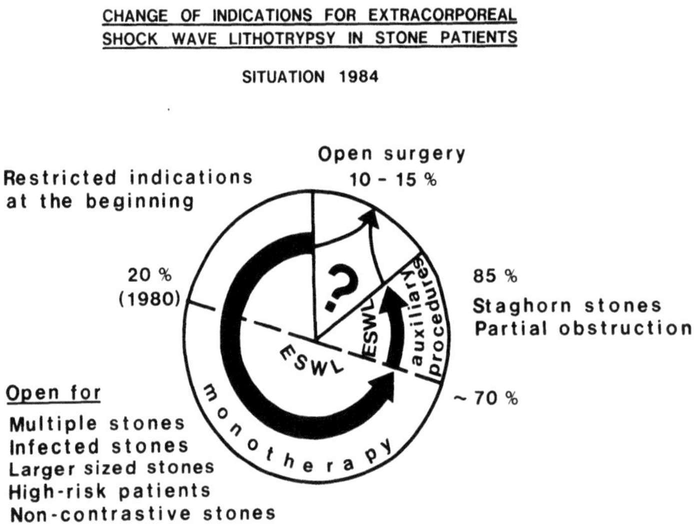

Fig. 19. Percentage of nonsurgically treatable stone patients including combined approaches with percutaneous nephrostomy and litholapaxy

V. Conclusion

Since the results presented here have meanwhile been reproduced at nine other ESWL centers, it may be assumed that as ESWL gains wider currency it will necessitate a fundamental change in current therapeutic guidelines – and this for a steadily increasing list of indications.

Whereas in the initial phase of clinical use only about 20% of no nonselected patient collective were eligible for ESWL, today about 70% of stone patients could be treated noninvasively by ESWL alone (Fig. 19). Taking into consideration the extended range of indications provided by the combination of ESWL with percutaneous nephrostomy and litholapaxy, no more than 10–15% of stone patients will have to undergo surgery in the future. This also means that the "endourologic techniques" will retain their importance, although in a reduced scope, and that only skill in all the methods of stone removal can ensure optimal therapy.

On the basis of present experience with the current range of indications for ESWL and the possibilities of extending its scope of applications by combining it with auxiliary semi-invasive techniques, a trend to centralize this therapeutic method so as to justify the expense for the sophisticated equipment is emerging. This demands the acceptance of unavoidable changes in the treatment of nephrolithiasis and should lead to a reconsideration of current organizational forms and educational concepts. Urologists should bear in mind that other medical disciplines would be only too happy to relieve us of these problems.

References

Alken P, Hutschenreiter G, Günther R, Marberger M (1981) Percutaneous stone manipulation. J Urol 125:463

Chaussy Ch (ed) (1982) Extracorporeal shock wave lithotripsy. New aspects in the treatment of kidney stone disease. Karger, Basel Munich New York

Chaussy Ch, Schmiedt E (1983) Shock wave treatment for stones in the upper urinary tract. Urol Clin North Am 10:743

Chaussy Ch, Eisenberger F, Wanner K, Forssmann B, Hepp W, Schmiedt E, Brendel W (1976) The use of shock waves for the destruction of renal calculi without direct contact. Urol Res 4:175

Chaussy Ch, Eisenberger F, Wanner K (1977) Die Implantation humaner Nierensteine – ein einfaches experimentelles Steinmodell. Urologe [Ausg A] 16:35

Chaussy Ch, Eisenberger F, Wanner K, Forssmann B (1978a) Extracorporale Anwendung von hochenergetischen Stoßwellen. Ein neuer Aspekt in der Behandlung des Harnsteinleidens. Akt Urol 9:95

Chaussy Ch, Wieland W, Jocham D, Eisenberger F, Forssmann B (1978b) Röntgenologische Steinortung im System der berührungsfreien Nierensteinzertrümmerung. Verh Dtsch Ges Urol 30:333

Chaussy Ch, Schmiedt E, Forssmann B, Brendel W (1979) Contact-free renal stone destruction by means of shock waves. Eur Surg Res 11:36

Chaussy Ch, Brendel W, Schmiedt E (1980a) Extracorporeally induced destruction of kidney stones by shock waves. Lancet II:1265

Chaussy Ch, Forssmann B, Brendel W, Jocham D, Eisenberger F, Hepp W, Gogge JM (1980b) Berührungsfreie Nierensteinzertrümmerung durch extracorporal erzeugte fokussierte Stoßwellen. In: Chaussy Ch, Staehler G (eds) Beiträge zur Urologie. Karger, Basel München

Chaussy Ch, Schmiedt E, Jocham D, Brendel W, Forssmann B, Moser E (1981) Berührungsfreie Nierensteinzertrümmerung durch Stoßwellen. Dtsch Ärztebl 18:881

Chaussy Ch, Schmiedt E, Jocham D, Brendel W, Forssmann B (1982b) First clinical experience with extracorporeally induced destruction of kidney stones by shock waves. J Urol 127:414

Chaussy Ch, Schmiedt E, Jocham D, Forssmann B, Brendel W, Walther V (1982a) Therapiemöglichkeiten des Harnsteinleidens mit extracoroporal erzeugten Stoßwellen. In: Pathogenese und Klinik des Harnsteines, Vol 8, Fortschritte der Urologie und Nephrologie. Steinkopff, Darmstadt

Chaussy Ch, Schmiedt E, Jocham D (1983) Nonsurgical treatment of renal calculi with shock waves. In: Roth RA, Finlayson B (eds) Stones – clinical management of urolithiasis. Williams and Wilkins, Baltimore, London

Eisenberger F, Schmiedt E, Chaussy Ch, Wanner K, Forssmann B, Hepp W (1977a) Aspekte zum derzeitigen Stand der berührungsfreien Harnsteinzertrümmerung. Dtsch Ärztebl 17:1145

Forssmann B, Hepp W, Chaussy Ch, Eisenberger F, Wanner K (1977) Eine Methode zur berührungsfreien Zertrümmerung von Nierensteinen durch Stoßwellen. Biomed Tech (Berlin) 22:164

Eisenberger F, Chaussy Ch, Wanner K (1977b) Extracorporale Anwendung von hochenergetischen Stoßwellen – Ein neuer Aspekt in der Behandlung des Harnsteinleidens. Akt Urol 8:3

Preventive Measures

H.-J. Schneider

I. The Role of Prevention in the Management of Urolithiasis

Modern *diagnostic aids* have nowadays rendered the detection of urinary calculi a fairly simple affair. This is true not only of actual detection but equally of the localization of calculi within the urinary tract and of the elucidation of their structure and chemical composition. Understanding the causation of such calculi may present considerably greater difficulties. Metabolic studies and dynamic loading tests of ever increasing specificity, together with determinations of crystallizing activity and of urodynamic parameters contribute day by day to the list of etiologic factors and relationships documented in connection with urolithiasis. It is upon this fund of knowledge that our attempts at treatment and prevention of urolithogenesis are essentially based.

Treatment is no longer limited to surgery. Although over one third of all urinary stones continue to be removed at operation, there is ever increasing scope for endoscopic and pharmacologic maneuvers (Table 1).

Recurrence prevention, socalled *metaphylaxis,* is also a field of expanding importance. If one succeeds in eliminating, or at any rate modifying, factors causal to stone formation, dramatic reductions in recurrence rate may be achieved (Table 2).

One well tested strategy for preventing recurrence is the institution of stone clinics at community level. These latter provide a link between research, clinical practice and prevention (Hoffmann et al. 1979; Hosking et al. 1983; Kal-

Table 1. The treatment of urolithiasis

1. Treat ureteric colic	
2. Promote expulsion of calculus	
3. Surgery:	– lithotomy – correct lithogenic tract abnormalities
4. Endoscopic maneuvers:	– percutaneous endoscopic nephrolithotomy – extract ureteric calculi by Zeiss loop – mechanical, electrohydraulic or ultrasound litholapaxy
5. Chemical litholysis:	– oral medication – locally by instrumentation
6. Extracorporeal shockwave lithotripsy	
7. Treat urinary tract infections	

Table 2. Factors involved in comprehensive metaphylaxis

1.	Way of life in general
2.	Occupation
3.	Health education and patient compliance
4.	Psychological attitude and councilling
5.	Practical techniques (measurement of urinary pH and specific gravity etc.)
6.	Diet
7.	Rest cures
8.	Drug treatment

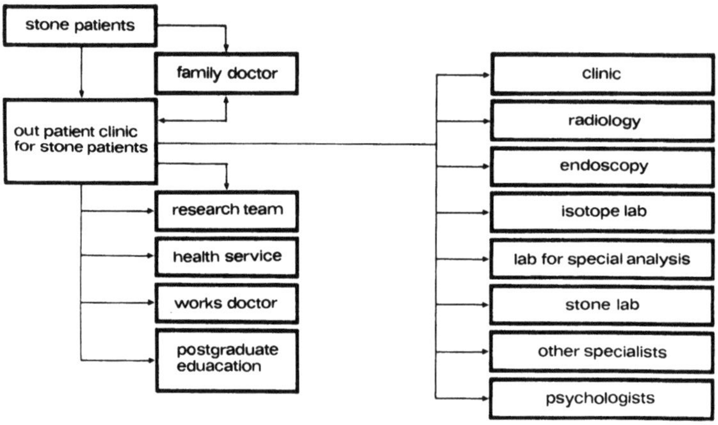

Fig. 1. The position of community stone clinic consultations within the framework of urolithiasis treatment (SCHNEIDER 1979)

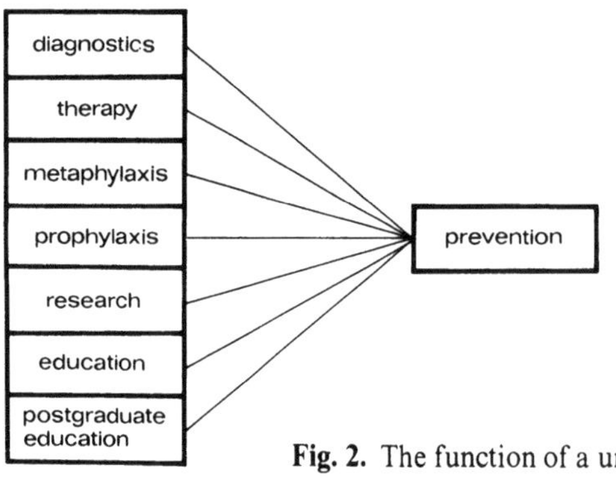

Fig. 2. The function of a urolithiasis outpatient unit (SCHNEIDER 1979)

LISTRATOS 1975; KARCHER 1962; OTTO-UNGER and MISSELWITZ 1978; OTTO-UNGER 1972; PEACOCK 1984; RUGENDORF 1975; SCHEWZOW et al. 1972; SCHNEIDER 1972a, b; SCHNEIDER 1974a, b; SCHNEIDER and HIENZSCH 1974; SCHNEIDER et al. 1969; SCHUBERT and SCHMECHEL 1975; SCHUELKE and SOPART 1980; TOTH 1976; ZECHNER 1981).

The overall import and role of a modern urolithiasis clinic is set out in Fig. 1 and 2. (SCHNEIDER 1979).

Fig. 3. Number of people at whom treatment, metaphylaxis and prevention are aimed in the GDR

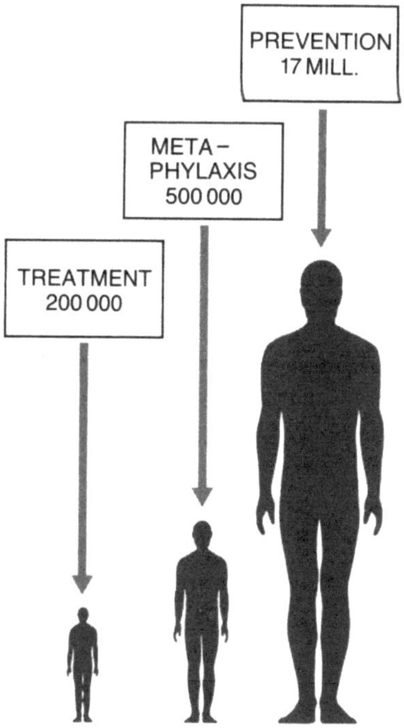

Despite remarkable advances in diagnosis, treatment and metaphylaxis, numerous countries throughout the world continue to experience an increasing incidence of urolithiasis. The function of *true prophylaxis* might be deemed to lie in protecting a healthy population from attack, in other words in reducing the frequency of new cases. According to DAHM and SCHORR (1980) prevention in the wider sense includes both the protection of those at risk and the avoidance of risk factors by those not, a priori, at risk. Such a strategy therefore includes a host of measures aimed at encouraging and maintaining high standards of health, at discouraging unhealthy practices and at recognizing and counteracting morbidity in its earliest manifestations. The constitution of the WHO defines health as a condition of complete physical, mental and social wellbeing (RENKER and PRESBER 1980).

The prevention of urolithiasis is still in its infancy. Initially it seemed that preventive measures would have to be aimed at entire populations. Since this is logistically impossible, a degree of selectivity soon becomes unavoidable. People at risk must be identified and arrangements made for their catchment, as well as for their protection from risk situations and risk factors. Figure 3 gives a quantitative idea of the numbers of people at whom treatment, metaphylaxis and prevention of urinary stones are aimed in the GDR (SCHNEIDER 1974b).

II. Risk Factors and Persons at Risk

1. Nutrition

As the standard of living and the consumption of luxury goods have risen throughout most European countries and the USA, so there has at the same time been a decrease in the general amount of exercise taken. A simultaneous increase in the incidence of urolithiasis may be connected with these factors. The same might be said of metabolic disorders, such as gout and diabetes, or of a general gain in average body weight. Many stone patients are obese, the mean weight excess among our own patients with uric acid stones being in the region of 14 kg (SCHNEIDER 1978). HORN et al. (1980) report a figure of 15.7 kg. 83% of 149 stone patients with a mean age of 52 years were overweight (by more than 10% of the Brocca index) and 62% were obese. Obesity and its related metabolic disorders should be regarded as risk factors for urolithiasis. According to HORN et al. (1980) 30–40% of the population in the GDR are obese. One very large group of people is thus defined, to whom preventive measures could be applied. Despite an increasing level of individual health concern among the population at large (HUETTNER 1979, 1976; HUETTNER et al. 1971) only little notice is taken of medical views on health education by those who enjoy good health. This is especially true of the obese and of the stone patients among them. Despite patient admonishment and continuing care the majority of these persons is quite unprepared to reduce their degree of overweight. Among the clinic group of HORN et al. (1980) 23% of 124 overweight stone patients continued to gain weight, 37% maintained their weight and only 40% had managed, three years later, to reduce their weight by a paltry average of 1.8 kg. Other outpatient units have reported similar depressing experiences, which should not, however, discourage one from continuing to attempt an overall modification of popular behavior. Such a strategy needs to be adhered to both in the consulting room and over the mass media, beginning at school age.

ROBERTSON et al. (1978, 1982) have termed urolithiasis a disease of plenty. In England urolithiasis is commonest in areas and among social strata with the highest expenditure on food. This finding is mirrored in the fact that the frequency of stone formation in Germany was at its lowest during war years and in their immediate aftermath (SCHUMANN 1963). A definite relationship has been established between the ingestion af animal protein and the excretion of uric acid (ZOELLNER 1976). ZECHNER (1981 a) is also of the opinion that an increasing financial outlay on food goes hand in hand with a rising rate of stone formation.

A study of 379 patients with stones revealed a significant increase in calcium-, phosphate- and uric excretion at low urinary pH among those persons of the highest income (ZECHNER 1981 b).

With increasing protein intake there is a rise in the urinary excretion of calcium by up to 23%, of oxalic acid by up to 24% and of uric acid by as much as 48% (ROBERTSON et al. 1979). Recurrent stone disease sufferers had a significantly higher overall animal protein intake than did stone free control subjects. By the same token the risk of calculus formation among vegetarians amounts to only 40 – 60% of that experienced by an age-, sex- and social class matched standard population (ROBERTSON et al. 1981, 1982).

The currently popular emphasis on animal protein as an answer to general overeating is thus quite inappropriate in terms of urolithiasis prevention. The correct solution lies in a balanced diet of just adequate energy content. In England, as elsewhere, foodstuffs of animal protein are becoming ever more expensive, and their consumption is decreasing. In this context ROBERTSON et al. (1979) have noted a steady decrease over the past five years in the number of patients admitted to hospital with an episode of stone disease. GROEBNER and ZOELLNER (1977) have suggested that persons with familial hyperuricemia or with gout should restrict their daily protein intake to 1 g/kg body weight. Studies by ZECHNER et al. (1981) also confirmed alcohol as a risk factor for urolithiasis. Among their 379 subjects urinary calcium and phospate excretion, serum uric acid and rate of stone formation increased with rising alcohol intake.

Whilst English vegetarians have an abnormally low frequency of stones, unbalanced vegetarian diets may have a negative effect on stone disease. Thus the urinary pH and uric acid saturation capacity are both considerably lower on a pure wheat diet than they are on a rice-based one (ANASUYA and RAO 1973). On the other hand, the high frequency of bladder calculi among village children in Thailand has been put down to the imbalance and inadequacy of their predominantly rice-based nutrition (BROCKIS et al. 1981; HALSTEDT and VALYASEVI 1972). The single most impressive prophylactic measure was a diet improved by introducing milk and increasing dietary phosphate. Food purine has only a minimal effect on uric acid excretion (ZOELLNER 1976), but the reverse is true of urinary calcium and oxalate; individuals at risk should avoid excesses of food rich in the latter substances (HESSE et al. 1982). Stone formers fed on 1.5 kg/day of spinach produced large whewellite conglomerates and microliths in a mainly crystalline urinary sediment, whilst control subjects on the same diet had only numerous small individual crystals (BERG et al. 1975). The prodigious intake of iced tea and fruit juices customary in the southern United States is also liable to increase urinary oxalate excretion (THOMAS and MALAGODI 1977; ARORA et al. 1984; FELLSTROEM et al. 1983; ROBERTSON and PEACOCK 1982). On the other hand the studies of CHURCHILL et al. (1984) suggest that tea drinking as such is not a risk factor for urolithiasis.

Because the rate of stone formation is considerably lower in dilute than in concentrated urine, attempts to increase diuresis take pride of place in any stone prevention strategy. In one study of 309 patients 12% gave a history of dehydration of various cause preceding their first episode of colic. 30% reported working conditions inimical to an adequate fluid intake (FUSS et al. 1979). One quarter of subjects drank less than 1 l/day and the histories of over 20% revealed inadequate physical activity. Ideally, fluid intake should be enough to guarantee a specific gravity of 1015 or less in the nocturnal urine. Such a regime poses considerable difficulties for some people, especially women and children. They need to become accustomed to drinking a wider variety of fluids and to having soup at mealtimes (SCHNEIDER 1973). For children OTTO-UNGER and MISSELWITZ (1979) have suggested the daily fluid intakes given in Table 3.

Table 3. Recommended daily fluid intake for children at risk of urolithiasis

Infants	800–1000 ml
Toddlers	1000–1500 ml
Playschool	1500–1800 ml
Schoolchildren	1800–2500 ml

The hardness of drinking water is not a risk factor. There is no, or at best an inverse, correlation with the frequency of stones (DONALDSON et al. 1979; SIERAKOWSKY et al. 1979). No scientific basis thus exists for recommending stone formers in areas with a hard supply to drink spa waters or rain water, any more than there does for recommending avoidance of fluorinated drinking water to prevent to the occurrence of phosphatic calculi (KOCVARA et al. 1982). There is an above average frequency of association between soft magnesium rich water and a raised regional stone prevalence (ILLIEVSKI and ILLIEVSKI 1984).

Water with a measurable magnesium content (eg. sea water) has, by contrast, been shown to have some prophylactic effect (SCHNEIDER and HORN 1968).

Various drinks and mineral waters exert specific effects on urine composition and pH (KLINGENBERG 1972; KOLLWITZ 1966). The acidifying action of certain spa waters and of "Pils" and "Kölsch" brands of beer is beneficial in cases of chronic urinary tract infection by urease positive organisms. Gout patients should exploit the alkalinizing action of orange juice and stout. Apple juice, raspberry and grape juices are without significant effect on urinary pH, whilst blackberry juice is mildly acidifying.

Both the quantity and the composition of daily diet may thus be seen to exert a powerful modifying effect on urine composition and consequently on stone formation (BACH 1982). Although inappropriate nutrition is a promotor of stone disease, it should not, however, be regarded as an initiator (SCHNEIDER and ALBERT 1967; SCHNEIDER and HIENSCH 1969). The principal role of nutritional measures is not in treatment but in prevention (HAENEL 1972). Whilst the urologist generally tends to underestimate the influence of diet on the course of urolithiasis, general practitioner, physician and patient alike may attach undue importance to it (ZIELINSKI 1972).

A comprehensive stone prevention program must include public education (aimed particularly at high risk groups) on sensible dietary habits and the avoidance of excess calory intake or nutritional imbalance (SCHOLZ et al. 1981). High risk groups comprise chiefly the obese, persons suffering from metabolic disorders, those with inadequate physical activity and individuals with a strong family history.

A high standard of public information might be hoped to lead people at large to recognise and accept a scientifically sound cuisine. Such a change in popular attitudes is fundamental to proper general nutrition and thus to the prevention of urolithiasis (RAPOPORT 1969).

2. Metabolic Disorders

Increased urinary elimination of uric acid may result in the formation not only of uric acid calculi, but also of calcium oxalate stones. It is for this reason that all gout patients, all those receiving cytotoxic therapy, diabetics, the obese and all persons exposed to environmental stress must be considered at risk. Cytotoxics should never be administered without regular serum uric acid estimations, and the latter are of equal importance during uricosuric therapy for gout. Since patients with calcium oxalate calculi include a greater proportion of latent hyperuricemics than does the general population, high risk subjects with normal serum uric acid levels should be subjected to a uric acid tolerance test (HESSE et al. 1980; OHLENSCHLAEGER and ULRICH 1976).

One third of all gout patients have uric acid lithiasis, and uric acid stones are approximately 100 times as common among these people as among persons with normal metabolism. The prevalence increases with rising uric acid levels (SINGER 1976). By contrast CURRIE and TURMER (1979) found uric acid stones in only 6% of their 604 gout patients. In this context the work of CIFUENTES DELATTE et al. (1973) is of more than passing interest. Their findings in 835 subjects with gout are summarised in Table 4.

Stone formation due to increased uric acid excretion should be combatted by an increased diuresis, by neutralizing an acid urine and by the administration of a xanthine oxidase inhibitor. Special attention must be paid to ensuring adequate dilution of nocturnal urine. Diabetics may form stones either because of an associated disorder of uric acid metabolism or as a consequence of chronic urinary tract infection. Depending on the cause they will therefore develop either uric acid stones or socalled infective calculi. In more recent years there have been sporadic reports of 2,8-dihyroxyadenine calculi, which tend to behave similarly to uric acid stones. JOOST et al. (1981) were able to demonstrate that these stones are due to a total deficiency of phophoribosyl transferase.

Table 4. Relationship between gout and uric acid lithiasis (n = 835) (CIFUENTES DELATTE et al. 1973)

	Normouricemia with uric ac. stones (n = 204)	Hyperuricemia with uric ac. stones (n = 76)	Gout with uric ac. stones (n = 160)	Gout without uric ac. stones (n = 478)
First attack of colic over 40 years before	38	38	34	–
More than ten episodes	30	30	42	–
High purine diet	65	72	68	70
Family history of urolithiasis	33	41	42	18
Family history of gout	8	10	42	29
Obesity	69	39	80	67
Diabetes	6	4	7	5

Hereditary renal hypouricemia due to an isolated renal tubular transport defect is a rare disorder associated with urinary stones. SPERLING (1984) has so far documented 7 families affected by this inborn error of metabolism.

Cystinuria is an inborn error of metabolism frequently complicated by and often presenting as urolithiasis. 83% of the patients (n = 255) in the series reported by KRIZEK (1981, 1983) had formed cystine stones.

Every attempt should be made to diagnose the condition prior to stone formation and to prevent the latter. In Czechoslovakia there is approximately one cystinuric per 75,000 population (KRIZEK 1981), in England one per 20,000, in Sweden one per 10,000 (WILLIAMS et al. 1980), in Japan one per 8,000 (HARUO ITO 1983). Only 10–15% of these patients reaches the seventh decade of life without an episode of stone disease. Initial screening must concentrate on children and extend to the adult relatives of proven cases. KRIZEK and VENDL (1978) have coined the term "active biochemical and genetic genealogy". The highest likelihood of finding further cystinurics will be among members of the same generation (siblings) (KUEKN and SCHORSCH 1981).

The WHO screening procedure is only recommended for metabolic disease occurring more commonly than 1 in 10,000 of the population. Nevertheless, the high complication rate due to urinary calculi and the extreme effectiveness of prophylaxis may justify whole population screening for cystinuria in countries where it is rarer. Suitable methods include simple spot testing in well baby clinics, using the nitroprusside reaction (MAASER et al. 1972) or the urocystine color reaction described by KALLISTRATOS et al. (1977) and by KINOSHITA et al. (1979). What is ideally required is a simple napkin or dipstick test. If any of these techniques gives a positive result, a formal quantitative urinary amino acid estimation should be ordered. Although the occurrence of typical cystine crystals is definite evidence of cystinuria, they occur in only one third of cystinurics and are not related to urine specific gravity (ALKEN and SCHAEFER 1978).

Familial xanthinuria with xanthine lithiasis is an exceptionally rare finding (CIFUENTES DELATTE and CASTRO-MENDOZA 1967; CASTRO-MENDOZA et al. 1972; CASTELLO et al. 1984), as is the induction of xanthine stones during allopurinol therapy (GREEN et al. 1969; LANDGREBE et al. 1975). In cases of normoxanthinuria purine restriction and urine alkalinization will be of no avail. Relatives of xanthinurics should merely be recommended to ensure a dilute urine by taking plentiful fluids (HARTUNG and LESKOVAR 1980). More specific preventive measures are seldom needed.

Two children with LESCH-NYHAN syndrome and xanthine lithiasis have been reported by BROCK et al. (1983).

75% of all uroliths consist of calcium oxalate. Urinary oxalate concentration represents the principal risk factor in affected persons (ACHILLES et al. 1977; WILLIAMS 1976). *Primary congenital hyperoxaluria* is extremely uncommon, and in such cases the only recommended prophylaxis against stone formation consists of high doses of vitamins B1 and B6 together with magnesium preparations and hydrochlorothiazide (CONSTABLE et al. 1978; HARRISON and ROSE 1978; LEUMANN et al. 1978; ROSE et al. 1982). In individual cases it may be possible to avoid further stone formation and the redevelopment of nephroalcinosis after renal transplantation (FREI et al. 1979; LEUMANN et al. 1978).

Hyperoxaluria due to increased oxalate intake or increased absorption in intestinal disorders is considerably more common and offers greater scope for effective prophylaxis. Hyperoxaluria should be suspected in persons with a habitually high oxalate intake, where there is known familial hyperoxaluria, in cases of chronic vitamin B6 deficiency and above all in persons suffering from chronic intestinal disorders (Crohn's disease) or who have undergone intestinal resections. The latter type is termed *intestinal hyperoxaluria* (ANDERSON and BOSAEUS 1981; CASPARY and TONISSEU 1978; DOWLING et al. 1971; SMITH and HOFMAN 1972).

Hyperoxaluria of this type is primarily due to fat malabsorption. Calcium becomes bound to fats or to bile acids and the consequence is the formation of soluble free oxalate ions in place of calcium oxalate. There is concomitant hypomagnesiuria and hypocitriuria, both facilitating stone formation (RUDMAN et al. 1980; SCHNEIDER and BOCKHORN 1979; SCHAEFER and GUTSCHE 1983). The same mechanism operates after gut resections following on injury or for the treatment of morbid obesity (BACKMANN and HOLLBERG 1976; CAPRON et al. 1977; CLAYMAN et al. 1978; DE WIND and PAYNE 1976; STAUFFER et al. 1973). The ensuing stones are usually of calcium oxalate, although reduced urine volume and intestinal alkali loss with compensatory urinary hydrogen ion excretion may result in uric acid lithiasis. The mean incidence of stones is 5% in inflammatory bowel disease, 10% following ileostomy and 20–50% following jejunoileal bypass (DOBBIUS 1984; NORDENWALL et al. 1983).

ANDERSON and JAGENBURG (1974), BOSSECKERT (1978) and RUDMAN et al. (1980) have recommended the following preventive regime:

1. A fluid intake adequate to secure an appropriate urine volume even in the presence of diarrhea.
2. A low oxalate diet, avoiding spinach, rhubarb, beetroot, celery, carrots, dandelion, mustard, tea, cocoa and chocolate.
3. Reduction in the intake of usual fats and their replacement with medium chain triglycerides.
4. Cholestyramine administration.
5. Oral calcium supplements.
6. Oral citrate supplements and intramuscular magnesium preparations.

The prevention of uric acid stones requires not only an adequate urine dilution but also the correct degree of urine alkalinity. Intestinal water loss and reduced urinary sodium/calcium ratio have been cited as the cause of stone formation in chronic purgative abusers (WOERSDOERFER and SCHREITER 1973).

Hypercalciuria alike is an undisputed risk factor for stone formation, albeit a great number of people have hypercalciuria without ever suffering from stones. A prevention program should be instituted for all patients whose disease leads to increased urinary calcium excretion associated with skeletal rarifaction, who have malignant disease or renal abnormalities.

Episodes of crystalluria or urolithiasis are notorious complications of long term immobilization (BERG et al. 1982). Hypercalciuria is most marked early on in any period of bedrest and is related to the absence of longitudinal skeletal loading, combined with reduced renal tubular reabsorption (BRAUNE and HARTA 1972; JURICEK et al. 1975; MILLARD et al. 1970; PACOVSKY 1975). Stones occur in only 2% of patients on bedrest for fractures, but among paraplegics or persons suffering from poliomyelitis this figure rises to 30% (BURCHARDT and HULAND 1978).

In the latter group the situation is frequently compounded by urinary tract infection alkalinizing the urine and by abnormal urodynamics within the tract. Urinary calcium excretion may rise beyond 600–800 mg/day.

The following preventive measures must be applied from the very beginning of any period of bedrest (GRIFFITH 1971; KOWALCZYK et al. 1975; MEISSNER 1975; SMITH and ROBERTSON 1969; STOEHR 1968):

1. Early partial or whole-body mobilization with weightbearing.
2. A high fluid intake supplemented by 1 g sodium chloride per day.
3. Administration of hydrochlorothiazide to reduce calcium excretion.
4. Maintain sterility of urine drainage systems, even if this requires long-term antibiotics.
5. Administer specific urease inhibitors (acetohyroxamic acid) in cases of chronic Proteus UTI (GRIFFITH and MUSHER 1963).
6. Urine acidification with careful monitoring of urinary acid-base balance (renal tubular acidosis).
7. Allopurinol to be given if uric acid excretion rises, aluminum hydroxide to reduce phosphate absorption.

Among toxic environmental promoters of urolithiasis chronic cadmium exposure is the chief offender (ANKE and SCHNEIDER (1979); ANKE et al. 1980; AXELSON 1963; FRIBERG et al. 1974; KASANTZIS 1979).

Cadmium induces renal damage, with consequent hypercalciuria. From an industrial medical point of view therefore, stone prevention involves maintaining adequate diuresis coupled with early detection of hypercalciuria and urinary microglobulin. No worker in whom the two latter appear should continue to be exposed.

3. Drugs

At one time stones were not uncommon following treatment with poorly soluble sulfonamides and this led to a recommendation for promoting diuresis during such therapy. Stone formation and massive crystalluria have also been observed following treatment with sulphamethoxazole/trimethoprim (ALFTHAN and LIEWENDAHL 1972; BUELOW et al. 1977; OEZGEN 1979) and, more bizarrely perhaps, following the treatment of glaucoma by carbonic anhydrase inhibitors (JUERGENSEN et al. 1975; GACA 1975; THOMAS 1976).

Sadly enough one continues to come across reports of severe urolithiasis and nephrocalcinosis in the wake of vitamin D or dihydrotachysterol treatment for hypocalcemia following thyroidectomy (DINKEL 1965; ECKE and MUELLER 1975; HEIDBREDER et al. 1974; LENK et al. 1976; STOCKER 1972). Where there is a genuine therapeutic requirement the following must be observed (GEBHARDT 1977):

1. Careful assessment of the indications.
2. Regular estimation of calcium levels, serum *and* urinary.
3. Dose to be modified according to response.
4. The patient must understand the signs and symptoms of overdosage.
5. Adequate diuresis must be secured if treatment is to be long term.

Hypercalciuria and stone formation may also occur during antituberculous therapy with preparations such as PAS-Calcium® (SCHOENE et al. 1969).

Stone formation occurring after long term oral contraception is probably unrelated to the mild hypercalciuria induced by such steroids, representing rather a secondary consequence of urinary tract infection (KLINGER et al. 1974, 1978, 1979). For this reason the control of urinary tract sepsis is central to stone prevention in women on oral contraception. Stones have also been recorded occurring during prolonged sodium bicarbonate or silicate ingestion for peptic ulcer (BERG et al. 1982; BURR 1976; CIFUENTES DELATTE et al. 1978; JOEKES et al. 1973; LAGERGREN 1962; SZABO-FOELDVARI 1975; THOMAS 1976).

4. Infection and Outflow Obstruction

The relationship between urinary tract infection and stone formation is subject to a variety of factors, all needing to be taken into account in stone prevention (Fig. 4).

Principal among these is urine alkalinization by urea splitting organisms. The activity of these results in optimal formation conditions for socalled in-

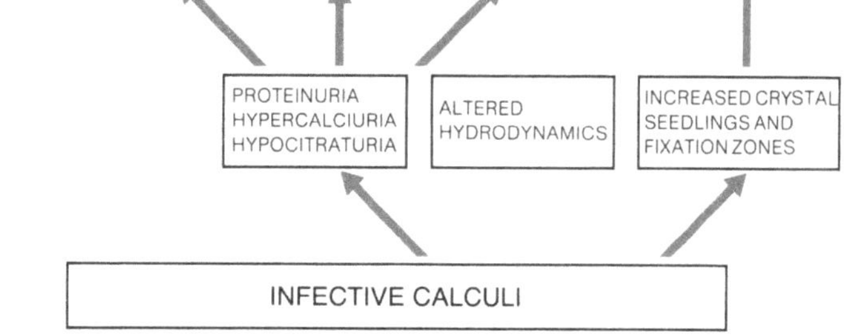

Fig. 4. Diagram of the causal interactions involved in infective stone formation (SCHNEIDER 1980b)

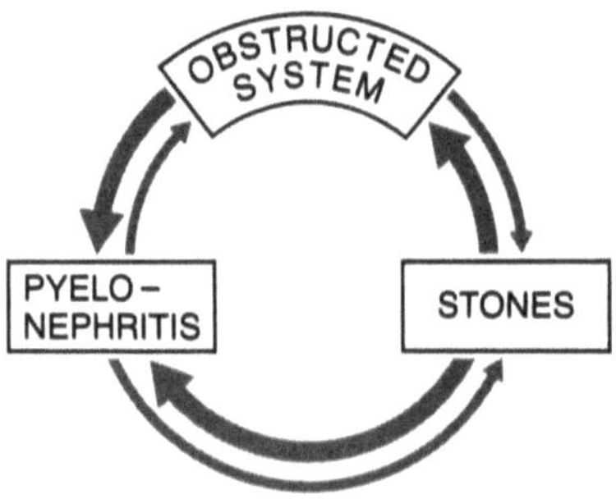

Fig. 5. Interactions of pyelonephritis, urine stasis and urolithiasis (SCHNEIDER 1980b)

fective stones of struvite and carbonate apatite. Thus it is that over 90% of patients with struvite calculi have a proteus UTI (BASTIAN et al. 1978). In one series of women with phosphatic staghorn calculi proteus infection (Proteus vulgaris, P. rettgeri, P. mirabilis and P. morgagni) was the single common pathogenetic feature (ABOULKER and BERNARD 1971). However, other organisms such as Ps. aeruginosa, staph. aureus and Klebsiella spp. are also capable of further alkalinizing an alkaline urine. Any urinary tract infection due to urease positive organisms harbors a grave risk of stone formation and demands not only specific antiinfective treatment but also all the general panoply of stone prevention (SMITH 1976). Thus specific chemotherapy should be supplemented by adequate urine dilution and acidification and by urease inhibitors (GRIFFITH et al. 1978, 1983).

BEHRENDT et al. (1977) have recommended the use of an indicator plate to provide a rapid and simple test for urea splitters in the urine. There is a close and frequently causal relationship between urinary tract infection and urine outflow obstruction, resulting in a complex interplay between pyelonephritis, urine stagnation and stone formation (Fig. 5). Urine stasis favors infection and the consequence is infective stones in an alkaline urine. Frequent episodes of struvite and carbonate apatite lithiasis in early childhood are generally considered to denote urogenital malformation, especially so in boys. VAHLENSIECK (1978) recorded abnormalities in 42% of his young stone patients. MINKOW (1978) and HOHMANN et al. (1977) found tract deformities in 25% of cases of infective calculi. According to BORGMANN and NAGEL (1982) outflow disorders and urodynamic abnormalities are the chief factor determining stone formation in childhood. Metabolic disorders are, by contrast, a rather rare cause of stone formation in children (SCHNEIDER and OTTO-UNGER 1979; SINNO et al. 1979). In this field, therefore, prevention includes early measures to correct abnormal outflow, if possible before the occurrence of secondary infection (SCHNEIDER and HIENZSCH 1975). These remarks should apply with equal force to bladder calculi occurring in elderly men with bladder neck obstruction.

3–30% of patients with permanent urinary diversions develop stones in the ileal loop or in their kidneys – the commonest complication of these procedures. Loop and kidney stones are of different causation and are releated to urine composition, stasis and urinary tract infection (SCHWILLE and SIGEL 1975). ZINGG et al. (1975) have suggested the following prevention protocol:

1. Meticulous surgical technique
2. Regular followup examinations over many years
3. Antiinfective measures

Hydrochlorothiazide offers some protection, whilst urine acidification or bicarbonate administration are of doubtful value and have their own inherent metabolic dangers, which may outweigh any stone preventing effect.

A foreign body within the urinary tract may provoke stone formation, and this is certainly true of suture material (SCHNEIDER 1972), catheters, cystostomy tubes etc. Incrustation will depend on the surface of the foreign material, on the crystallizing potential of the urine and on the rate of flow. For this reason one should prefer catheters and tubes with the smoothest possible surface (siliconised) while aiming for the lowest possible urinary specific gravity. Foreign bodies should spend as little time as possible within the urinary tract and infection is to be excluded. In our own hands prophylactic doses of methylene blue (AHMED and TAWASAKI 1978; BOYCE et al. 1967; SMITH 1972; SUTOR 1970) have merely resulted in the blue staining of incrustations, but not in their prevention (SCHNEIDER et al. 1977).

5. Occupation and Environment

The links between stones and occupation, general life style and place of residence (rural or metropolitan) have been discussed at length in chapter "Epidemiology of Urolithiasis" (Volume "Urolithiasis: Etiology, Diagnosis"). The current situation is one in which the discrepancy between the demands of technologic and scientific advance for ever increasing emphasis on mental work and of a minimal amount of physical exercise can no longer be made good by leisure pursuits and sports. If this is viewed in the context of inappropriate or exessive nutrition, it will soon become clear where general stone prevention might begin.

Studies at a steelworks have shown it to be office employees who develop stones, not the blast furnace workers with their strenuous physical exertion and high rate of fluid loss (FRANK et al. 1975). The ratio was 3.7 : 1.2, similar observations being reported by ZIELINSKI (1972). The example cited by HERING (1977) of a blast furnace liner with a high rate of oxalate stone formation cannot be considered pathognomonic for the simple reason that he had a strong family history and was on record as passing stones regularly before he ever worked on a blast furnace.

The main thrust of prevention must be aimed at those of sedentary and predominantly mental occupation. These people should be encouraged to drink greater quantities of fluid, take part in workplace exercises and, ideally, spend their leisure hours in some form of group physical or sporting activity. It emerged from one study by ZECHNER et al. (1981) that 50% of stone patients never engaged in sports and 41% did so only occasionally.

People who travel to countries hotter than they are used to respond quite differently to socalled high temperature workers. Additional fluid losses and the fear of catching gastrointestinal disorders from drinks may occasionally lead to urines of exceptionally high specific gravity. To this is added a certain amount of nervous stress inherent in any sojourn abroad. We therefore recommend anyone travelling to a hot climate to take detailed advice from their local stone clinic.

In recent years stress has been suggested as a causal factor for a number of disorders, including urolithiasis. Urolithogenic trends in metabolic responses and an increased incidence of urolithiasis both occur in persons of stressful occupation, apparently confirming the hypothesis (BRUNDIG et al. 1980; 1981 a, b; 1982; BRUNDIG and SCHNEIDER 1981). The same conclusion seems inescapable from the work of TOGGENBURG et al. (1981) on immigrant workers in Switzerland. 20% of their clinic material consisted of immigrants, 81% of whom had had their first stone episode after immigrating. This considerably elevated stone incidence persists only for the first two years after arrival in Switzerland and is entirely accounted for by calcium oxalate calculi located in the ureter.

Experience in our own stone clinic outpatient sessions has highlighted the difficulties in seeking to influence the stress pattern of an individual patient's life. The best one can achieve is to draw the attention of people in high pressure occupations to the negative ways in which they react to stressful situations or to the expectation thereof. By understanding the pathogenetic mechanism and its dangers they may themselves arrive at means of compensating (ULSHOEFER et al. 1982).

Members of families with an increased incidence of urolithiasis also face an excess risk. It is rarely that one identifies genuine genetic factors and in most cases the causes are probably to be found in the shared environmental and nutritional factors operating within a family group. For this reason the entire family of stone patients should be drawn into the councelling process at the local stone clinic. At marriage guidance level attention must be drawn to the heritability of certain metabolic causes of urolithiasis. Cystinuria is the classical example.

6. Calculating the Risk of Stone Formation

Stones occur when several risk factors operate simultaneously, so that an overall probability of stone episodes could be calculated from the individual factors. ROBERTSON et al. (1978) have presented a suitable equation for the overall relative probability that an individual will form stones, and this is discussed in detail in the chapter by ROBERTSON and PEACOCK in the volume "Urolithiasis: Etiology, Diagnosis".

Such formulae might enable one to assess both the risk to individual stone patients and the effectiveness of treatment. Furthermore they should be useful in screening to identify individuals at risk of stone disease.

Despite being common in clinical usage the calcium/magnesium and sodium/calcium ratio are of little true prognostic value, since they are too far removed from the true determinants of urolithogenesis.

First attempts at a comprehensive classification of risk levels are due to KALLISTRATOS (1975), who proposed a quotient for urinary crystallizing potential with stone promoting factors in the numerator and litholytic factors in the denominator. ACHILLES et al. (1976, 1984), ROBERTSON (1976) and ROBERTSON et al. (1978, 1983) approached the problem from the point of view of the interrelationships between lithogenic and litholytic urine constituents. From the activity products for calcium oxalate they derive a mathematical term for the thermodynamic probability of urolithogenesis. MARSHALL and ROBERTSON (1976) drew attention to the value of nomograms derived from theoretical calculations for rapid estimation of urine supersaturation and of activity products. Nowadays one uses simple creatinine or citrate based ratios to separate the healthy from persons at risk, since such a criterion offers an excellent compromise between information content and diagnostic expense (HERING et al. 1981; LESKOVAR et al. 1979; TISELIUS and LARSSON 1981; TISELIUS et al. 1978; TISELIUS 1982, 1983).

Creatinine offers the advantage as a reference value that errors in urine collection, individual quirks of fluid intake and body size are all taken into account.

BERG et al. (1982) studied a group of 82 patients with recurrent calcium oxalate stones and 95 control subjects in order to determine the practical usefulness of various lithogenic/litholytic factor quotients. The study enabled the juxtaposition of computations based on discriminant analysis on the one hand and complex salt chemistry on the other. In view of the well established circadian rhythms in urinary concentration and excretion patterns, standard 0–6 am urine collections were used throughout.

The computations are based on the means of 16 parameters, including obligatory urinary excretion products, pH, urine volume and age of the subject. As expected there is considerable overlap between the distributions within either group. Better discrimination is afforded (Fig. 6) by the calcium/citrate ratio and the term:

$$\frac{[\text{calcium}] \times [\text{oxalate}] \times \text{urine volume}}{[\text{citrate}]}$$

The best distinction between the two groups was given by a discriminant function of 13 variables, corrected for linear combinations and weighted according to the degree of indispensibility evident on multivariant analysis. Even if this set of variables was subsequently reduced to four (age, calcium, magnesium and citrate) the appropriate discriminant function still gave excellent separation of groups (Fig. 7).

The appearance in the discriminant function X (Fig. 8) of age alongside the concentrations of calcium, magnesium and citrate suggests that increased risk of stone formation cannot be seen in isolation from age. This concept would correspond with the finding by ZECHNER et al. (1981) in their study of social distribution among stone patients that old age pensioners were overrepresented in terms of the Austrian national standard risk.

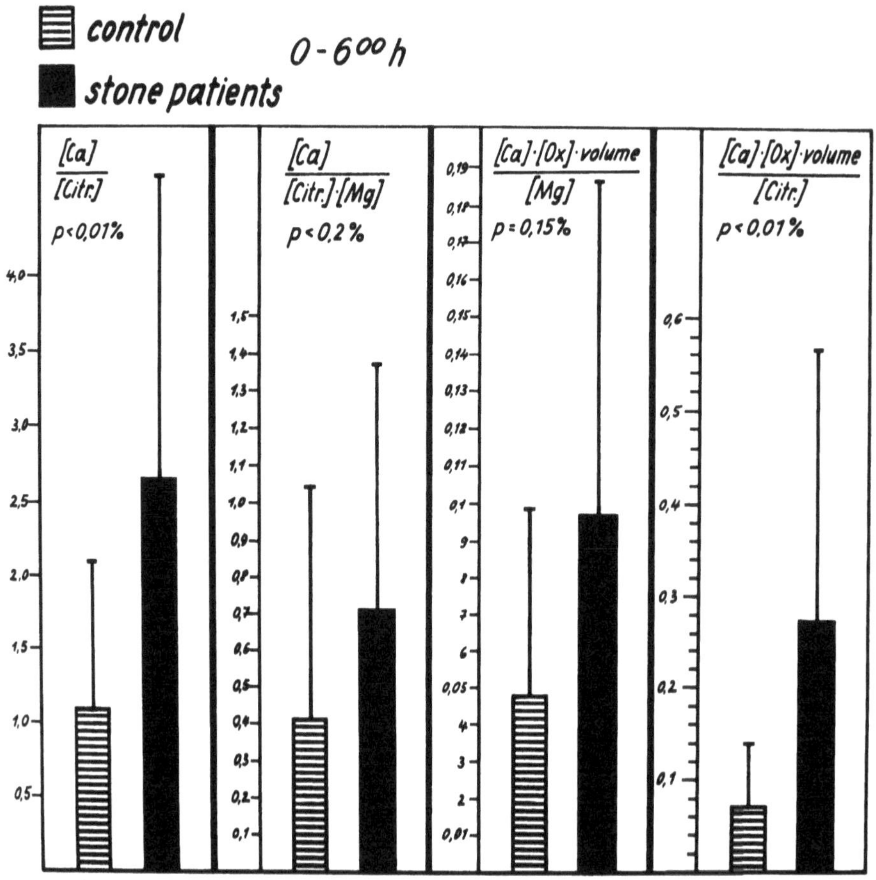

Fig. 6. Mean values and scatter of quotients calculated from the patient cohort of BERG et al. (1982)

Risk of misclassification was taken to denote the quality of separation achieved. 60 of 82 recurrent stone patients appeared to the right of the arithmetic mean, i.e. their status as stone patients was confirmed. Likewise, 76 of the 95 controls were confirmed to be normal.

The frequency distribution for individual values within the cohort is shown in Fig. 8. Even if the analysis is restricted to the three parameters calcium, magnesium and citrate, the corresponding discriminant function still gives a satisfactory accuracy of separation between groups, thus further approaching the requirements of clinical practice:

$$X = 1.78 \times 10^{-1} \times (X_{[Ca]}) + 2.72 \times 10^{-1} \times (X_{[Mg]}) - 1.21 \times 10^{-1} \times (X_{[cit.]})$$

These studies were restricted to a limited number of variables, and in the future additional factors such as ionised calcium, glycosaminoglycans, urinary proteolytic activity etc. may be included to improve predictive power.

Another approach lies in direct measurement of urinary crystallizing potential or of the inhibiting effect of individual test urines on a standard system.

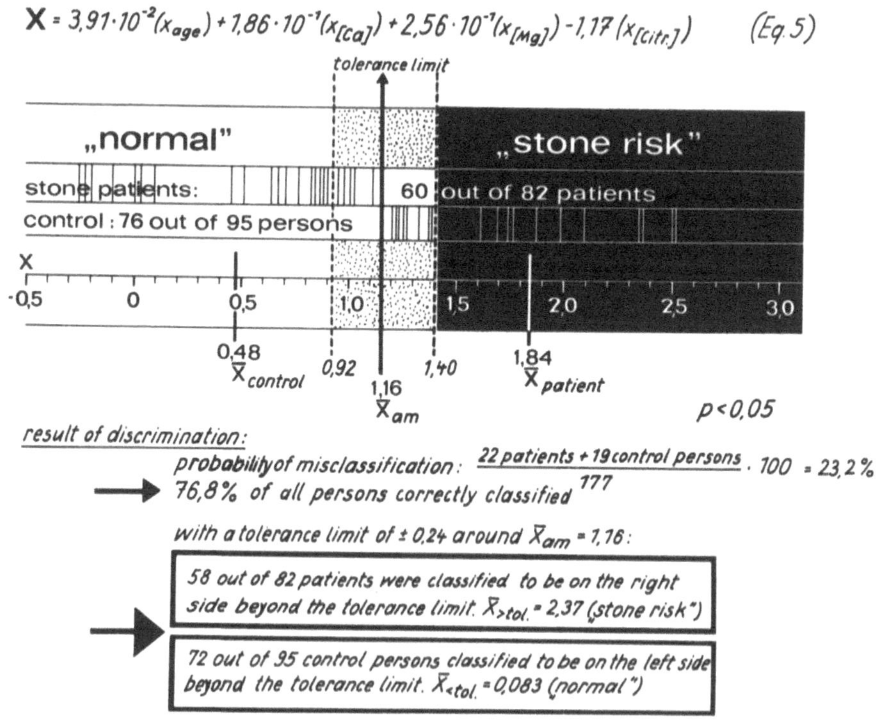

Fig. 7. Discriminant function with four variables and discriminance of individual proband parameters (BERG et al. 1982)

From data in the literature on diffusion and crystallization in gels it is easy to devise a simple gel model by means of which the inhibiting capacity of a urine sample, and therefore its corresponding crystallization tendency can be determined (ACHILLES et al. 1980, 1983; ROEHRBORN et al. 1984; SCHNEIDER et al. 1983, 1984).

An agar coated microscope slide is used as a reaction area, in which wells and channels of uniform volume have been punched with a special instrument. Calcium chloride and ammonium oxalate are pipetted into wells opposite urine or test solution (Fig. 9). Starting solutions diffuse toward one another, and after 24 hours incubation a macroscopically visible band of calcium oxalate crystals is precipitated, its breadth and density depending on the concentration of inhibitors in the test urine. These changes can be measured as photometric extinction and expressed mathematically as an inhibition index (Fig. 10).

The term inhibiting activity is used here as a global expression of the effect of urine on calcium oxalate crystallization. This gel model thus differs from so-called risk indices which, however many factors they include, remain unable to embrace the full complexity of urine crystallization and inhibition.

Further simplification of the system (preloaded gels and starting solutions, elimination of photometry by using colored crystals) would enable its routine clinical use in the identification of patients at risk and in monitoring the effectiveness of prophylactic maneuvers.

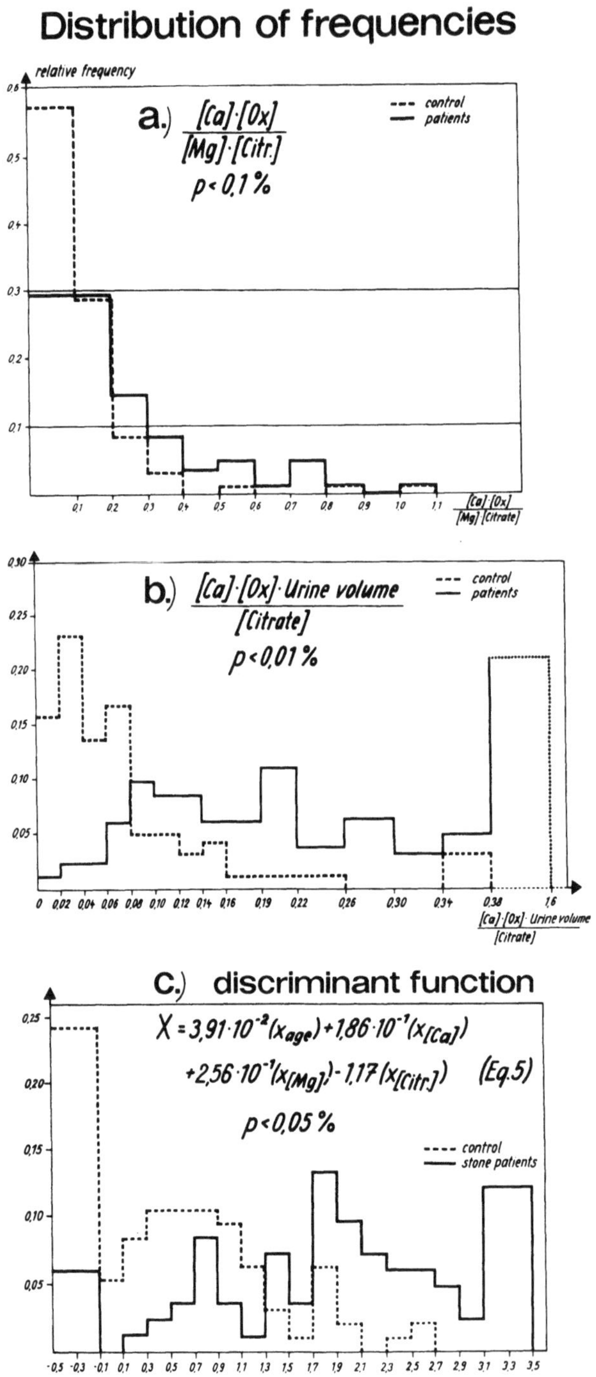

Fig. 8. Frequency distribution of individual values within the cohort (BERG et al. 1982)

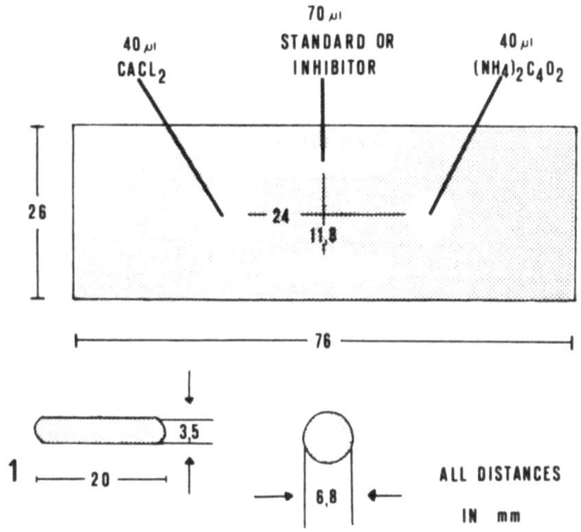

Fig. 9. Schematic drawing of gel diffusion slide, showing the effect of inhibitor on calcium oxalate crystal formation

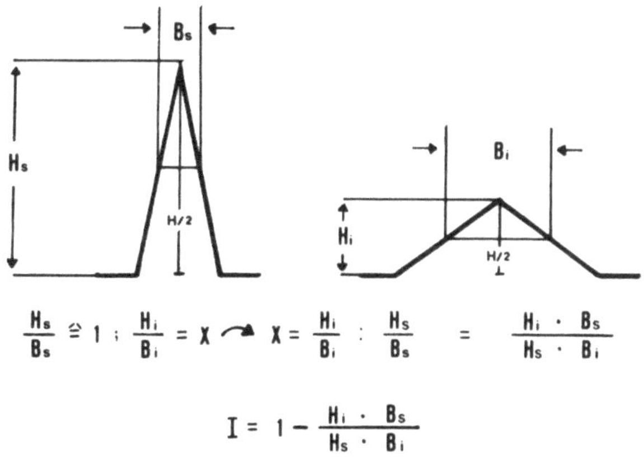

Fig. 10. Diagram of gel extinction curve and derivation of the inhibition index

H: Height B: Breadth (H/2) I: Inhibition Index
s: Standard (distilled water / NaCl 0,9%) i: Inhibitor

III. Health Education and Behavior Patterns

With an incidence of barely 1% and a prevalence of 5% of the whole population urolithiasis is not merely a medical problem: It has equally become one affecting national economic and social policy, and assumes proportions similar to diabetes mellitus in terms of health economics. Stone disease is described both as a modern day endemic and as a disease of plenty, both terms which imply statements about frequency and etiology of the disease.

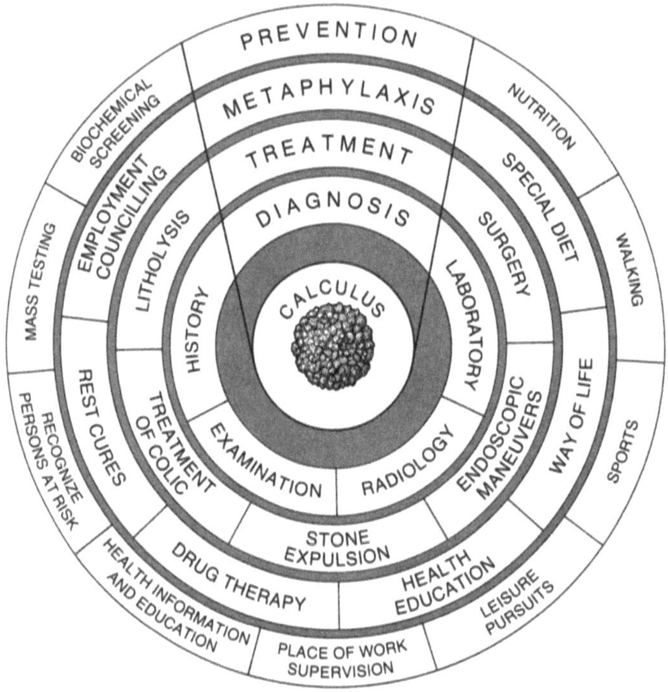

Fig. 11. Interrelationship of diagnosis, treatment, metaphylaxis and prevention of urolithiasis (SCHNEIDER 1974b)

Both the respectable results of modern surgery, including new techniques such as remote renal stone destruction, and the ability of metaphylaxis to reduce the recurrence rate from 50 to 10% remain but partial successes. The rate at which new cases accrue continues its inexorable rise, and for this reason true prevention must occupy a dominant position in any overall anti-urolithisiasis program. At the time of writing we are still far from achieving this goal. Before a positive answer can be given to the provocative question, whether we in fact have any true urolithiasis prevention schemes (SCHNEIDER 1974b), two important sets of problems must first be solved (Fig. 11).

1. Prevention is only likely to be effective when based on an exact understanding of pathogenesis. It is precisely the multifactorial etiology of urolithiasis that continues to evade such an exact understanding.
2. It is extremely difficult to influence the behaviour of basically healthy persons, as evidenced by experience with obesity, smoking and alcohol.

The following approach is recommended on the basis of over twenty years consulting room experience in community stone clinics:

1. A general prevention program must emanate from the urolithiasis outpatient clinic, where doctors, nurses and paramedical staff have the greatest expert knowledge of stone disease. Such staff will be in a position to write information leaflets, discuss the subject on radio and television, give lectures and li-

aise with family practitioners and works medical officers. The latter in turn have the greatest power to influence the health care habits of their local population. It is the close ties between research establishments and highly sophisticated diagnostic and treatment facilities that put the chief of a urolithiasis unit in the strongest position to run a general prevention program.

2. The individual level of health consciousness has been rising in the population at large. Doctors can no longer be the sole source of health education aimed at increasing a sense of self-responsibility among members of the public. The mass media, state institutions, large organisations and the mouthpieces of public opinion all have an important role to play. Unfortunately their effectiveness is as yet inadequate, as the man in the street proves extremely difficult to wean from cherished but misguided habitudes. More publicity must be given to the pathophysiology of stone disease. Our own experience shows that the individual is more likely to comply with the dietary and long term medication requirements of metaphylaxis, the better he understands the relationship between his disease and the measures prescribed.

3. Any stone prevention program aimed at the whole population must be extremely general and will be limited to promulgating the virtues of correct nutrition and adequate physical activity. More intensive attention needs to be focussed on individuals and groups at high risk, always bearing in mind that the etiologic factors are only partly understood and that our knowledge of them is ever on the increase. The principal task is to recognise local groups of people and individuals at risk, to recruit them into prevention schemes and to influence the way they live.

The steadily rising number of new cases suggests that present day stone prevention is having little effect. The recognition of this fact does nothing to absolve one from an obligation to devote more effort to this cause.

40 years ago chest physicians saw no solution to the tuberculosis problem, yet we now know that their relentless dedication to the aim of eradicating it has been largely crowned with success.

References

Aboulker P, Bernard E (1971) Phosphathaltige Nierenbeckenausgußsteine mit gramnegativer Begleitinfektion bei Frauen. XV. Internationaler Urologenkongreß Tokio. Urologe [Ausg A] 10:46–48

Achilles W, Ulshöfer B (1985) Calculations of complex chemical equilibria in urine: Estimate of stone-formation risks and derivation of prophylactic measures. In: Schwille PO, Smith LH, Robertson WD, Vahlensieck W (eds) Urolithiasis and Related Clinical Research. Plenum Press, New York London, S 777–780

Achilles W, Cumme GA, Scheffel M (1976) Investigation of complex chemical equilibria in urinary systems with respect to calcium oxalate formation. In: Fleisch H, Robertson WG, Smith LH, Vahlensieck W (eds) Urolithiasis Research. Plenum Press, New York London, p 229–232

Achilles W, Mergner Ch, Simon M, Berg W, Schneider H-J (1980) Ein neues optisches Mikroverfahren zur Bestimmung von Kristallisationsgeschwindigkeiten. VI. Jenaer Harnsteinsymposium. Wissenschaftliche Beiträge der Friedrich-Schiller-Universität, Jena, S 61–68

Achilles W, Mergner Ch, Simon M (1983) An optical micromethod for the determination of relative crystallisation rates of calcium oxalate in gels: Method and preliminary results. Urol Res 11:87–91

Ahmed K, Tawashi R (1978) Methylene blue as an inhibitor of stone formation. Urol Res 6:77–80

Alfthan OS, Liewendahl K (1972) Investigation of sulfonamide crystalluria in man. Scand J Urol Nephrol 6:44–46

Alken P, Schäfer A (1978) Kristallurie bei Cystinsteinpatienten. In: Vahlensieck W, Gasser G (Hrsg) Pathogenese und Klinik der Harnsteine VI. Steinkopff, Darmstadt, S 183–191

Anasuya A, Rao BSN (1973) Studies on the role of nutritional factors in urinary lithiasis. Uric acid excretion and its solubility in urine on wheat and rice diets. Invest Urol 10:426–428

Andersson H, Bosaeus J (1981) Hyperoxaluria in malabsorptive states. Urol Int 36:1–9

Andersson H, Jagenburg R (1974) Fat-reduced diet in the treatment of hyperoxaluria in patients with ileopathy. Gut 15:360–364

Anke M, Schneider H-J (Hrsg) (1979) Int. Cadmium-Symposium. Wissenschaftliche Beiträge der Friedrich-Schiller-Universität, Jena

Anke M, Grün M, Kronemann H, Schneider H-J (1980) Die Diagnose der Kadmiumbelastung beim Menschen. Wiss Z Karl-Marx-Universität Leipzig 29:515–522

Arora B, Selby PL, Peacock M, Robertson WG (1984) The effect of an increased intake of various constituents of a high animal protein diet on the risk of calcium oxalate stone formation. In: Schwille PO, Smith LH, Robertson WD, Vahlensieck W (eds) Urolithiasis and Related Clinical Research. Plenum Press, New York London, S 85–88

Axelson B (1963) Urinary calculus in long term exposure to cadmium. Int Congr Occup Health 14:939–946

Bach D (1982) Die Stoffwechseluntersuchung beim Harnsteinpatienten. Z Urol Nephrol 75: 545–552

Bach D, Rohde M, Schneeberger W, Hamm W, Dewes W, Vahlensieck W, Zilitzen W (1978) Circadiane Ausscheidung von Calcium, Magnesium und Harnsäure im Urin von Calciumsteinträgern unter Standardkost. In: Vahlensieck W, Gasser G (Hrsg) Pathogenese und Klinik der Harnsteine VI. Steinkopff, Darmstadt, S 274–279

Backman L, Hollberg D (1976) The incidence of kidney stones after small intestinal bypass operations for treatment of obesity. In: Fleisch H, Robertson WG, Smith LH, Vahlensieck W (eds) Urolithiasis Research. Plenum Press, New York London, p 401–403

Bastian HP, Vahlensieck W, Brühl P (1978) Die Bedeutung der Harnwegsinfektion für die Nephrolithiasis. 29. Kongreß Dt. Ges. Urol. Thieme, Stuttgart, S 317

Behrendt WA, Bichler KH, Schulze HS, Ideler V (1977) Ein verbessertes diagnostisches Schnellverfahren zur Erkennung von Infektionen mit harnstoffspaltenden Keimen im Urin. In: Gasser G, Vahlensieck W (Hrsg) Pathogenese und Klinik der Harnsteine V. Steinkopff, Darmstadt, S 218–220

Berg W, Schneider HJ, Vogel E (1975) Die Oxalatausscheidung im Harn bei oraler Oxalsäure- und Magnesiumzufuhr. Dtsch Z Verdau Stoffwechselkr 35:241–245

Berg W, Börner R, Brundig P, Schneider H-J (1982) Diagnostischer Wert von Gefährdungsformeln für die Erfassung von Bildungsrisiken bei der Kalziumoxalatlithiasis. VII. Jenaer Harnsteinsymposium, Wissenschaftliche Beiträge der Friedrich-Schiller-Universität, Jena, S 125–133

Bisaillon S, Tawashi R (1975) Growth of calcium oxalate in gel system. J Pharm Sci 64:958–962

Borgmann V, Nagel R (1980) Analyse von 171 Fällen von Urolithiasis im Kindesalter. Z Kinderchir 29:48–56

Boshamer K (1961) Morphologie und Genese der Harnsteine. In: Alken, Dix, Weyrauch, Wildbolz (Hrsg) Handbuch der Urologie, Bd. X. Springer Berlin Göttingen Heidelberg, S 1–171

Bosseckert H (1978) Gastroenterologische Erkrankungen in Beziehung zum Urogenitalsystem. Z Urol Nephrol 71:657–661

Boyce WH, McKinney WM, Long TT, Drach GW (1967) Oral administration of methylene blue to patients with renal calculi. J Urol 97:783–785

Braune R, Harta G (1972) Zur Urolithogenese bei Querschnittslähmungen. Zentralbl Chir 97:242–250
Brock WA, Golden J, Kaplan W (1983) Xanthine calculi in the Lesch-Nyhan syndrome. J Urol 130:157–161
Brockis JG, Bowyer RC, Ryan G, Tayler TA, Kamordi T, Rizal A (1981) Endemic bladder stones in Indonesia. In: Smith LH, Robertson WG, Finlayson B (eds) Urolithiasis: Clinical and Basic Research. Plenum Press, New York London, S 329–332
Brühl P, Bastian HP (1976) Nephrolithiasis und Harnwegsinfektion. Therapiewoche 26:5941–5945
Brundig P, Schneider HJ (1981) Stressinduzierte Veränderungen der Magnesiumausscheidung und der Magnesiumkonzentration im Urin bei Kalziumoxalatsteinpatienten und bei Normalpersonen. IV. Hohenheimer Magnesiumsymposium 1980. Magnes Bull 3:69–73
Brundig P, Berg W, Naumann J, Hoppe H, Cumme GA, Achilles W, Schneider H-J (1980) Kalzium-Oxalat-Aktivitätsprodukte und diskriminanzanalytische Verrechnungen von Harnparametern als Grundlage eines Kalzium-Oxalat-Screening-Programmes. Urologe [Ausg A] 19:54–56
Brundig P, Schneider HJ, Berg W (1981) Stress und Harnsteinbildungsrisiko. I. Der Einfluß von Stress auf lithogene Harnsubstanzen. Urol Int 36:199–207
Brundig P, Schneider HJ, Berg W (1981) Stress und Harnsteinbildungsrisiko. II. Der Einfluß von Stress auf litholytische Harnsubstanzen. Urol Int 36:265–273
Brundig P, Berg W, Schneider H-J (1982) Die Veränderungen der Kalziumoxalat-Aktivitätsprodukte unter Streßbedingungen bei Kalziumoxalatsteinpatienten und Normalpersonen. Wissenschaftliche Beiträge der Friedrich-Schiller-Universität Jena, S 253–257
Bülow H, Klee WE, Hotzel A, Frohmüller H (1977) Zur Frage einer Harnsteinbildung nach Trimethoprim/Sulfamethoxazol-Therapie. In: Gasser G, Vahlensieck W (Hrsg) Pathogenese und Klinik der Harnsteine V. Steinkopff, Darmstadt, S 116–118
Burchhardt P, Huland H (1978) Renal calculus dissolution in immobilized patients. Eur Urol 4:420–423
Burr RG (1976) The determination of silicates in urinary calculi. Clin Chim Acta 69:259–265
Capron JP, Dupas JL, Delamarre (1977) Lithisiase renale oxalique et lithiase vesiculaire après resection iliale pour maladie de Crohn. Gastroenterol Clin Biol 1:165–169
Caspary WF, Tonissen J (1978) Enterale Hyperoxalurie. I. Intestinale Oxalsäureresorption bei gastroenterologischen Erkrankungen. Klin Wochenschr 56:607–615
Castro-Mendoza HJ, Cifuentes Delatte L, Rapado Erratzi A (1972) Una nueva observacion de xantinuria familiar. Rev Clin Esp 124:341–352
Churchill DN, Morgan J, Gault MH (1985) Tea drinking – a risk factor for urolithiasis? In: Schwille PO, Smith LH, Robertson WD, Vahlensieck W (eds) Urolithiasis and Related Clinical Research. Plenum Press, New York London, p 93–96
Cifuentes Delatte L, Castro-Mendoza H (1967) Xanthinuria familiar. Rev Clin Esp 28:244–256
Cifuentes Delatte L, Rapado A, Abehsera A, Troba ML, Cortes M (1973) Uric acid lithiasis and gout. In: Cifuentes Delatte L, Rapado A, Hodgkinson A (eds) Urinary Calculi. Karger, Basel, p 115–118
Cifuentes Delatte L, Medina J, Santos U, Rodriguez (1978) Lithiasis urinary de silice ($SiO_2 \cdot nH_2O$) en los animales y en la espedie humana. Rev Clin Esp 151:343–348
Clayman RV, Buchwald H, Varco RL, Dewolf WC, Williams RD (1978) Urolithiasis in patients with a jejunoileal bypass. Surg Gynecol Obstet 147:225–230
Constable AR, Joekes AM, Kasidas GP, Regan PO, Rose GA: Plasma level and renal clearance of oxalate in normal subjects and in patients with primary hyperoxaluria and/or chronic renal failure. In: Vahlensieck W, Gasser G (eds) Pathogenese und Klinik der Harnsteine VI. Steinkopff, Darmstadt, S 207–213
Costello J, Al-Dabagh E, Bentley M, Watson A, Keogh B (1985) Familial xanthinuria in a large kidred: Purine metabolites in plasma and urine of xanthinurics, siblings and normal subjects. In: Schwille PO, Smith LH, Robertson WD, Vahlensieck W (eds) Urolithiasis and Related Clinical Research. Plenum Press, New York London 681–684
Currie WJC, Turmer P (1979) The frequency of renal stones within Great Britain in a gouty and non-gouty population. Brit J Urol 51:337–341

Dahm J, Schorr R (1980) Zu einigen Auswirkungen eines hohen Niveaus der Prophylaxe auf die ambulante medizinische Betreuung. Z Ärztl Fortbild (Jena) 74:1140–1143

DeWind LT, Payne JH (1976) Intestinal bypass surgery for morbid obesity: Long-term results. JAMA 15:2298–2301

Dinkel H (1965) Nephrocalcinosis und Dihydrotachysterin-Medikation. Dtsch Med Wochenschr 90:1569–1572

Dobbins J (1985) Nephrolithiasis associated with intestinal disease. In: Schwille PO, Smith LH, Robertson WD, Vahlensieck W (eds) Urolithiasis and Related Clinical Research. Plenum Press, New York London, 119–126

Donaldson D, Pryce JD, Rose GA, Toey JE (1979) Tap water calcium and its relationship to renal calculi and 24 h urinary calcium output in Great Britain. Urol Res 7:273–276

Dowling RH, Rose GA, Sutor DJ (1971) Hyperoxaluria and renal calculi in ileal disease. Lancet I:1103–1105

Ecke M, Müller GW (1975) Entwicklung von Harnsteinen unter medikamentöser Therapie. IV. Jenaer Harnsteinsymposium, Wissenschaftliche Beiträge der Friedrich-Schiller-Universität Jena, S 231–232

Fellström B, Danielson BG, Karlström B, Lithell H, Ljunghall S, Vessby B (1983) The influence of a high dietary intake of purine-rich animal protein on urinary urate excretion and supersaturation in renal stone disease. Clinical Sci 64:399–405

Frank D, Schneider H-J, Hesse A (1975) Untersuchungen zum Harnsteinleiden bei Hitzearbeitern. Dt Gesundh-Wes 30:716–720

Frei D, Binswanger U, Keusch G, Bringer J, Largiader F (1979) Intakte Nierentransplantatfunktion 3 Jahre nach Organübertragung bei primärer Oxalose. Schweiz Med Wochenschr 109:979–983

Friberg L, Piscator M, Nordberg GF, Kjellström T (1974) Cadmium in the environment. 2. Ed. CRC-Press, Cleveland, p 106–107

Fuss M, Simon J, Fontinoy N, Coussaert E (1979) High fluid–low calcium intake: Not all renal stone formers adhere to this simple treatment. Eur Urol 5:97–99

Gaca A (1975) Arzneimittelinduzierte Konkrementbildung. IV. Jenaer Harnsteinsymposium, Wissenschaftliche Beiträge der Friedrich-Schiller-Universität, Jena, S 233–234

Gebhardt K (1977) Jatrogene Nierensteinbildung und Niereninsuffizienz durch Langzeittherapie mit Kalzinosefaktoren (Dihydrotachysterin, Vit. D). Z Ärztl Fortbild (Jena) 71:447–449

Green ML, Fujimoto WJ, Seegmiller JE (1969) Urinary xanthine stone – a rare complication of allopurinol therapy. N Engl J Med 280:426–428

Griffith DP (1971) Control of hypercalcuria in the immobilized patient. J Urol 105:698–701

Griffith DP, Musher DM (1973) Prevention of infected urinary stones by urease inhibition. Invest Urol 11:228–233

Griffith DP, Gibson JR, Clinton CW, Musher DM (1978) Acetohydroxamic acid: clinical studies of a urease inhibitor in patients with staghorn renal calculi. J Urol 119:9–12

Griffith DP, Mac Cue Pat, Hai Lee, Benson J, Carlton CE (1983) Stone cancer. Palliative treatment with acetohydroxamic acid. World J Urol 1:170–175

Gröbner W, Zöllner N (1977) Harnsäuresteine und Ernährung. Akt Ernähr 2:82–86

Haenel H (1972) Moderne Ernährung und ihr Einfluß auf sogenannte Volkskrankheiten. II. Jenaer Harnsteinsymposium, Wissenschaftliche Beiträge der Friedrich-Schiller-Universität, Jena S 117–126

Halstead SB, Valyasevi A (1972) Current epidemiology of bladder stone disease studies in the Thailand endemic area. In: van Reen R (ed) Proceedings WHO, Regional Symposium on vesical calculi disease. Bangkok, S 17–22

Harrison AR, Rose GA (1978) Reversal of chronic renal failure from primary hyperoxaluria on treatment with pyridoxine. In: Vahlensieck W, Gasser G (eds) Pathogenese und Klinik der Harnsteine VI. Steinkopff, Darmstadt, S 298–301

Hartung R, Leskovar P (1980) Xanthinstein. In: Vahlensieck W (Hrsg) Urolithiasis, Bd. 5. Springer, Berlin Heidelberg New York, S 53–57

Heidbreder E, Hennemann H, Heidland A (1974) Hypercalciurie – Nephrocalcinose – Kalklithiasis der Niere. Dtsch Med Wochenschr 99:586–590

Hering F (1977) Calciumoxalatnephrolithiasis als Berufskrankheit. Urologe [Ausg A] 16:227–229

Hering F, Pyhel N, Ratajczak H, Friedrich R, Lutzeyer W (1981) Kalkulation der relativen Übersättigung – Entscheidungshilfe bei der Therapieplanung. In: Vahlensieck W, Gasser G (Hrsg) Pathogenese und Klinik der Harnsteine VIII. Steinkopff, Darmstadt, S 345–349

Hesse A, Hicking W, May P (1980) Harnsäurestein. In: Vahlensieck W (Hrsg) Urolithiasis, Bd 5. Springer, Berlin Heidelberg New York, S 1–39

Hesse A, Schneider H-J, Berg W, Hienzsch E (1977) Erarbeitung eines Ca-Oxalatstein-Screening-Programms auf der Grundlage biochemischer Meßdaten. In: Gasser G, Vahlensieck W (Hrsg) Pathogenese und Klinik der Harnsteine V. Steinkopff, Darmststadt, S 278–285

Hesse A, Cumme GA, Hoppe H, Achilles W, Berg W, Brundig P, Schneider H-J (1978) Untersuchungen zum Harnsteinbildungsrisiko. V. Jenaer Harnsteinsymposium, Wissenschaftliche Beiträge der Friedrich-Schiller-Universität, Jena, S 83–87

Hesse A, Strenge A, Bach D, Vahlensieck W (1982) Einfluß von Nahrungsbelastungen auf die Ausscheidung von Oxalsäure, Calcium und Harnsäure. In: Gasser G, Vahlensieck W (Hrsg) Pathogenese und Klinik der Harnsteine IX. Steinkopff, Darmstadt, S 67–75

Hoffmann L, Becher R, Erdmann Th (1979) Untersuchungen zur Harnsteinprophylaxe und -metaphylaxe und zum Gesundheitsverhalten der Patienten mit Harnsteinleiden, I, II. Z Ärztl Fortbild (Jena) 73:I S 1115–1117, II S 1166–1169

Hoffmann L, Becher R, Erdmann Th (1979) Über die Zuverlässigkeit und aktive Mitarbeit der Patienten bei der Metaphylaxe des Harnsteinleidens. Z Urol Nephrol 72:269–275

Horn G, Weiß K-B, Kaszubowski U (1980) Wert der Diätetik und allgemeiner Ernährungsrichtlinien in der Harnsteinmetaphylaxe. Z Urol Nephrol 73:539–547

Hosking DH, Erickson StB, van Den Berg J, Wilson M, Smith H (1983) The stone clinic effect in patients with idiopathic calcium urolithiasis. J Urol 130:1115–1118

Hüttner J (1972) Soziologische Merkmale und Gesundheitsverhalten des Harnsteinträgers. II. Jenaer Harnsteinsymposium, Wissenschaftliche Beiträge der Friedrich-Schiller-Universität, Jena, S 144–151

Hüttner H (1976) Zur Gesundheitserziehung in der Allgemeinpraxis. Z Ärztl Fortbild (Jena) 70:1242–1243

Hüttner H, Hüttner J, Kopske Chr (1971) Arzt und Gesundheitserziehung. Z Ärztl Fortbild (Jena) 65:1144–1147

Illievski PM, Illievska SS (1985) Drinking water quality and urolithiasis. In: Schwille PO, Smith LH, Robertson WD, Vahlensieck W (eds) Urolithiasis and Related Clinical Research. Plenum Press, New York London, p. 105–110

Joekes AU, Rose GA, Sutor J (1973) Multiple renal silica calculi. Br Med J 5846:146–147

Joost J, Schabel F, Doppler W (1981) Complete adenine phosphoribosyltransferase, deficiency with 2,8-dihydroxyadenine stone formation. Fortschr Urol Nephrol 16:58–65

Jürgensen UJ, Schwaar R, Waltz J, Austenat J (1975) Harnsteinbildung bei Nephramidtherapie. Dtsch Ges Wesen 30:364–367

Juricek V, Kolas O, Sramek F (1975) Der Einfluß langdauernder Immobilisation auf den Kalzium- und Phosphormetabolismus und die Steinbildung. IV. Jenaer Harnsteinsymposium, Wissenschaftliche Beiträge der Friedrich-Schiller-Universität, Jena, S 180–183

Kallistratos G (1975) Aufbau einer Harnsteinprophylaxe. Urologe [Ausg A] 3:95–101

Kallistratos G (1975) Aufbau einer Nierensteinprophylaxe durch Beeinflussung einiger pathophysiologischer Vorgänge. In: Vahlensieck W, Gasser G (Hrsg) Pathogenese und Klinik der Harnsteine III. Steinkopff, Darmstadt, S 169–182

Kallistratos G, Ponteliadis C, Marketos S (1977) Zystinurienachweis mit Hilfe des „Urocystin"-Tests. In: Gasser G, Vahlensieck W (Hrsg) Pathogenese und Klinik der Harnsteine V. Steinkopff, Darmstadt, S 210–212

Karcher G (1962) Die Prophylaxe des Harnsteinleidens. Landarzt 38:1409–1412

Kazantzis G (1975) The effect of cadmium on the human kidney. In: Anke M, Schneider H-J (eds) Internationales Kadmiumsymposium, Wissenschaftliche Beiträge der Friedrich-Schiller-Universität, Jena, S 117–121

Kinoshita K, Takemoto M, Itatani H, Yachiku S, Kotake T, Sonoda T (1979) A new screening method for cystinuria. Urol Int 34:369–373

Klingeberg J (1972) Die Beeinflussung der aktuellen Harnreaktion durch verschiedene Getränke im Rahmen der Harnsteintherapie und -prophylaxe. Urologe [Ausg B] 12:155–157

Klinger G, Hesse A, Schneider H-J (1974) Zur Frage einer Bedeutung hormonaler Kontrazeptiva für die Entstehung von Harnsteinen. Zentralbl Chir 96:248–253
Klinger G, Berg W, Schneider H-J, Stelzner A (1979) Untersuchungen zur Langzeitwirkung verschiedener hormonaler Kontrazeptiva auf die Ausscheidung von Natrium, Kalium, Kalzium, Magnesium, Chlorid, Harnsäure, Zitronensäure, Oxalsäure, Sulfat und Lysozym im 24-Stunden-Urin. Z Urol Nephrol 72:393–398
Klinger W, Oettel M, Gruhn J, Chemnitius K-H, Hübler D, Hesse A, Schneider H-J (1978) Untersuchungen zur Wirkung von Sexualsteroiden auf die Harnsteinbildung. V. Jenaer Harnsteinsymposium, Wissenschaftliche Beiträge der Friedrich-Schiller-Universität, Jena, S 117–120
Kocvara S, Dubansky A, Zdimera A, Pribyl O (1982) Fluoruntersuchungen von Harnsteinen. VII. Jenaer Harnsteinsymposium, Wissenschaftliche Beiträge der Friedrich-Schiller-Universität, Jena, S 63–65
Kollwitz A-A (1966) Harnveränderungen durch Gaben von Mineralquellen bei gesunden Versuchspersonen. Urol Int 21:193–208
Kowalszyk J, Klecz K, Zielinski J, Czopik J (1975) Die Harnsteinkrankheit bei Paraplegie. Z Urol Nephrol 68:799–805
Krizek V (1981) Epidemiologische und genealogische Studie der Zystinurie und Zystinsteinkrankheit anhand von 255 Fällen. In: Vahlensieck W, Gasser G (Hrsg) Pathogenese und Klinik der Harnsteine VIII. Steinkopff, Darmstadt, S 61–67
Krizek V (1983) Zystinurie und Zystinsteinkrankheit. 25-jährige Erfahrungen bei 255 Fällen Urologe [Ausg B] 23:320–322
Krizek V, Vendl L (1978) Urolithiasis cystinurica bei Kindern. V. Jenaer Harnsteinsymposium, Wissenschaftliche Beiträge der Friedrich-Schiller-Universität, Jena, S 195–199
Kühn H-D, Schorsch H (1981) Die Behandlung der Zystinsteinpatienten. Z Urol Nephrol 74:349–354
Lagergren C (1962) Development of silica calculi after oral administration of magnesium trisilicate. J Urol 87:994–996
Landgrebe AR, Nyhan WL, Coleman M (1975) Urinary tract stones resulting from the excretion of oxypurinol. N Engl J Med 292:629–694
LeGeros RZ, Morales P (1973) Renal stone crystals grown in gel system. Invest Urol 11:12–14
Lenk S, Brien G, Bick C (1976) Harnsteinbildung durch Dihydrotachysterolüberdosierung. Z Ärztl Fortbild (Jena) 70:470–471
Leskovar P, Hartung R, Riedel J (1979) Kann allein aus der Harnanalyse auf ein erhöhtes Steinbildungsrisiko bei Steinpatienten geschlossen werden? Med Welt 30:937–941
Leumann EP, Wegmann W, Lagiader F (1978) Prolonged survial after renal transplantation in primary hyperoxaluria of childhood. Clin Nephrol 9:29–34
Maaser M, Hesse A, Linke E, Klare B, Schneider H-J (1972) Möglichkeiten der Screening-Untersuchungen bei der Zystinurie. Dtsch Gesundh Wesen 27:1119–1121
Marshall RW, Robertson G (1976) Nomograms for the estimation of the saturation of urine with calcium oxalate, calcium phosphate, magnesium ammonium phosphate, uric acid, sodium acid urate, ammonium acid urate and cystine. Clin Chim Acta 72:353–359
Martelli A, Buli P, Cortecckia V (1981) Acetohydroxamic acid therapy in infected renal stones. Urology 17:320–322
Matouschek E, Huber R-D (1981) Urolithiasis. Pathogenese, Diagnostik, Therapie. Schattauer, Stuttgart New York
Meißner R (1975) Harnsteinbildung bei Immobilisation nach orthopädischen Operationen. IV. Jenaer Harnsteinsymposium, Wissenschaftliche Beiträge der Friedrich-Schiller-Universität, Jena, S 173–176
Millard FJC, Nassim JR, Woollen JM (1970) Urinary calcium excretion after immobilization and spinal fusion in adolescents. Arch Dis Child 45:399–403
Minkov N (1978) Zur Frage der Ätiopathogenese der Urolithiasis im Kindesalter. V. Jenaer Harnsteinsymposium, Wissenschaftliche Beiträge der Friedrich-Schiller-Universität, Jena, S 148–151
Murakami HIM, Miyauchi T, Mori I, Yamaguchi K, Usui T, Shimazaki J (1983) The incidence of cystinuria in Japan. J Urol 129:1012–1015
Nordenvall B, Backman L, Larssom L, Tiselius H-G (1983) Urine composition following jejunoileal bypass. Eur Urol 9:35–39

Ohlenschläger G, Ulbrich H (1976) Ambulante und klinische Erfahrungen mit einem neuen Harnsäurebelastungstest. Therapiewoche 26:1254–1257

Otto-Unger G (1972) Harnsteindispensaire bei Kindern. II. Jenaer Harnsteinsymposium, Wissenschaftliche Beiträge der Friedrich-Schiller-Universität, Jena, S 182–185

Otto-Unger G (1978) Pädiatrische Aspekte zum Harnsteinleiden des Kindes. V. Jenaer Harnsteinsymposium, Wissenschaftliche Beiträge der Friedrich-Schiller-Universität, Jena, S 129–135

Otto-Unger G, Misselwitz J (1978) Empfehlungen eines Screenings auf Stoffwechselstörungen beim Harnsteinleiden im Kindesalter. V. Jenaer Harnsteinsymposium, Wissenschaftliche Beiträge der Friedrich-Schiller-Universität, Jena, S 240–243

Otto-Unger G, Misselwitz J (1979) Empfehlungen für die unspezifische Rezidivprophylaxe der Urolithiasis im Kindesalter. Dtsch Ges Wesen 34:2141–2143

Pacovsky V (1975) Kalziummetabolismus bei Immobilisation. IV. Jenaer Harnsteinsymposium, Wissenschaftliche Beiträge der Friedrich-Schiller-Universität, Jena, S 170–172

Peacock M (1984) Institution and management of a stone clinic. In: Schwille OP, Smith LH, Robertson WD, Vahlensieck W (eds) Urolithiasis and Related Clinical Research. Plenum Press, New York London (in press)

Rapoport MS (1969) Medizinische Biochemie, 5. Auflage. Verlag Volk und Gesundheit, Berlin, S 956–960

Renker K, Presber W (1980) Die WHO-Definition der Gesundheit und die Rehabilitation Geschädigter. Z Ärztl Fortbild (Jena) 74:1137–1139

Robertson GW, Peacock M, Heyburn PJ, Hanes FA, Rutherford A, Clementson E, Swaminathan R, Clark PB (1979) Should recurrent calcium oxalate stone formers become vegetarians? Br J Urol 51:427–431

Robertson WG, Peacock M (1982) The pattern of urinary stone disease in Leeds during the period 1960–1980. In: Gasser G, Vahlensieck W (eds) Pathogenese und Klinik der Harnsteine IX. Steinkopff, Darmstadt, S 8–14

Robertson WG, Peacock M (1982) The pattern of urinary stone disease in the United Kingdom in relation to animal protein intake during the period 1960–1980. Urol Int 37:394–399

Robertson WG, Peacock M (1983) Review of risk factors in calcium oxalate urolithiasis. World J Urol 1:114–118

Robertson WG, Morgan DB, Marshall DH, Peacock M, Nordin BEC (1978) Risikofaktoren bei der Kalziumsteinbildung. V. Jenaer Harnsteinsymposium, Wissenschaftliche Beiträge der Friedrich-Schiller-Universität, Jena, S 45–52

Robertson WG, Peacock M, Heyburn PJ, Speed R, Hanes F (1978) The role of affluence and diet in the genesis of calcium-containing stones. In: Vahlensieck W, Gasser G (eds) Pathogenese und Klinik der Harnsteine VI. Steinkopff, Darmstadt, S 5–14

Robertson WG, Peacock M, Marshall PH, Speed R (1981) The prevalence of urinary stone disease in practising vegetarians. In: Vahlensieck W, Gasser G (eds) Pathogenese und Klinik der Urolithiasis VIII. Steinkopff, Darmstadt, S 6–14

Robertson WG, Peacock M, Marshall DH (1982) Prevalence of urinary stone disease in vegetarians. Eur Urol 8:334–339

Röhrborn C, Schneider H-J, Rugendorff EW (1985) Determination of stone-forming risks by measuring crystallization inhibitor activity in urine with a gel model. In: Schwille PO, Smith LH, Robertson WD, Vahlensieck W (eds) Urolithiasis and Related Clinical Research. Plenum Press, New York London, p 879–882

Rose GA, Arthur LJH, Kasidas GP, Scott IV (1982) Primary hyperoxaluria in a neonate. In: Gasser G, Vahlensieck W (eds) Pathogenese und Klinik der Harnsteine IX. Steinkopff, Darmstadt, S 8–14

Rudman D, Dedonis JL, Fountain MT, Chandler JB, Gerron GG, Fleming GA, Kutner MH (1980) Hypocitraturia in patients with gastrointestinal malabsorption. N Engl. J. Med. 303:657–661

Schäfer F, Gutsche B (1983) Klinische und tierexperimentelle Untersuchungen zur pathogenetischen Bedeutung von Dünndarmerkrankungen bzw. -resektionen für das Harnsteinleiden. Z Urol Nephrol 76:433–437

Schewzow IP, Towstoles KP, Chidekel BS, Fenomenow RN (1972) Dispensairebetreuung der Harnsteinkranken. II. Jenaer Harnsteinsymposium, Wissenschaftliche Beiträge der Friedrich-Schiller-Universität, Jena, S 165–170
Schneider H-J (1971) Das Harnsäuresteinleiden, Klinik – Therapie – Prophylaxe. Z Inn Med 26:272–277
Schneider H-J (1972a) Harnsteindispensaire: Bedeutung und erreichter Stand in der Deutschen Demokratischen Republik. Z Urol Nephrol 65:527–532
Schneider H-J (1972b) Harnsteindispensaire: Ihre Beurteilung durch den Steinträger. Z Ärztl Fortbild (Jena) 66:477–478
Schneider H-J (1973) Urometrie in der Harnsteindispensaire. Dtsch Ges Wesen 28:1478–1479
Schneider H-J (1974a) Dispensairebetreuung durch den Facharzt für Allgemeinmedizin. Dtsch Ges Wesen 29:1434–1435
Schneider H-J (1974b) Gibt es eine echte Prophylaxe des Harnsteinleidens? Urologe [Ausg A] 13:161–165
Schneider H-J (1978) Möglichkeiten einer Harnsteinprophylaxe. Z Ärztl Fortbild (Jena) 72:1164–1169
Schneider H-J (1979) Organisation, Aufgaben und Wirkung einer Harnsteinambulanz. Therapiewoche 29:2188–2198
Schneider H-J (1980a) Harnsteinleiden, 3. Auflage. VEB Verlag Volk und Gesundheit, Berlin
Schneider H-J (1980b) Steinbildung und Harnwegsinfekt. In: Hautmann R, Lutzeyer W (Hrsg) Harnsteinfibel. Deutscher Ärzteverlag, Köln, S 77–86
Schneider H-J (1980c) Steinbildung und Nierenerkrankungen. In: Hautmann R, Lutzeyer W (Hrsg) Harnsteinfibel. Deutscher Ärzteverlag, Köln, S 98–113
Schneider H-J, Albert L (1967) Wert und Grenzen diätetischer Maßnahmen beim Harnsteinleiden. Z Ärztl Fortbild (Jena) 61:958–961
Schneider H-J, Bockhorn V (1979) Stoffwechseluntersuchungen bei extravesikaler Harnableitung unter Verwendung von Dünndarm. Z Urol Nephrol 72:365–374
Schneider H-J, Hienzsch E (1969) Die Bedeutung der Ernährung für die Entstehung von Harnsteinen und die Stellung der Diätetik in der modernen Therapie der Urolithiasis. Dtsch Z Verdau Stoffwechselkr 29:401–406
Schneider H-J, Hienzsch E (1974) Fortschritte in der Dispensairebetreuung Harnsteinkranker. Z Urol Nephrol 67:749–757
Schneider H-J, Horn G (1968) Trinkkuren mit Meerwasser. Z Urol Nephrol 61:753–760
Schneider H-J, Otto-Unger G (1978) Das Harnsteinleiden in Kindesalter. Z Ärztl Fortbild (Jena) 72:1164–1169
Schneider H-J, Horn G, Tscharnke J (1969) Erfahrungen mit einer Dispensairesprechstunde für Harnsteinpatienten. Z Urol Nephrol 62:241–248
Schneider H-J, Albert L, Hesse A (1972) Der Einfluß des Nahtmaterials auf die experimentelle Blasensteinbildung. Z Exp Chir Transplant Künstliche Organe 5:356–360
Schneider H-J, Hesse A, Berg W, Lange U, Hartmann U, Hensel K (1977) Einfluß der Nahrung auf die Zusammensetzung von Fremdkörpersteinen im Tierexperiment III. Z Urol Nephrol 70:357–362
Schneider H-J, Röhrborn C, Rugendorff EW (1983) A gel model for measuring crystallization inhibitor activities in calcium oxalate urolithiasis. World J Urol 1:155–158
Schneider H-J, Bothor C, Berg W, Börner RH, Jacob M (1983) A gel model for measuring crystallization inhibitor activities. Urol Int 37:33–38
Schöne D, Hausschild G, Wässer St (1969) Hypercalciurie unter PAS-Calcium-Medikation als pathogenetischer Faktor der Urolithiasis. Dtsch Med Wochenschr 94:1491–1493
Scholz D, Schwille PO, Sigel A (1981) Ernährungsgewohnheiten von Patienten mit Urolithiasis. In: Vahlensieck W, Gasser G (Hrsg) Pathogenese und Klinik der Harnsteine. Steinkopff, Darmstadt, S 83–87
Schubert J, Schmechel C (1975) Das Harnsteinleiden im Kindesalter aus urologischer Sicht. Z Ärztl Fortbild (Jena) 69:1064–1067
Schülke J, Sopart H-J (1980) Erfahrungen bei der Dispensairebetreuung von Harnsäuresteinpatienten. Z Urol Nephrol 73:241–245
Schumann HJ (1963) Die Häufigkeit der Urolithiasis im Sektionsgut des Pathologischen Instituts St. Georg, Leipzig. Zentralbl Allg Pathol 105:88–94

Schwille PO, Sigel A (1975) Kriterien der Harnsteindiathese nach Ileum-Conduit-Operationen. IV. Jenaer Harnsteinsymposium, Wissenschaftliche Beiträge der Friedrich-Schiller-Universität, Jena, S 221–222

Scott R, Paterson PJ, Burns R, Fell GS, Ottoway JM (1979) The effects of treatment of the hypercalciuria of chronic Cadmium poisoning. Urol Res 7:285–289

Singer P (1976) Die Gicht (Arthritis urica). Med Actuell 2:63–66

Sinno K, Boyce WH, Resnick MJ (1979) Childhood urolithiasis. J Urol 121:662–664

Smith LH (1976) Renal lithiasis and infection. In: Thomas WC (ed) Renal calculi. C. C. Thomas Publisher, Springfield, p 77–96

Smith LH, Hofmann AF (1972) Acquired hyperoxaluria, urolithiasis, and intestinal disease: a new digestive disorder? N Engl J Med 286:1371

Smith MJV (1972) Concretion and methylene blue. J Urol 107:164–168

Smith PH, Robertson WG (1969) Stone formation in the immobilized patient. In: Hodgkinson A, Nordin BEC (eds) Renal stone research symposium. Churchill, London, p 85–92

Sperling O (1985) Urolithiasis in hereditary renal hyperuricemia. In: Schwille PO, Smith LH, Robertson WD, Vahlensieck W (eds) Urolithiasis and Related Clinical Research. Plenum Press, New York London, p 13–16

Stauffer JQ, Humphreys MH, Weir GJ (1973) Acquired hyperoxaluria with regional enteritis after ileal resection. Ann Int Med 79:383

Stocker WG (1972) Nil nocere; Nephrokalzinose nach langfristiger Dihydrotachysterin-Medikation (A. T. 10). MMW 114:653–656

Stöhr Chr (1968) Verhütung von Steinbildungen im Harnsystem der Querschnittsgelähmten. MMW 110:2308–2310

Sutor DJ (1970) The possible use of methylene blue in the treatment of primary hyperoxaluria. Br J Urol 42:389–392

Szabo-Földvari E (1975) Spezielle Fälle iatrogener Harnsteinbildung. IV. Jenaer Harnsteinsymposium, Wissenschaftliche Beiträge der Friedrich-Schiller-Universität, Jena, S 243–244

Thomas WC (1976) Renal calculi, A guide to management. C. C. Thomas Publisher, Springfield, p 62–65

Thomas WC, Malagodi MH. Dietary habits in patients with calcareous calculi. In: van Reen, R (ed) Idiopathic urinary bladder stone disease. Washington, p 311–320

Tiselius H-G (1982) An improved method for the routine biochemical evaluation of patients with recurrent calcium oxalate stone disease. Clin Chim Acta 122:409–418

Tiselius H-G (1983) Different estimates of the risk of calcium oxalate crystallization in urine. Eur Urol 9:231–234

Tiselius HG, Almgard LE, Larsson L, Sörba B (1978) A biochemical basis for grouping of patients with urolithiasis. Eur Urol 4:241–249

Toggenburg H, Horica Ch, Bandhauer K (1981) Das Harnsteinleiden bei Gastarbeitern – eine epidemiologische Studie. In: Vahlensieck W, Gasser G (Hrsg) Pathogenese und Klinik der Harnsteine VIII. Steinkopff, Darmstadt, S 15–19

Toth C (1976) Betreuung der Harnsteinkranken in unserem Arbeitsbereich. Z Urol Nephrol 69:427–431

Ümmuhan, Özgen (1979) Sulfonamidharnsteine. Med Diss Würzburg

Ulshöfer B, Paar G, Cramer B (1982) Harnsteinmanifestation und Stress. In: Gasser G, Vahlensieck W (Hrsg) Pathogenese und Klinik der Harnsteine IX. Steinkopff, Darmstadt, S 46–51

Vahlensieck W (1978) Therapie und Rezidivprophylaxe des kindlichen Harnsteinleidens. V. Jenaer Harnsteinsymposium, Wissenschaftliche Beiträge der Friedrich-Schiller-Universität, Jena, S 136–144

Wiederhold E, Schneider H-J, Hesse A (1974) Postoperative Infusionen bei Harnsteinpatienten unter Einsatz von Mannitol und Furosemid in einer Gegenüberstellung. Z Urol 67:99–109

Williams HE (1976) Oxalic acid: absorption excretion and metabolism. In: Fleisch H, Robertson WG, Smith LH, Vahlensieck W (eds) Urolithiasis Research. Plenum Press, New York London, p 181–184

Woersdoerfer O, Schreiter F (1973) Laxantienabusus und Urolithiasis. Akt Urol 4:265–268
Zechner O (1981) Offene Fragen der Harnsteinrezidivprophylaxe. Z Urol Nephrol 74:401–405
Zechner O (1981) Richtlinien zur Rezidivprophylaxe von Harnsteinen. Wien Klin Wochenschr 93:619–624
Zechner O, Latal D, Pflüger H, Schreiber V (1981) Nutritional risk factors in urinary stone disease. J Urol 125:51–54
Zechner O, Latal D, Pflüger H, Schreiber V (1981) Die soziale Infrastruktur von Harnsteinpatienten. Wien Klin Wochenschr 93:635–638
Zielinski J (1972) Bemerkungen zum Diätproblem bei Harnsteinkranken. II. Jenaer Harnsteinsymposium, Wissenschaftliche Beiträge der Friedrich-Schiller-Universität, Jena, S 127–130
Zingg E, Mayor G, Keller U, Schmucki O (1975) Die Steinbildung bei definierter Harnableitung. IV. Jenaer Harnsteinsymposium, Wissenschaftliche Beiträge der Friedrich-Schiller-Universität, Jena, S 215–220
Zöllner N (1976) Influence of diet on urinary uric acid excretion. In: Fleisch H, Robertson WG, Smith LH, Vahlensieck W (Hrsg) Urolithiasis Research. Plenum Press, New York London, S 155–163

Subject Index

W. Leistenschneider, R. Nagel

Atlas of Prostatic Cytology

Techniques and Diagnosis

Foreword by G. Dhom

Translated from the German by R. Mills, D. Winter

1985. 325 color and black and white illustrations, 27 tables.
X, 227 pages. ISBN 3-540-13954-0
Distribution rights for Japan: Igaku Shoin, Tokyo

Contents: Introduction. - The Technical Bases of Aspiration Biopsy. - Cytological Microscopy. - Normal Findings. - Atypia. - Secondary Findings. - Artefacts. - Primary Diagnosis of Carcinoma. - Grading of Prostatic Carcinoma. - Treatment Control by Means of Regression Grading. - Sarcomas. - Secondary Tumors of the Prostate. - Prostatitis. - DNA Cytophotometry. - Results of the Measurement of Nuclear DNA by Single-cell Scanning Cytophotometry in Prostatic Carcinoma. - References. - Subject Index.

This monograph fulfills the double mission of describing all tried and proven methods of cytological evaluation of the prostate known to date which are relevant for the clinic and independent practice, and of providing instruction in the basic techniques required for the application of this approach. The full potential of prostatic cytology is clearly and impressively demonstrated.
One of the book's decisive advantages is its comprehensive treatment of both primary diagnosis and, especially, of follow-up of the therapeutic success afforded by different forms of treating advanced, inoperable prostatic carcinoma with the aid of cytological methods. This is the first work to include all these aspects.
It is also the first time that the basic principles and results of DNA cytophotometry and a discussion of secondary tumors of the prostate have been published in this form.
Inflammatory diseases of the prostate gland (prostatitis), which have been accorded little space in previous publications, and the wide range of cytomorphological forms in which they are present, are discussed in detail. Each section of the book also contains new, standardized methods of classification.
The distinguishing feature of the volume is its magnificent illustrations which are all of high informative value and almost all in color.

Springer-Verlag
Berlin Heidelberg
New York Tokyo

K. Korth

Percutaneous Surgery of Kidney Stones

Techniques and Tactics

Foreword by W. Mauermayer

1984. 65 figures, 3 color plates. X, 96 pages
ISBN 3-540-13572-3

The noted urologic surgeon K. Korth has drawn upon his experience with hundreds of percutaneous renal lithotomies to provide a uniquely comprehensive introduction to this important operative technique. He covers all aspects of the operation, including the equipment involved, selection and positioning of the patient, operative strategy and execution, as well as eventual pitfalls and how to avoid them. Each step is fully illustrated with line drawings, photographs, sonograms and x-ray photographs.
Dr. Korth devotes particular attention to the all-important placement of the percutaneous canal. The tactical considerations involved (size, shape and location of the stones) plus the tricks on which the success of the operation often depends are described for you in detail without unnecessary theoretical ballast. The author also outlines additional percutaneous kidney operations in the appendix, such as the lancing of subpelvic ureteral structures, resection of papillary tumors, and intrarenal marsupialization of renal cysts. Clear, concise, authoritative - **Percutaneous Surgery of Kidney Stones** is your guide to a surgical technique whose efficacy has been proved over and over again.

W. Mauermayer

Transurethral Surgery

With contributions by K. Fastenmeier, G. Flachenecker, R. Hartung, W. Schütz

Translated from the German by A. Fiennes

Foreword by W. E. Goodwin

1983. 240 figures, 14 color plates.
XXIX, 473 pages. ISBN 3-540-11869-1

"Surgical techniques are described in a number of steps... this enables even a novice to understand the various procedures. (Dr. Mauermayer) also describes many tried and proven 'clinical secrets,' which are illustrated by means of numerous outstanding drawings. A number of excellent color illustrations at the end of the book demonstrate his impressive cystoscopic photography."
Journal of Urology

Urodynamics

Upper and Lower Urinary Tract II

Editors: **W. Lutzeyer, J. Hannappel,**

1985. 243 figures, 22 tables. XI, 343 pages.
ISBN 3-540-15357-8

Contents: Workshop on Upper Urinary Tract Urodynamics: Myogenic Control for the Upper Tract. Hydrodynamics and Mechanics of the Upper Tract. - Upper and Lower Urinary Tract Urodynamics - Reviewing the Aachen 1971 Meeting: Lower Tract Urodynamics. Upper Tract Urodynamics. - Subject Index.

This volume reviews the essential results of clinical and research urodynamics during the past 12 years. It is based on a follow-up meeting held to review the development since the historical 1971 Aachen meeting. Speakers who had lectured in 1971 or who had made significant contributions to urodynamics critically examine the validity of previous statements and the clinical applicability of their findings. This follow-up review is preceded by reports from a special workshop on mycogenic control, hydrodynamics and mechanics of the upper urinary tract.

Springer-Verlag
Berlin Heidelberg
New York Tokyo

Springer

MIX
Papier aus verantwortungsvollen Quellen
Paper from responsible sources
FSC® C105338

If you have any concerns about our products,
you can contact us on
ProductSafety@springernature.com

In case Publisher is established outside the EU,
the EU authorized representative is:
Springer Nature Customer Service Center GmbH
Europaplatz 3, 69115 Heidelberg, Germany

Printed by Libri Plureos GmbH
in Hamburg, Germany